LOCALIZATION IN CLINICAL NEUROLOGY

LOCALIZATION IN CLINICAL NEUROLOGY

Paul W. Brazis, M.D.
Carolina Neurological and Neurosurgical Service,
Florence, South Carolina; formerly Assistant Professor of
Neurology, Loyola University of Chicago Stritch School
of Medicine, Maywood, Illinois, and Staff Physician,
Veterans Administration Hospital, Hines, Illinois

Joseph C. Masdeu, M.D.
Associate Professor of Neurology, Albert Einstein College
of Medicine of Yeshiva University, New York, New
York; Head, Neurology Section, North Central Bronx
Hospital, Montefiore Hospital and Medical Center, New
York, New York

José Biller, M.D.
Assistant Professor of Neurology, University of Iowa
College of Medicine, Iowa City, Iowa

Doug
Carlson
June
1985

Little, Brown and Company
Boston / Toronto

To Elizabeth, Paul, Erica, José, Maria-Luisa, Mercedes, Celika, Sofía, Gabriel, and Rebecca

CONTENTS

PREFACE

This book may seem to be born out of time. Is there still a role for clinical localization in neurologic practice in the CT era? Not uncommonly, medical students echo the widespread opinion that the practice of neurology has been reduced to trying to guess what the CT scan or magnetic resonance imaging will show. As clinical neurologists, we wish this were true! Instead of spending long hours interviewing and examining patients, we would put them through the marvel machines and speedily obtain all the diagnostic information needed for their treatment. Unfortunately, the machines are not sufficient. The new techniques have meant a giant advance in our diagnostic armamentarium, but by no means have they lessened the need for accurate clinical diagnostic evaluation. Brain tumors and other lesions that distort the anatomy of the nervous system or neighboring tissues can now be localized with much greater precision than in the past. However, such lesions may go undetected on imaging procedures unless those procedures focus on the region responsible for the patient's symptoms. Furthermore, neuroimaging may disclose anatomic anomalies not germane to the patient's presenting problem and often of no clinical import. These may be pursued relentlessly unless a thorough understanding of the clinical picture places them in proper perspective.

Nonetheless, CT has had an enormous impact on our understanding of the clinical expression of different brain lesions. Properly used, the anatomic information provided by CT has clarified a number of issues regarding localization, particularly the clinical expressions of acute lesions and their evolution over time and the manifestations of space-occupying lesions such as hydrocephalus and brain tumors. Many of the references in this book reflect the contributions of the newer neuroimaging techniques to the field of clinical localization. The advances in this field over the past few years have been remarkable. The present volume resulted from our interest in documenting the new and emphasizing the old in clinical neurologic localization, at a time when this art continues to play a central role in the evaluation of patients with neurologic disease. A number of works in recent years have dealt with the manifestations of disease in different parts of the nervous system. Books on the peripheral nervous system and the cerebral hemispheres are not lacking, but there is a real dearth of texts providing a comprehensive discussion of localization in clinical neurology. Because many excellent accounts are available on ancillary diagnostic means used in the work-up of patients with neurologic disease, we have focused on anatomic diagnosis as inferred from the patient's history and physical findings.

This book was written with the clinician in mind. Manifestations of neurologic disease that are helpful for localization have been emphasized rather than the myriad "reflexes" with high-sounding eponyms that have accumulated throughout the years in the literature of neurology. We hope that not only the physician in training or practice but also other health care professionals who deal with neurologically impaired patients will find helpful information in the present volume.

We thank Drs. Frank A. Rubino and Sudhansu Chokroverty, who first taught us the importance of neuroanatomic localization, and Dr. Robert Tentler, through whom we discovered that clinical neurology could be fun. We thank also Drs. Herman D. Barest, Herman Buschke, Richard Mayeux, Isabelle Rapin, Naemi Stilman, Leon J. Thal, James F. Toole, and Daniel Wagner for their assistance in reviewing some of the chapters, and for their encouragement. For their support, we are indebted to the Neurology Resident staffs of Loyola University Medical Center and the Albert Einstein College of Medicine. Finally, we express appreciation to Mrs. Helen Hlinka for her secretarial help.

P. W. B.
J. C. M.
J. B.

LOCALIZATION IN CLINICAL NEUROLOGY

Chapter 1

THE LOCALIZATION OF LESIONS AFFECTING THE PERIPHERAL NERVES

Paul W. Brazis

PRINCIPAL SIGNS AND SYMPTOMS
OF PERIPHERAL NERVE DISEASE

Disorders affecting mixed peripheral nerves cause various symptoms and signs corresponding in anatomic distribution to regions supplied by each particular nerve. To make a correct topographic diagnosis of peripheral nerve lesions, the clinician must know thoroughly the area of sensory supply of each nerve, the muscles it innervates, any muscle stretch reflex subserved by the nerve, and the area of sudomotor (sweating) function served by the nerve [9, 16, 18, 26]. Certain nerves are purely motor, some are purely sensory, and others are mixed. The symptoms and signs of a peripheral nerve lesion include the following disturbances:

Sensory Disturbances. With division of a sensory nerve, all modalities of cutaneous sensibility are lost only over the area exclusively supplied by that nerve (the autonomous zone). This zone is surrounded by an intermediate zone, which is the area of the nerve's territory overlapped by the sensory supply areas of adjacent nerves. The full extent (autonomous plus intermediate) of the nerve's distribution constitutes the maximal zone. In clinical diagnosis, the autonomous zone of sensory loss for each nerve must be specifically sought to make an accurate topographic localization. In general, with peripheral nerve lesions the area of light touch sensory loss is greater than the area of pinprick sensory loss.

Pain and paresthesias may also help in localizing a peripheral nerve lesion, but these subjective sensations frequently radiate beyond the distribution of the damaged nerve (e.g., proximal arm pain in the carpal tunnel syndrome).

Motor Disturbances. Interruption of the motor fibers in a motor or mixed nerve leads to lower motor neuron paresis or paralysis of the muscles innervated by that nerve. Atrophy of specific muscle groups and characteristic deformities follow.

The actions of agonist muscles, which have the same or similar mechanical effects on a joint, and antagonist muscles, which have the opposite effect, should be considered in testing the strength of a particular muscle. The action of a powerful agonist may conceal weakness in a smaller muscle (e.g., the pectoralis may compensate for subscapular muscle weakness). A nerve often supplies several muscles with a similar action, and a lesion of that nerve will result in weakness of the muscle group.

Disturbances of Muscle Stretch Reflexes. As a consequence of sensorimotor loss, the muscle stretch reflex subserved by each nerve damaged is decreased or absent.

Vasomotor, Sudomotor, and Trophic Disturbances. The skin subserved by the affected nerve may become thin and scaly. The nails may become curved, with retardation of nail and hair growth in the affected area. The affected area of skin may become dry and inelastic and cease sweating. Because the analgesic cutaneous area is liable to injury, ulcers may develop.

Although ancillary procedures (e.g., electromyography and nerve stimulation studies, muscle and nerve biopsy, sweat tests) may aid greatly in topographic diagnosis, the following discussion will stress only the bedside diagnosis and localization of individual peripheral nerve abnormalities.

MONONEURITIS MULTIPLEX

Mononeuritis multiplex (mononeuropathy multiplex) refers to involvement of several isolated nerves. The nerves involved are often widely separated (e.g., right median and left femoral nerve). These multiple neuropathies will result in sensory and motor disturbances that are confined to the individual nerves affected. Mononeuritis multiplex is usually due to a disseminated vasculitis that affects individual nerves (for example, vasculitis in diabetes mellitus or polyarteritis nodosa).

POLYNEUROPATHY

In polyneuropathy the essential feature is impairment of function of many peripheral nerves simultaneously, resulting in a symmetrical, usually distal, loss of function. The characteristic features include muscle paresis with or without atrophy, sensory disturbances, autonomic and trophic changes, and hyporeflexia or areflexia, especially affecting the distal extremities. In general, the legs are affected before the arms. Polyneuropathy may be due to many systemic processes and may be mainly sensory, mainly motor, or both sensory and motor. It may also affect predominantly nerve fibers of a particular caliber. Thick fibers are more affected in the neuropathy of Friedreich's ataxia or vitamin B_{12} deficiency, whereas thin fibers are more involved in the Riley-Day syndrome or in familial amyloidosis of the Andrade type.

LESIONS OF INDIVIDUAL NERVES

Dorsal Scapular Nerve (C4–C5)

ANATOMY. The dorsal scapular nerve (a purely motor nerve) arises mainly from the C5 spinal nerve within the substance of the scalenus medius muscle. The nerve courses downward behind the brachial plexus deep to the levator scapulae muscle (which it supplies) and terminates by piercing the deep surfaces of the rhomboids (major and minor). The rhomboids normally elevate and adduct the medial border of the scapula (they are antagonists of the serratus anterior) and, along with the levator scapulae, rotate the scapula so that the inferior angle moves medially. The rhomboids are tested by having the patient press his elbow backward against resistance while his hand is on his hip [16].

NERVE LESIONS. Because it is derived from the proximal plexus, affection of the dorsal scapular nerve in an upper brachial plexopathy suggests a proximal lesion. The nerve may also be entrapped within the substance of the scalenus medius muscle [13]. Dorsal scapular nerve lesions result in lateral displacement of the vertebral borders of the scapula, which is rotated with the inferior angle displaced laterally. Rhomboid atrophy is concealed by the overlying trapezius muscle. Rhomboid paresis is evident if the elbow can only weakly be pressed back against resistance (keeping the hand on the hip). Weakness is also evident when the patient attempts to push the palm of his hand backward against resistance with his arm folded behind his back.

Subclavian Nerve (C5–C6). This purely motor nerve emerges from the upper trunk of the brachial plexus and descends in the posterior cervical triangle to innervate the subclavian muscle. This muscle depresses and draws medially the lateral end of the clavicle. Lesions of the subclavian nerve cause no important clinical disturbances.

Long Thoracic Nerve (C5–C7)

ANATOMY. This purely motor nerve arises from the C5–C7 roots shortly after they emerge from the intervertebral foramina. After passing through the scalenus medius muscle the upper two roots are joined by a contribution from the C7 root. The nerve runs posterior to the brachial plexus and then crosses the outer border of the first rib to reach the serratus anterior muscle. The nerve further descends along the lateral thoracic wall, sending individual filaments to muscle slips of the serratus.

The serratus anterior muscle fixes and stabilizes the scapula against the chest wall and is tested by observing for scapular winging (the vertebral border of the scapula stands away from the thorax, forming a "wing") while the patient pushes the extended arms against a fixed object (e.g., a wall) [16].

NERVE LESIONS. The long thoracic nerve is injured alone most frequently as a result of pressure on the shoulder (e.g., sudden trauma or carrying heavy objects on the shoulder) [10]. Nerve paralysis usually causes no deformity of the scapula when the arm is at rest. If, however, the patient is asked to push the arm forward against resistance or hold the arms up in front of the body, the scapula becomes winged (*"winged scapula"* or *"scapula alata"*), especially in its lower two-thirds. The patient often complains of weakness of the shoulder and fatigue on raising the arm above the head.

Suprascapular Nerve (C5–C6)

ANATOMY. This nerve is a branch of the upper trunk of the brachial plexus. The nerve passes downward beneath the trapezius to the upper border of the scapula, where it passes through the suprascapular notch. This notch is bridged by the superior transverse scapular ligament, forming an osseo-fibrous foramen through which the nerve passes to enter the supra-spinous area beneath the supraspinatus muscle. The nerve gives off branches to the supraspinatus and to the capsule of the shoulder joint and then courses around the free lateral border of the spine of the scapula to supply the infraspinatus muscle.

The supraspinatus muscle normally abducts the humerus (mainly the first 15 degrees of abduction), whereas the infraspinatus is mainly an external rotator of the upper arm.

NERVE LESIONS. The nerve may be injured in proximal upper brachial plexopathies and is also subject to damage in the supraclavicular region. Entrapment lesions may occur in the suprascapular foramen [27]. This entrapment will cause pain in the shoulder region that is aggravated by shoulder girdle movements, and also weakness and eventual atrophy in the two spinati muscles. Supraspinatus paresis results in weakness of arm abduction, whereas infraspinatus paresis results in impaired external rotation at the shoulder joint.

The branch to the infraspinatus muscle may be damaged in isolation by entrapment of the suprascapular nerve at the spinoglenoid notch by a hypertrophied inferior transverse scapular ligament [1]. This results in shoulder pain, which is elicited by external rotation of the shoulder joint associated with weakness and wasting of the infraspinatus.

Subscapular Nerves (C5–C7)

ANATOMY. These purely motor nerves arise as branches of the posterior cord of the brachial plexus. The upper subscapular nerves supply the subscapularis, whereas the lower subscapular nerves supply the teres major.

NERVE LESIONS. Subscapular nerve palsies usually occur with posterior cord brachial plexus lesions. The arm will be somewhat externally rotated with some paresis of internal rotation, although the latissimus dorsi and pectoralis major muscles are usually able to compensate well for this paresis. The patient may complain of difficulty in scratching his lower back.

Thoracodorsal Nerve (C6–C8)

ANATOMY. This purely motor nerve, also known as the nerve to the latissimus dorsi, is a branch of the posterior cord of the brachial plexus and usually emerges from the plexus in close association with the subscapular nerves. The nerve runs along the posterior axillary wall to reach and innervate the deep surface of the latissimus dorsi muscle. This muscle (along with the teres major) adducts and internally rotates the arm and depresses the raised arm. It is best tested by having the patient adduct the horizontally raised upper arm against resistance or by palpating the muscle bellies when the patient coughs [16].

NERVE LESIONS. Lesions of this nerve usually occur with damage to the posterior cord or proximal parts of the brachial plexus. Nerve lesions cause little deformity or atrophy, but proximal arm adduction is compromised. A combined movement comprising extension, adduction, and internal rotation in which the dorsum of the hand is placed on the opposite buttock usually best reveals latissimus paresis.

Anterior Thoracic Nerves (C5–T1)

ANATOMY. These purely motor nerves (also called the pectoral nerves) are divided into the lateral anterior thoracic nerve (C5–C7), a branch from the anterior divisions of the upper and middle trunks of the brachial plexus, and the medial anterior thoracic nerve (C8–T1), a branch of the proximal section of the medial cord of the plexus. After these nerves descend posterior to the clavicle, the lateral nerve supplies the clavicular and upper sternocostal portion of the pectoralis major, and the medial division supplies the lower sternocostal portion of this muscle and the pectoralis minor.

The pectoralis major is an adductor and medial rotator of the humerus. It is tested by having the patient hold the arm in front of the body. The two portions can be seen and palpated when the patient resists attempts by the examiner to force the arm laterally [2].

NERVE LESIONS. Lesions of these nerves are of relatively little clinical importance except in corroborating brachial plexus damage. Adduction and medial rotation of the upper arm are weak, and the patient will notice difficulty in using the arm in climbing.

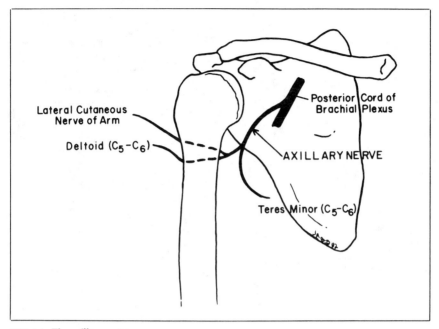

FIG. 1-1. *The axillary nerve.*

Axillary Nerve (C5–C6)

ANATOMY. The axillary (circumflex) nerve (Fig. 1-1), a mixed nerve, arises as one of the terminal branches of the posterior cord of the brachial plexus from spinal segments C5 and C6. The nerve descends on the subscapularis muscle behind the axillary artery and then winds around the surgical neck of the humerus accompanied by the posterior circumflex humeral artery. The nerve passes deep to the deltoid and teres minor muscles, supplying both. It sends sensory branches to the capsule of the shoulder joint *(articular branch)* and to the skin of the upper lateral aspect of the arm superficial to the deltoid muscle *(lateral cutaneous nerve of the arm).*

The teres minor muscle is a lateral rotator of the shoulder joint. The central part of the deltoid muscle is tested by having the patient abduct the upper arm against resistance (15–90 degrees), the anterior part is tested by elevating the arm forward against resistance (up to 90 degrees), and the posterior part is tested by having the patient retract the abducted upper arm against resistance.

NERVE LESIONS. Lesions of the posterior cord of the brachial plexus will affect this nerve as well as the radial nerve. The nerve is most often in-

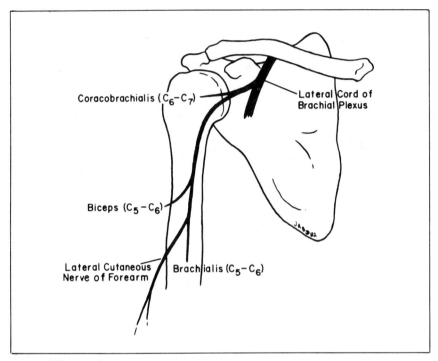

FIG. 1-2. *The musculocutaneous nerve.*

jured as it winds around the lateral aspect of the humerus in a relatively exposed position and also when the shoulder joint is dislocated or when the scapula is fractured [2]. These lesions usually cause a sensorimotor nerve palsy, but a purely motor palsy is possible with nerve lesions at the humeral head. A purely sensory loss with no motor defects is also possible [2]. In nerve lesions, the deltoid muscle becomes atrophic, causing a flattening or concavity of the shoulder contour. Teres minor paresis is usually not demonstrable on clinical examination because other muscles can perform its functions. Deltoid paralysis results in difficulty in abducting the arm, but this function can be compensated by other muscles of the shoulder girdle. An axillary cutaneous sensory defect is located on the outer aspect of the upper arm and is maximal on the patch of skin above the deltoid attachment.

Musculocutaneous Nerve (C5–C7)

ANATOMY. This mixed nerve (Fig. 1-2) arises from the lateral cord of the brachial plexus and proceeds obliquely downward between the axillary artery and the median nerve. The nerve pierces the coracobrachialis muscle and descends further between the biceps and brachialis muscles (it supplies all three of these muscles). It then continues distally as the lateral cutaneous nerve of the forearm after it pierces the deep fascia over the anterior elbow. The coracobrachialis muscle is a forward elevator of the arm, the brachialis (which occasionally also receives innervation from the radial nerve) is an elbow flexor, and the biceps is an elbow flexor and forearm supinator (especially when the elbow is flexed at 90 degrees). The biceps is tested by having the patient flex the supinated arm against resistance [16]. The biceps reflex is subserved by the musculocutaneous nerve.

The autonomous zone of the lateral cutaneous nerve of the forearm (a narrow band along the radial forearm) will show sensory loss. This zone of cutaneous sensory loss may extend from the elbow to the wrist and cover the entire lateral forearm from the dorsal to the ventral midline.

NERVE LESIONS. Nerve damage may result from lesions of the lateral cord of the brachial plexus. Because the nerve is deep and is protected between the entry site into the coracobrachialis and the elbow, lesions here are relatively uncommon. A purely sensory syndrome may result when the lateral cutaneous nerve of the forearm is damaged in the lateral cubital fossa or forearm.

With lesions of this nerve, atrophy of the biceps and brachialis results in wasting of the ventral aspect of the upper arm. Loss of coracobrachialis function is difficult to detect clinically. With biceps weakness, flexion of the elbow is weak (especially when the forearm is in supination), and the biceps reflex is lost.

Median Nerve (C5–T1)

ANATOMY. The mixed median nerve (Fig. 1-3) is formed in the axilla by the joining of the lateral cord of the brachial plexus (spinal segments C5–C7) with the medial cord (spinal segments C8–T1). The nerve then descends down the medial side of the arm in close association with the brachial artery to the cubital fossa. From there, the median nerve enters the forearm between the two heads of the pronator teres muscle and gives off the *anterior interosseous nerve*, after which it dips under the sublimies bridge. It then courses deep to the flexor retinaculum at the wrist *(carpal tunnel)* to reach the hand. At a variable distance above the flexor retinaculum, the median nerve provides a *palmar cutaneous branch*, which crosses the flexor retinaculum either subcutaneously or through the superficial ligament fibers to supply the skin over the thenar eminence and proximal palm on the radial aspect of the hand. The median

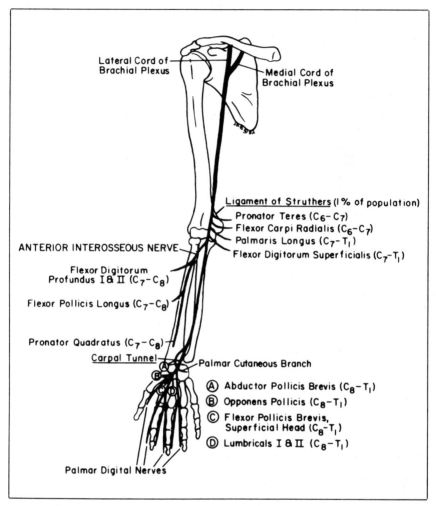

FIG. 1-3. *The median nerve.*

nerve passes through the carpal tunnel accompanied by the flexor tendons of the digits and emerges to divide into its terminal branches. These terminal branches include branches to the thenar muscles and the *palmar digital nerves,* which innervate the skin of the palmar aspect of the thumb, second, third, and half of the fourth finger, the palm overlying the corresponding metacarpophalangeal joints, and the posterior middle and distal phalanges of the second, third, and half of the fourth finger.

The median nerve gives off no muscular branches until it reaches the elbow. As it passes between the heads of the pronator teres muscle, it supplies the following muscles:

1. *Pronator teres* (C6–C7), a forearm pronator. It is tested by having the patient pronate the forearm against resistance.
2. *Flexor carpi radialis* (C6–C7), a radial flexor of the hand. This is tested by having the patient flex and abduct the hand at the wrist against resistance.
3. *Palmaris longus* (C7–T1), a flexor of the wrist.
4. *Flexor digitorum superficialis* (C7–T1), a flexor of the middle phalanges of the second, third, fourth, and fifth fingers. It is tested by having the patient flex the finger at the interphalangeal joint against resistance with the proximal phalanx fixed.

After it passes between the two heads of the pronator teres, the median nerve gives off the purely motor *anterior interosseous nerve*, which innervates the following three muscles:

1. *Flexor pollicis longus* (C7–C8), a flexor of the terminal phalanx of the thumb that is tested by having the patient flex the distal phalanx of the thumb against resistance while the proximal phalanx is fixed.
2. *Flexor digitorum profundus I and II* (C7–C8), a flexor of the terminal phalanges of the second and third fingers. It is tested by having the patient flex the distal phalanx of the second and third fingers against resistance with the middle phalanx fixed.
3. *Pronator quadratus* (C7–C8), a forearm pronator.

At the distal end of the carpal tunnel, the nerve divides into its terminal branches. The motor branches innervate the first and second lumbricals and the thenar muscles, which include the following:

1. *Abductor pollicis brevis* (C8–T1), an abductor of the metacarpal of the thumb. It is tested by having the patient abduct the thumb at right angles to the palm against resistance.
2. *Opponens pollicis* (C8–T1), a muscle that brings the metacarpal of the thumb into opposition. It is tested by having the patient touch the base of the little finger with the thumb against resistance.
3. *Superficial head of the flexor pollicis brevis* (C8–T1), a flexor of the proximal phalanx of the thumb.
4. *Lumbricals I and II* (C8–T1), flexors of the proximal and extensors of the

two distal phalanges of the second and third fingers. They are tested by having the patient extend the finger at the proximal interphalangeal joint against resistance with the metacarpophalangeal joint fixed and hyperextended.

The finger flexor reflex (C8-T1) is in part innervated by the median nerve.

It is important to be aware of potential variations in the innervation of the intrinsic hand muscles. Anomalous communications in the hand are sometimes referred to as *Riche-Cannieu anastomoses* [3, 20, 23] and are thought to involve communications between the motor branch of the median nerve and the deep ulnar nerve branch in the radial aspect of the hand. For example, the adductor pollicis and first dorsal interosseous muscles may be exclusively supplied by the median nerve and thus will be involved in median nerve lesions and spared in ulnar lesions. Also, the abductor pollicis brevis and the flexor pollicis brevis may be exclusively supplied by the ulnar nerve.

NERVE LESIONS

LESIONS IN THE AXILLA AND UPPER ARM. Lesions at this level [22] will result in paresis or paralysis of all the muscles innervated by the median nerve with a sensory loss in the distribution of both the palmar cutaneous and palmar digital branches. There will be atrophy of the thenar eminence affecting especially the abductor pollicis brevis and the opponens pollicis. Because of the atrophy of the thenar eminence with recession of the metacarpal bones of the thumb to the plane of the other metacarpal bones, the hand takes on an abnormal appearance called *simian hand* or *ape hand*. This appearance results from the unopposed action of the extensor pollicis longus (radial nerve) and the adductor pollicis (ulnar nerve). Because the second finger cannot be flexed and the third finger can be flexed only partially, when the person attempts to make a fist these fingers remain extended. The hand then takes on the appearance of that of a clergyman saying benediction *(benediction hand)*.

Because all of the median muscles are affected, there will be paresis of forearm pronation, of radial wrist flexion, of distal flexion of the thumb, of palmar abduction and opposition of the thumb, and of flexion of the second and to a lesser extent, the third fingers.

LESIONS AT THE LIGAMENT OF STRUTHERS. In approximately 1 percent of the population, an anomalous spur of bone occurs 3 to 5 cm above the medial epicondyle on the anteromedial humerus. A fibrous tunnel may be formed by a ligament *(ligament of Struthers)* that connects this spur to the medial epicondyle. The median nerve may be compressed here by this ligament, causing motor and sensory signs and symptoms as described in Lesions in the Axilla and Upper Arm (above) [29].

THE PRONATOR SYNDROME. The median nerve may be entrapped or constricted where it passes between the two heads of the pronator teres muscle and under the fibrous arch of the flexor digitorum superficialis *(pronator syndrome)* [17]. Nerve injury is especially likely to occur if the nerve passes deep to a hypertrophied pronator teres. This syndrome has the following characteristics:

1. Pain in the proximal forearm, especially on resistance to pronation of the forearm and on flexion at the wrist.
2. Tenderness on deep pressure over the pronator teres muscle.
3. Frequently, lack of involvement of the pronator teres, flexor carpi radialis, palmaris longus, and flexor digitorum muscles because nerve branches to these muscles often depart from the median nerve proper before the site of nerve compression.
4. Sparing of the muscles innervated by the anterior interosseous nerve if this nerve takes a high origin from the median trunk.
5. Paresthesias and sensory loss in the median field of innervation (both palmar and digital cutaneous areas).
6. Atrophy and paresis of the median thenar musculature.

THE ANTERIOR INTEROSSEOUS NERVE SYNDROME (KILOH-NEVIN SYNDROME). Isolated lesions of this nerve [5, 19, 25] are not uncommon and may be due to trauma, to a fibrous band constricting the nerve, or to an accessory head of the flexor pollicis longus *(Gantzer's muscle)* entrapping the nerve. This pure motor syndrome consists of several characteristics.

1. Mild paresis of forearm pronation (due to pronator quadratus weakness).
2. Paresis of flexion of the terminal phalanges of the second and third fingers (due to paresis of the flexor digitorum profundus I and II).
3. Paresis of flexion of the terminal phalanx of the thumb (due to paresis of the flexor pollicis longus).
4. A characteristic *pinch attitude* of the hand on attempting to make a full circle by applying the pulp of the thumb to that of the index finger with firm pressure. This results from weakness of the flexor pollicis longus and the flexor digitorum profundus. There is hyperextension of the interphalangeal joint of the thumb, inability to flex the thumb and index distal phalanges, and proximal approximation of the thumb on the index finger.
5. Normal sensation.

THE CARPAL TUNNEL SYNDROME. The median nerve is particularly vulnerable to compression as it passes into the hand between the carpal bones and the transverse carpal ligament (carpal tunnel). This syndrome usually consists of four main symptoms.

1. Bouts of pain or paresthesia in the wrist and hand that are often most severe and troublesome during the hours of sleep. Although these symptoms are usually localized to the wrist or median innervated fingers, they may spread upward into the forearm.
2. Paresis and atrophy of the abductor pollicis brevis and opponens pollicis muscles. Because the opponens pollicis is occasionally anomalously supplied by the ulnar nerve, this muscle may be spared.
3. Sensory loss on the lateral palm, the palmar aspect of the first three and a half fingers, and the dorsal aspect of the terminal phalanges of the second, third, and half of the fourth fingers. This sensory loss is usually most prominent in the appropriate fingertips. (Because the palmar cutaneous nerve takes its origin proximal to the wrist joint, sensation on the thenar eminence and proximoradial palm is spared. Thus, if this area shows a sensory loss, the lesion is proximal to the wrist joint).
4. Increased sensitivity of the damaged nerve fibers to mechanical deformation. Because of this, various clinical tests may help to detect a lesion at the carpal tunnel. Percussion over the nerve tunnel may elicit a tingling sensation in the median distribution *(Tinel's sign)*. When a blood pressure cuff is applied to the arm and compression is above systolic pressure, median paresthesias and pain may be aggravated *(cuff compression test of Gilliatt and Wilson)*. Flexion of the wrists for 1 minute may aggravate paresthesias and pain *(Phalen's sign)*, as may hyperextension of the wrist.

LESIONS WITHIN THE HAND. Injury to the deep palmar branches of the median nerve in the distal carpal canal or at the thenar eminence will produce a pure motor syndrome with weakness and wasting of the thenar muscles (abductor pollicis brevis, opponens pollicis, and superficial head of the flexor pollicis brevis) with no sensory abnormalities.

Ulnar Nerve (C7–T1)

ANATOMY. This mixed nerve (Fig. 1-4) is the main branch of the medial cord of the brachial plexus and is derived from the seventh and eighth cervical and first thoracic spinal roots. It crosses the axilla beneath the pectoralis minor muscle and continues to the upper arm, where it lies

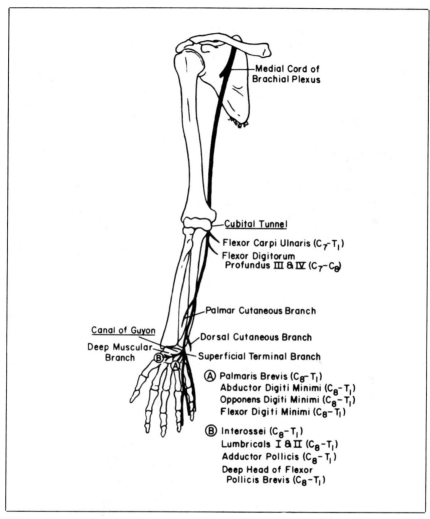

FIG. 1-4. *The ulnar nerve.*

medial to the brachial artery. In the distal arm it enters a groove between the medial humeral epicondyle and the olecranon process. It then passes between the humeral and ulnar heads of the flexor carpi ulnaris to rest upon the flexor digitorum profundus. The aponeurosis between the olecranon and medial epicondyle forms the roof of an osseofibrous canal *(the cubital tunnel),* the floor of which is formed by the medial ligament of the elbow joint. Immediately distal to the elbow joint the nerve gives off its first two muscular branches, the flexor carpi ulnaris and the flexor digitorum profundus III and IV.

FLEXOR CARPI ULNARIS (C7-T1). An ulnar flexor of the wrist. It is tested by having the patient flex and adduct the hand at the wrist against resistance.

FLEXOR DIGITORUM PROFUNDUS III AND IV (C7-C8). A flexor of the terminal phalanges of the fourth and fifth fingers. It is tested by having the patient flex the distal interphalangeal joint against resistance while fixing the third phalanx.

The ulnar nerve then descends beneath the flexor carpi ulnaris and in the middle of the forearm gives off the *palmar cutaneous branch*, which supplies the skin over the hypothenar eminence. It then gives off a *dorsal cutaneous branch*, which supplies the dorsal ulnar aspect of the hand and the dorsal aspect of the fifth finger and half of the fourth finger. The ulnar nerve proper then enters the wrist lateral to the tendon of the flexor carpi ulnaris muscle. In the hand it gives off the *superficial terminal branch*, which is a sensory branch to the skin of the distal part of the ulnar aspect of the palm and the palmar aspect of the fifth and half of the fourth finger, and then passes between the pisiform carpal bone medially and the hook of the hamate carpal bone laterally *(canal of Guyon)* as the deep muscular branch. This deep branch supplies several muscles:

1. *Palmaris brevis* (C8-T1). A cutaneous muscle at the proximal border of the ulnar aspect of the hand.
2. *Abductor digiti minimi* (C8-T1). An abductor of the fifth finger. It is tested by having the patient abduct the fifth finger against resistance while the volar aspect of the hand is on a flat surface.
3. *Opponens digiti minimi* (C8-T1). An opposer of the fifth finger.
4. *Flexor digiti minimi* (C8-T1). A flexor of the fifth finger. It is tested by having the patient flex the fifth finger at the metacarpophalangeal joint against resistance.
5. *Lumbricals III and IV* (C8-T1). Flexors of the metacarpophalangeal joints and extensors of the proximal interphalangeal joints of the fifth and fourth fingers. It is tested by having the patient extend the proximal interphalangeal joint against resistance with the metacarpophalangeal joint hyperextended and fixed.
6. *Interosseous muscles* (C8-T1). Flexors of the metacarpophalangeal joints and extensors of the proximal interphalangeal joints. The four dorsal interossei are finger abductors, whereas the three palmar interossei are finger adductors. They are tested by spreading or abducting the fingers against resistance.
7. *Adductor pollicis* (C8-T1). An adductor of the metacarpal of the thumb.

It is tested by having the patient adduct the thumb at right angles to the palm against resistance.

8. *Deep head of the flexor pollicis brevis* (C8–T1). A flexor of the first phalanx of the thumb.

NERVE LESIONS

LESIONS ABOVE THE ELBOW. Lesions of the ulnar nerve above the elbow (e.g., a lesion of the medial cord of the brachial plexus) will produce the following signs:

Abnormal Appearance of the Hand. There will be atrophy and flattening of the hypothenar eminence and interossei. The hand will often have a "claw-hand" deformity *(main en griffe),* in which the fifth, fourth, and, to a lesser extent, the third fingers are hyperextended at the metacarpophalangeal joints and flexed at the interphalangeal joints. The hyperextension at the metacarpophalangeal joints is due to paralysis of the interossei and ulnar lumbricals, which results in unopposed action of the long finger extensors (extensor digitorum); the flexion at the interphalangeal joints is due to pull exerted by the long flexor tendons.

Paresis or Paralysis of Ulnar Flexion. This applies to ulnar flexion of the wrist, of the terminal phalanges of the fourth and fifth fingers, and at the metacarpophalangeal joints of the second to fifth fingers. Ulnar paresis or paralysis also affects extension at the interphalangeal joints of the second to fifth fingers, adduction and abduction of the second to fifth fingers, and abduction and opposition of the fifth finger. As a result of adductor pollicis affection, *Froment's prehensile thumb sign (signe du journal)* may be present (when a sheet of paper is grasped between the thumb and index finger and pulled, the proximal phalanx of the thumb is extended and the distal phalanx is flexed if an ulnar nerve lesion is present).

In 15 to 31 percent of subjects, a median-ulnar communication exists *(Martin-Gruber anastomosis)* [15, 28] in which axons descending in the median nerve cross through the forearm to join the ulnar nerve at the wrist. The median fibers ultimately innervate the intrinsic hand muscles, especially the first dorsal interosseous, adductor pollicis, and hypothenar muscles. Thus, if a patient has an ulnar neuropathy above the forearm, these muscles may be spared or minimally involved if a median-ulnar communication is present.

Sensory Findings. Because all three sensory branches of the ulnar nerve are affected (palmar, dorsal, and superficial terminal cutaneous branches), paresthesias and sensory loss occur on the dorsal and palmar surfaces of the fifth and ulnar half of the fourth finger and the ulnar portion of the hand to the wrist.

LESIONS AT THE ELBOW (CUBITAL TUNNEL SYNDROME). The ulnar nerve is frequently compressed at the elbow in the cubital tunnel [6] because this tunnel narrows during movement, especially elbow flexion. Nerve entrapment is due to thickening of the aponeurotic arch between the two heads of the flexor carpi ulnaris or bulging of the medial collateral ligament of the elbow joint (floor of the cubital tunnel). The syndrome produced will be the same as that described in Lesions Above the Elbow, above.

LESIONS AT THE WRIST AND IN THE HAND. An ulnar lesion at the wrist will cause the same motor findings as a lesion at a more proximal level, except that the flexor carpi ulnaris and the flexor digitorum profundus III and IV will be spared. The sensory findings will depend on the location of the nerve lesion with respect to the sites of origin of the palmar and dorsal cutaneous branches. If the lesion is distal to these two branches, the sensory loss will be restricted to the distal palm and the palmar surfaces of the fifth and medial fourth finger (the area of supply of the superficial terminal cutaneous branch). The proximal palmar area and the entire dorsum of the hand will then be spared.

Lesions of the ulnar nerve in the hand have been divided by Ebeling et al. [4] into three groups:

1. Compression of the nerve as it enters the hand. All of the ulnar-innervated muscles of the hand are affected, and because the lesion is proximal to the superficial terminal cutaneous nerve, there will be sensory loss on the distal palm and the palmar surfaces of the fifth finger and medial half of the fourth finger.
2. Compression of the proximal part of the terminal motor branch (usually due to nerve compression within the canal of Guyon or pisohamate tunnel). In these pure motor lesions all of the hand muscles innervated by the ulnar nerve are affected. Because the lesion is distal to the superficial terminal cutaneous branch, there is no sensory loss.
3. Distal compression of the terminal motor branch of the ulnar nerve. This pure motor lesion is distal to the site of origin of the motor fibers to the hypothenar muscles and is also distal to all sensory branches. It will thus result in paresis and atrophy of the interossei, the medial two lumbricals, and the adductor pollicis muscles only.

Radial Nerve (C5–C8)

ANATOMY. This mixed nerve (Fig. 1-5) is derived from the posterior cord of the brachial plexus and is composed of fibers from spinal levels C5 to C8. This nerve descends posterior to the axillary artery and between the

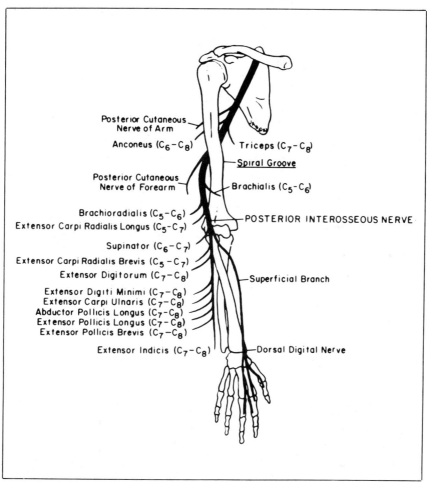

Posterior Cutaneous
Nerve of Arm

Anconeus (C_6–C_8)

Triceps (C_7–C_8)

Spiral Groove

Posterior Cutaneous
Nerve of Forearm

Brachialis (C_5–C_6)

Brachioradialis (C_5–C_6)
Extensor Carpi Radialis Longus (C_5–C_7)

POSTERIOR INTEROSSEOUS NERVE

Supinator (C_6–C_7)
Extensor Carpi Radialis Brevis (C_5–C_7)
Extensor Digitorum (C_7–C_8)

Superficial Branch

Extensor Digiti Minimi (C_7–C_8)
Extensor Carpi Ulnaris (C_7–C_8)
Abductor Pollicis Longus (C_7–C_8)
Extensor Pollicis Longus (C_7–C_8)
Extensor Pollicis Brevis (C_7–C_8)

Extensor Indicis (C_7–C_8)

Dorsal Digital Nerve

FIG. 1-5. *The radial nerve.*

long and medial heads of the triceps. It then continues distally in the spiral groove of the humerus (in contact with the bone or separated from it by some fibers of the medial head of the triceps).

In the axilla, the nerve gives rise to the *posterior cutaneous nerve of the arm,* which supplies the skin over the posterior aspect of the arm as far down as the olecranon. A secondary sensory branch, the *posterior cutaneous nerve of the forearm,* arises either within or proximal to the spiral groove and innervates the skin on the distal extensor aspect of the arm and the extensor aspect of the forearm up to the wrist. Within or proximal to the spiral groove, two motor branches are given off. They supply two muscles:

1. *Triceps* (C6–C8), a forearm extensor subserving the triceps reflex. The muscle is tested by having the patient extend the forearm at the elbow against resistance.
2. *Anconeus* (C6–C8), a forearm extensor.

After its course in the spiral groove, the radial nerve reaches the lateral aspect of the humerus and pierces the lateral intermuscular septum to occupy a position in front of the lateral condyle of the humerus between the brachialis and brachioradialis muscles. Here it supplies the following muscles:

1. *Brachialis* (C5–C6), an elbow flexor. It is also innervated by the musculocutaneous nerve.
2. *Brachioradialis* (C5–C6), a forearm flexor. It is tested by having the patient flex the forearm against resistance with the forearm midway between pronation and supination. This muscle subserves the radial reflex.
3. *Extensor carpi radialis longus* (C6–C7), a radial extensor of the hand. It is tested by having the patient extend and abduct the hand against resistance.

The radial trunk then bifurcates into a superficial branch and a deep branch. The *superficial branch* passes over the origin of the extensor carpi radialis brevis and down the forearm under the brachioradialis. It emerges in the distal forearm and, as the *dorsal digital nerve*, supplies the skin on the medial aspect of the back of the hand and the dorsum of the first four fingers (the autonomous zone of supply is the skin over the first interosseous space).

The *deep branch* passes through the fibrous edge of the extensor carpi radialis through a slit in the supinator muscle *(arcade of Frohse)* to the posterior forearm. In the forearm it is in contact with the interrosseous membrane and is referred to as the *posterior interosseous nerve*. This purely motor nerve innervates the following muscles:

1. *Supinator* (C6–C7), a forearm supinator that is tested by having the patient supinate the forearm against resistance.
2. *Extensor carpi radialis brevis* (C5–C7), a radial extensor of the hand.
3. *Extensor digitorum* (C7–C8), an extensor of the metacarpophalangeal joints of the second through the fifth fingers. It is tested by having the patient extend the metacarpophalangeal joints against resistance.

4. *Extensor digiti minimi* (C7–C8), an extensor of the metacarpophalangeal joint of the fifth finger.
5. *Extensor carpi ulnaris* (C7–C8), an ulnar extensor of the hand that is tested by having the patient extend and adduct the hand at the wrist against resistance.
6. *Abductor pollicis longus* (C7–C8), an abductor of the metacarpal of the thumb. It is tested by having the patient abduct the carpometacarpal joint in a plane at right angles to the palm.
7. *Extensor pollicis longus* (C7–C8), an extensor of the thumb. It is tested by extending the thumb at the interphalangeal joint against resistance.
8. *Extensor pollicis brevis* (C7–C8), an extensor of the thumb that is tested by having the patient extend the thumb at the metacarpophalangeal joint against resistance.
9. *Extensor indicis* (C7–C8), an extensor of the second finger.

NERVE LESIONS

LESIONS IN THE AXILLA. Lesions of the posterior cord of the brachial plexus or high axillary lesions affect all of the sensory and motor branches of the radial nerve. Symptoms include:

Abnormal Appearance of the Hand. Characteristically, the hand hangs in flexion *(wrist drop).* There is wasting of the dorsal arm (triceps) and muscle mass on the posterior surface of the forearm.

Motor Loss. There is paresis or paralysis of extension of the elbow, extension of the wrist, supination of the forearm, extension of all five metacarpophalangeal joints, and extension and abduction of the interphalangeal joint of the thumb. Elbow flexion tends to be weak.

Hyporeflexia or Areflexia of the Triceps (C6–C8) and Radial (C5–C6) Reflexes.

Sensory Loss. There are paresthesias and sensory loss on the entire extensor surface of the arm and forearm and on the back of the hand and dorsum of the first four fingers.

LESIONS WITHIN THE SPIRAL GROOVE OF THE HUMERUS. Lesions at this location are usually due to humeral fractures or compressive lesions *(Saturday night palsy).* These patients will have the same symptoms as those described for Lesions in the Axilla (above) except for the following modifications:

1. Sensibility on the extensor aspect of the arm is spared because this nerve usually arises high in the axilla.
2. Sensibility on the extensor aspect of the forearm may or may not be spared depending on the site of origin of this nerve from the radial nerve proper.

3. The triceps muscle (and therefore the triceps reflex) is spared because the branches to this muscle have a proximal origin.

Lesions distal to the spiral groove and distal to the site of origin of the brachioradialis and extensor carpi radialis longus (prior to the bifurcation of the nerve) have symptoms that are similar to those seen with a spiral groove lesion with the following exceptions:

1. The brachioradialis and extensor carpi radialis longus muscles are spared.
2. The radial reflex is spared.
3. Sensibility on the extensor surface of the forearm (posterior cutaneous nerve of the forearm) is more likely to be spared.

LESIONS AT THE ELBOW. The posterior interosseous nerve (deep motor branch of the radial nerve) may be injured or entrapped at the elbow. Entrapment may be caused by:

1. A constricting band at the radiohumeral joint capsule.
2. The sharp edge of the extensor carpi radialis brevis muscle [7].
3. A fibrotendinous arch where the nerve enters the supinator muscle (arcade of Frohse) [24].
4. Its occurrence within the substance of the supinator muscle (supinator channel syndrome).

When the posterior interosseous nerve is damaged at these locations, the supinator muscle and the superficial sensory branch of the radial nerve are often spared. These patients have atrophy and paresis of the extensor carpi ulnaris, extensor digitorum, extensor digiti minimi, abductor pollicis longus and brevis, and extensor indicis. Because the extensor carpi radialis is unaffected while the extensor carpi ulnaris is paretic, the wrist will deviate radially, especially when the patient attempts to make a fist. The patient will have difficulty in extending the metacarpophalangeal joints of all five fingers, extending the wrist in an ulnar direction, extending the interphalangeal joint of the thumb, and abducting the thumb. The superficial cutaneous branch may be injured anywhere along its location in the forearm, resulting in a pure sensory syndrome (paresthesias and sensory loss) that affects the radial part of the dorsum of the hand and the dorsal aspect of the first three and a half fingers. (The autonomous zone of sensory loss will occur on the area of skin covering the first interosseous space.) Paresthesias and sensory loss confined to the radial side of the thumb (*cheiralgia paresthetica*) may occur with a lesion of the distal dorsal digital nerve (in the thumb).

Medial Cutaneous Nerves of the Arm and Forearm (C8–T1)

ANATOMY. These two purely sensory branches arise from the medial cord of the brachial plexus. The medial cutaneous nerve of the arm supplies the skin of the axilla and medial part of the arm. The medial cutaneous nerve of the forearm divides above the elbow into anterior and posterior divisions that supply the skin of the anteromedial and posteromedial forearm, respectively, down to the wrist.

NERVE LESIONS. Injuries to these nerves may occur in the axilla, affecting the medial cord of the brachial plexus. A sensory loss will occur in the distribution of the individual nerve branches.

Iliohypogastric (T12–L1), Ilioinguinal (L1), and Genitofemoral (L1–L2) Nerves

ANATOMY AND NERVE LESIONS. The mixed *iliohypogastric nerve* arises from the anterior rami of spinal root segments T12 and L1. The nerve runs across the psoas muscle and then behind the kidney, crossing the quadratus lumborum muscle and reaching the iliac crest. It then pierces the internal oblique and transversus abdominis muscles, both of which it supplies. It terminates in the *lateral cutaneous branch,* a sensory nerve that supplies the skin over the outer buttock and hip, and the *anterior cutaneous branch,* a sensory branch that supplies the anterior abdominal wall above the pubis.

This nerve may be injured in the lumbar plexus, at the posterior or anterior abdominal wall, or distally near the inguinal ring. Lesions of this nerve result in little motor deficit but lead to pain or sensory loss in the area of cutaneous supply of the nerve.

The mixed *ilioinguinal nerve* arises from the anterior ramus of the first lumbar spinal segment within the psoas muscle. It runs laterally and downward parallel with the iliohypogastric nerve to reach the iliac crest. This nerve, like the iliohypogastric, supplies the internal oblique and transversus abdominis muscles. After it pierces and supplies these two muscles, it enters the inguinal canal and passes to the superficial inguinal ring, from which its sensory fibers emerge. These fibers are distributed to the skin of the medial thigh below the inguinal ligament as well as to the skin of the symphysis pubis and the external genitalia.

This nerve may be injured in the lumbar plexus, at the posterior abdominal wall, at the anterior abdominal wall, or within the inguinal canal. Lesions of this nerve cause the *ilioinguinal syndrome,* which consists of pain and sensory loss in the inguinal region. Motor findings are negligible.

The *genitofemoral nerve,* a predominantly sensory nerve, arises from the first and second lumbar segments within the substance of the psoas muscle. It transverses the psoas muscle and, near the inguinal ligament, divides into two branches; the *genital branch* (mainly L1) enters the deep inguinal ring, traverses the inguinal canal, and ends in the cremaster muscle and skin of the scrotum (or labia majus) and adjacent medial thigh. The *femoral branch* (mainly L2) passes behind the inguinal ligament near the femoral artery and supplies the skin over the femoral triangle.

Injury to this nerve may occur in the lumbar plexus, within the abdomen, or in the femoral or inguinal region. Injury will cause pain and sensory loss in the area of cutaneous supply of the nerve. The cremasteric reflex, which is subserved by this nerve, may be lost on the side of the nerve lesion.

Femoral Nerve (L2−L4)

ANATOMY. This mixed nerve (Fig. 1-6) arises within the substance of the psoas muscle from the posterior rami of the second, third, and fourth lumbar segments. The nerve runs in the groove between the psoas and iliacus muscles (flexors of the thigh, both of which it supplies) and descends beneath the inguinal ligament (lateral to the femoral artery) to enter the thigh. Just distal to the inguinal ligament within the femoral triangle, it separates into the anterior and posterior divisions. The *anterior division* divides almost immediately into a *muscular branch* (to the sartorius muscle, a flexor and evertor of the thigh) and into a sensory branch, the *medial cutaneous nerve of the thigh* (which supplies the skin of the anterior and medial aspects of the thigh). The *posterior division* immediately divides into the sensory *saphenous nerve* and into *muscular branches.* The muscular branches of the posterior division of the femoral nerve supply the following muscles:

1. *Pectineus muscle* (L2–L3), an adductor, flexor, and evertor of the thigh.
2. *Quadriceps femoris muscle* (L2–L4), an extensor of the leg. It is tested by having the patient extend the leg against resistance with the extremity flexed at the hip and knee. This muscle is also, particularly through the rectus femoris, an extensor of the thigh. The tendon of this muscle subserves the patellar reflex.

The *saphenous nerve* descends to the knee in the adductor canal, accompanied by the femoral artery, and becomes cutaneous between the tendons of the sartorius and gracilis muscles. It then joins the great saphenous vein and proceeds to the medial aspect of the leg. It supplies

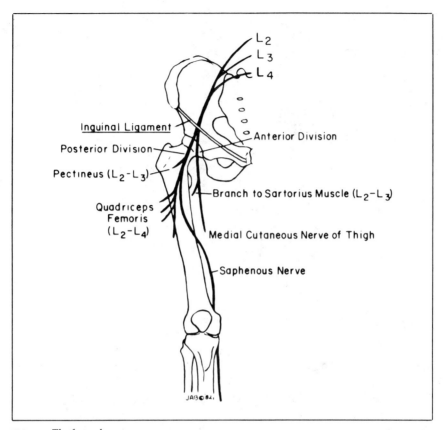

FIG. 1-6. *The femoral nerve.*

the skin over the medial aspect of the lower leg as far as the medial malleolus.

NERVE LESIONS. A proximal lesion of the femoral nerve (e.g., at the lumbar plexus or within the pelvis) [21] will result in the following signs:

1. Atrophy. There will be wasting of the musculature of the anterior part of the thigh.
2. Motor signs. There will be weakness or paralysis of hip flexion (iliacus, psoas, and rectus femoris muscles) and an inability to extend the leg (quadriceps femoris). With paralysis of the sartorius muscle, lateral thigh rotation may be impaired.
3. Sensory symptoms and signs. Sensory loss, paresthesias, and occa-

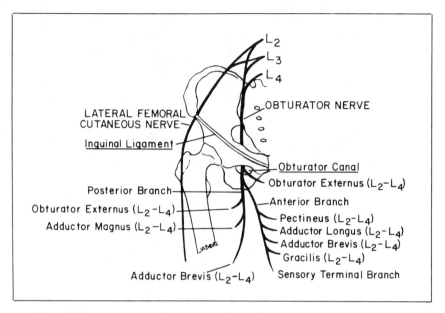

FIG. 1-7. *The obturator nerve and lateral femoral cutaneous nerve.*

sionally pain will occur on the anteromedial thigh and inner leg as far as the ankle.

4. Reflex signs. The patellar reflex will be depressed or absent.

Lesions at the inguinal ligament will result in similar findings, but thigh flexion will be spared because of the more proximal origin of the femoral nerve branches to the iliacus and psoas muscles. A pure motor syndrome (quadriceps atrophy and paresis) may result from lesions within the femoral triangle that affect the posterior division of the femoral nerve distal to the origin of the saphenous branch. A pure sensory syndrome (pain, paresthesias, and sensory loss) may result when the saphenous nerve alone is damaged. This nerve is most susceptible to injury where it pierces the aponeurotic roof of the adductor canal above the knee. In this syndrome, the only sign is a sensory disturbance that affects the medial side of the lower leg.

Obturator Nerve (L2–L4)

ANATOMY. This mixed nerve (Fig. 1-7) arises from the anterior primary rami of the second, third, and fourth lumbar segments within the substance of the psoas muscle. The nerve courses along the pelvis and enters the *obturator canal*. Within the obturator canal it supplies the obturator externus muscle and then divides into two branches, the anterior and posterior branches, which descend into the medial thigh. The mixed *anterior division* supplies the pectineus, adductor longus and adductor brevis (adductors of the thigh), and the gracilis (an internal rotator of the thigh and flexor of the knee) and ends in a sensory *terminal branch* that supplies the skin over the medial thigh. The motor *posterior division* supplies the obturator externus, adductor magnus, and adductor brevis muscles (adductors of the thigh). Motor function subserved by the obturator nerve is evaluated by having the patient adduct the extended leg against resistance.

NERVE LESIONS. The obturator nerve may be damaged within the lumbar plexus, near the sacroiliac joint, on the lateral pelvic wall, or within the obturator canal. Nerve damage results in wasting of the musculature of the inner aspect of the thigh, paresis of adduction of the thigh, and a sensory disturbance affecting the medial aspect of the thigh.

Lateral Femoral Cutaneous Nerve (L2–L3)

ANATOMY. This purely sensory nerve (Fig. 1-7) is derived from the primary rami of the second and third lumbar segments within the substance of the psoas muscle. It penetrates the psoas and crosses the iliacus muscle to the anterior superior iliac spine. It then passes medial to the spine beneath the inguinal ligament and enters the thigh beneath the fascia lata. The nerve runs downward and divides into two branches; the *anterior division,* which supplies the skin of the anterior thigh to the knee, and the *posterior division,* which supplies the skin of the upper half of the lateral aspect of the thigh.

NERVE LESIONS. The nerve is most often damaged within the abdomen or in the inguinal region. Compression or angulation of the nerve by the inguinal ligament near the anterior superior iliac spine may result in pain and paresthesias on the lateral or anterolateral aspect of the thigh. These paresthesias are associated with sensory loss in the cutaneous distribution of the lateral femoral cutaneous nerve *(meralgia paresthetica,* or *Bernhardt-Roth syndrome)* [12]. This sensory syndrome occurs especially in obese individuals who wear constricting garments (e.g., corsets) and may be bilateral.

Gluteal Nerves (L4–S2)

ANATOMY AND NERVE LESIONS. These purely motor nerves (Fig. 1-8) include the superior gluteal (from rami L4–S1) and inferior gluteal (from rami

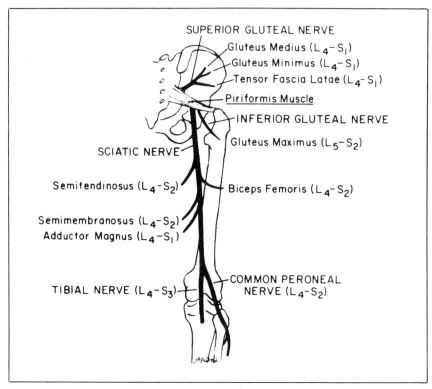

FIG. 1-8. *The sciatic nerve proper, superior gluteal nerve, and inferior gluteal nerve.*

L5–S2) nerves, which supply the musculature of the buttocks. The *superior gluteal nerve* leaves the pelvis by way of the greater sciatic notch above the piriformis muscle *(suprapyriform foramen)* to supply the gluteus medius (L4–S1), gluteus minimus (L4–S1), and tensor fasciae latae (L4–S1) muscles, which are abductors and internal rotators of the thigh. These muscles are especially important in maintaining the horizontal plane of the pelvis during walking. Lesions of the superior gluteal nerve may occur within the lumbosacral plexus, pelvis, greater sciatic foramen, or buttock. On walking, the pelvis will tilt toward the side of the unaffected raised leg *(Trendelenburg's sign)*. There will be paresis or paralysis of thigh abduction and medial rotation.

The *inferior gluteal nerve* leaves the pelvis by way of the greater sciatic notch below the piriformis muscle *(infrapyriform foramen)*, at which point it is near the sciatic nerve and posterior cutaneous nerve of the thigh. This nerve sends its branches to the gluteus maximus muscle (L5–S2), the main hip extensor, which is tested by having the patient extend the thigh against resistance.

The inferior gluteal nerve may be injured within the lumbosacral plexus, pelvis, greater sciatic foramen, or buttock. Nerve palsy results in paresis or paralysis of hip extension, which is most noticeable when the patient attempts to climb stairs.

Posterior Femoral Cutaneous Nerve (S1–S3)

ANATOMY AND NERVE LESIONS. This purely sensory nerve arises from the anterior primary rami of the first through third sacral segments. It leaves the pelvis through the greater sciatic notch and descends downward into the buttock deep to the gluteus muscle. It supplies the skin of the posterior thigh and popliteal fossa.

Damage to this nerve (which may occur in the sacral plexus, greater sciatic foramen, or buttock) results in a sensory disturbance in the cutaneous area of supply of the nerve.

Pudendal Nerve (S1–S4)

ANATOMY AND NERVE LESIONS. This nerve originates from the anterior rami of the first through fourth sacral segments. It leaves the pelvis through the greater sciatic notch below the piriformis muscle *(infrapyriform foramen)* and reaches the perineum. This mixed nerve supplies motor branches to the perineal muscles and external anal sphincter and sensory branches to the skin of the perineum, penis (or clitoris), scrotum (or labia majus), and anus.

Lesions of this nerve will produce a sensory disturbance in the cutaneous area of supply of these nerves and difficulty with bladder and bowel control.

Sciatic Nerve (L4–S3) and Its Branches

SCIATIC NERVE PROPER. This mixed nerve (Fig. 1-8) is derived from the fourth and fifth lumbar and the first, second, and third sacral spinal segments. The nerve emerges from the sacral plexus and leaves the pelvis through the greater sciatic foramen below the piriformis muscle *(infrapyriform foramen)*. The nerve then curves laterally and downward beneath the gluteus maximus muscle; in the posterior aspect of the thigh it innervates the semitendinosus (L4–S2), semimembranosus (L4–S2), and biceps femoris (L4–S2) muscles (i.e., the hamstring muscles, which are flexors of the knee joint) and the adductor magnus (L4–S1) muscle, an adductor of the thigh (which is also supplied by the obturator nerve). The nerve proceeds downward in the thigh, and at the apex of the popliteal fossa it divides into its two terminal branches, the *tibial* (medial

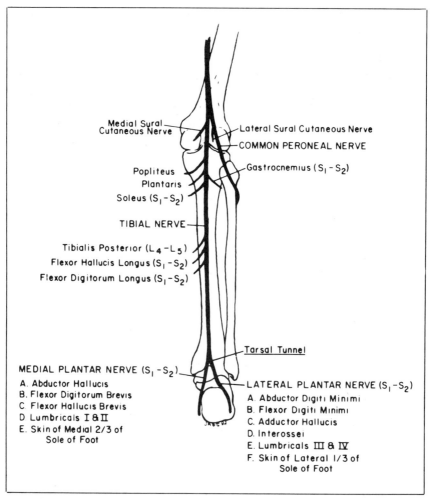

FIG. 1-9. *The tibial nerve.*

popliteal) *nerve* (L4–S3) and the *common peroneal* (lateral popliteal) *nerve* (L4–S2).

TIBIAL NERVE. The tibial nerve (Fig. 1-9) crosses the middle of the popliteal space and courses down the back of the leg. In the popliteal fossa it gives off the *medial sural cutaneous nerve.* This branch supplies the skin on the calf and then joins the lateral sural cutaneous nerve (a branch of the common peroneal) at the level of the Achilles tendon, forming the *sural nerve.* The sural nerve supplies the skin on the lateral heel and lateral aspect of the foot and small toe.

In the distal popliteal fossa the tibial nerve sends branches to the gastrocnemius (S1–S2) and soleus (S1–S2) muscles, which are the main plantar flexors of the foot, and to the popliteus and plantaris muscles. The nerve then descends in a plane between the gastrocnemius and soleus muscles posteriorly and the tibialis posterior anteriorly. It here gives off branches to three muscles:

1. *Tibialis posterior* (L4–L5), a plantar flexor of the foot and invertor of the foot. It is tested by having the patient invert the foot against resistance or walk on his toes.
2. *Flexor hallucis longus* (S1–S2), a plantar flexor of the foot and a plantar flexor of all the toes except the large toe. It is tested by having the patient flex the toes against resistance.
3. *Flexor digitorum longus* (S1–S2), a plantar flexor of the foot and a plantar flexor of the terminal phalanx of the toes except the great toe. It is tested by having the patient plantar flex the great toe against resistance.

The nerve then passes inferior to the medial malleolus along with the tendons of the tibialis posterior, flexor hallucis longus, and flexor digitorum longus muscles and the posterior tibial artery and vein. At this location the lanciniate ligament roofs over these structures to form a fibroosseous tunnel (the *tarsal tunnel*). Within the tunnel the nerve divides into the medial plantar, the lateral plantar, and the medial calcaneal nerves. The *medial plantar nerve* (S1–S2) supplies the skin of the medial two-thirds of the sole of the foot and innervates the abductor hallucis, flexor digitorum brevis, flexor hallucis, and the first two lumbricals of the foot. The *lateral plantar nerve* (S1–S2) carries sensation to the lateral third of the foot and innervates the abductor digiti minimi, flexor digiti minimi, adductor hallucis, interossei, and the third and fourth lumbricals of the foot. The *medial calcaneal* branch supplies the skin of the medial aspect of the heel.

COMMON PERONEAL NERVE. The common peroneal nerve (Fig. 1-10) gives off the *lateral sural cutaneous nerve* in the popliteal fossa. This branch joins the medial sural cutaneous nerve (from the tibial nerve) to form the sural nerve. In the popliteal fossa the common peroneal also gives off the *lateral cutaneous nerve of the calf,* which descends along the lateral head of the gastrocnemius to supply the skin on the lateral aspect of the leg below the knee. The common peroneal nerve then rounds the head of

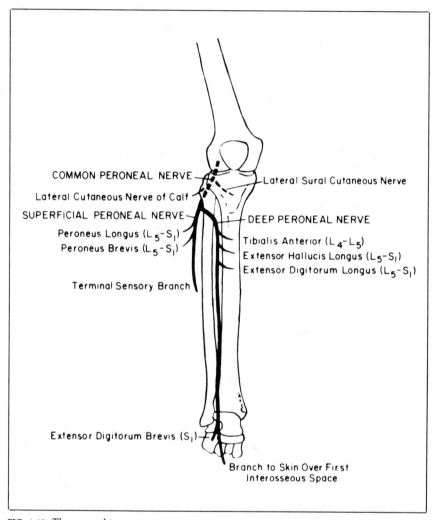

FIG. 1-10. *The peroneal nerve.*

the fibula and enters the substance of the peroneus longus muscle, where it divides into two branches, the deep peroneal (anterior tibial) nerve and the superficial peroneal nerve. The *deep peroneal nerve* gives motor branches to four muscles:

1. *Tibialis anterior* (L4–L5), a dorsiflexor and invertor of the foot. It is tested by having the patient dorsiflex the foot against resistance or walk on his heels.

2. *Extensor hallucis longus* (L5–S1), an extensor of the great toe and dorsi-flexor of the foot. It is tested by having the patient dorsiflex the distal phalanx of the big toe against resistance.
3. *Extensor digitorum longus* (L5–S1), an extensor of the four lateral toes and dorsiflexor of the foot. It is tested by having the patient dorsiflex the toes against resistance.
4. *Extensor digitorum brevis* (S1), an extensor of the large toe and three medial toes. It is tested by having the patient dorsiflex the proximal phalanges of the toes against resistance.

The terminal branch of the deep peroneal nerve passes under the tendon of the extensor hallucis longus on the dorsum of the foot and, after supplying the extensor digitorum brevis, innervates the skin on the first interosseous space and the adjacent skin of the sides of the first and second toes.

The *superficial peroneal nerve* supplies the peroneus longus and brevis muscles (L5–S1), which are plantar flexors and evertors of the foot. It is tested by having the patient evert the foot against resistance. The nerve terminates as a *sensory terminal branch*, which innervates the skin of the lateral distal portion of the lower leg and the dorsum of the foot and toes (except the first interosseous space).

In 20 to 28 percent of individuals, the lateral part of the extensor digitorum brevis (which extends the fourth and fifth digits) is supplied by an *accessory anomalous deep peroneal nerve* [14], which is a branch of the superficial peroneal nerve. This branch reaches the extensor digitorum brevis by winding around the lateral malleolus.

NERVE LESIONS

LESIONS OF THE SCIATIC NERVE PROPER. The sciatic nerve is frequently damaged in the sacral plexus, the pelvis, the gluteal region, or at the sciatic notch. These high sciatic lesions result in the following signs:

1. *Deformity.* A *flail foot* will be present because of paralysis of the dorsi-flexors and plantar flexors of the foot. When the leg is passively lifted, the foot will be plantar flexed and inverted (*foot drop*) but will also dorsiflex loosely when the foot is passively moved back and forth.
2. *Atrophy.* There will be wasting of the hamstrings and all muscles below the knee.
3. *Motor signs.* There will be paresis or paralysis of knee flexion (hamstrings), foot eversion (peronei), foot inversion (tibialis anterior), foot dorsiflexion (tibialis anterior and anterior leg musculature), foot plantar flexion (gastrocnemius and soleus), toe dorsiflexion (extensors of the toes), and toe plantar flexion (plantar flexors of the toes).

4. *Reflex signs.* There will be a decrease or absence of the Achilles reflex (S1–S2), which is subserved by the tibial nerve.
5. *Sensory signs.* There will be sensory changes (paresthesias and sensory loss) on the outer aspect of the leg and dorsum of the foot (common peroneal distribution) and on the sole and inner aspect of the foot (tibial nerve). The skin of the medial leg as far as the medial malleolus will be spared because it is innervated by the saphenous nerve (a branch of the femoral nerve). The patient may complain of pain and tenderness along the course of the nerve, especially paravertebrally, or in the buttock and posterior thigh. Tests that stretch the sciatic nerve (e.g., Lasegue's test, Gower's test) will accentuate this pain.
6. *Trophic changes.* Loss of hair, changes in the toenails, and changes in skin texture may occur in the distal leg below the knee.

The sciatic nerve proper may also be damaged just above the apex of the popliteal space. The findings will be the same as those seen with a more proximal sciatic lesion except that the hamstring muscles will be spared.

LESIONS OF THE TIBIAL NERVE. The tibial nerve is likely to be damaged in the popliteal space, within the tarsal tunnel, or within the foot *(abductor hallucis syndrome).*

1. *Lesions at the popliteal fossa.* Lesions of the tibial nerve at this location will result in paresis or paralysis of plantar flexion and inversion of the foot, plantar flexion of the toes, and movements of the intrinsic muscles of the foot. Sensory impairment will be located on the sole and lateral border of the foot.
2. *Lesions within the tarsal tunnel.* At the proximal end of the tarsal tunnel the trunk of the tibial nerve may be compressed by any process that causes narrowing of the tunnel [8, 11]. Because the medial plantar, lateral plantar, and medial calcaneal nerves branch distal to this location, there will be sensory symptoms (usually pain and paresthesias) and sensory loss affecting the skin of the sole and medial heel of the foot.

    Sensory symptoms are usually precipitated by standing or walking or by pressure applied below the medial malleolus. Motor deficits are minimal, but atrophy and paresis will be present on examination of the intrinsic muscles of the foot.
3. *Lesions within the foot.* The medial plantar or lateral plantar nerves may be damaged within the foot. This damage will result in pain, paresthesias, and sensory loss in the distribution area of the individual nerve (e.g., the medial two-thirds of the sole of the foot in medial plantar

nerve lesions). There may be localized tenderness over the individual nerve and some intrinsic muscle atrophy and paresis. The medial plantar nerve may be compressed by the calcaneonavicular ligament where the nerve pierces the abductor hallucis muscle. A plantar digital nerve may be compressed where it courses distally between the heads of the adjacent metatarsal bones. Pain in the third metatarsal space is the usual result. This pain is referred to as *Morton's metatarsalgia*.

LESIONS OF THE COMMON PERONEAL NERVE

1. *Lesions at the fibular head.* The majority of peroneal palsies occur at the level of the fibular head, where the nerve is quite superficial and susceptible to injury. The deep branch of the nerve is affected more commonly than the whole nerve, although the superficial branch alone may also be affected. When both branches (deep and superficial) are affected, there will be paresis or paralysis of toe and foot dorsiflexion and of foot eversion. There will also be a sensory disturbance that affects the entire dorsum of the foot and toes and the lateral distal portion of the lower leg. When only the deep branch of the peroneal nerve is affected, a deep peroneal nerve syndrome (see following paragraph) will occur.

2. *The anterior tibial (deep peroneal) nerve syndrome.* This nerve may be injured in isolation at the fibular head or more distally in the leg. Nerve injury results in a motor deficit (paresis or paralysis of toe and foot dorsiflexion); sensory deficit is limited to the web of skin located between the first and second toes. If an accessory (anomalous) deep peroneal nerve is present, the extensor digitorum brevis muscle, or at least the lateral portion of this muscle, will be spared.

   The deep peroneal nerve may also be compressed at the ankle *(anterior tarsal tunnel syndrome)*. This compression results in paresis and atrophy of the extensor digitorum brevis muscle alone. The terminal sensory branch to the skin web between the first and second toes may or may not be affected by lesions at this location.

3. *The superficial peroneal nerve syndrome.* The superficial peroneal nerve may be paralyzed in isolation by lesions at the fibular head or by lesions more distally in the leg. There will be paresis and atrophy of the peronei (foot eversion) and a sensory disturbance affecting the skin of the lateral distal portion of the lower leg and dorsum of the foot. The web of skin between the first and second toes will be spared (this is the area of supply of the deep peroneal nerve). If an accessory deep peroneal nerve is present, the lateral part of the extensor digitorum

36

brevis muscle will be paretic and atrophic. The sensory portion of the superficial peroneal nerve may be affected in isolation, causing a purely sensory syndrome.

REFERENCES

1. Aiello, I., et al. Entrapment of the suprascapular nerve at the spinoglenoid notch. *Ann. Neurol.* 12:314, 1982.
2. Blom, S., and Dahlback, L. O. Nerve injuries in dislocations of the shoulder joint and fractures of the neck of the humerus. A clinical and electromyographical study. *Acta Chir. Scand.* 136:461, 1970.
3. Cannieu, J. M. A. Note sur une anastomose entre la branche profonde du cubital et le median. *Bull. Soc. d'Anat. Physiol. Bordeaux* 18:339, 1897.
4. Ebeling, P., Gilliatt, R. W., and Thomas, P. K. A clinical and electrical study of ulnar nerve lesions of the hand. *J. Neurol. Neurosurg. Psychiatry* 23:1, 1960.
5. Farber, J., and Bryan, R. The anterior interosseous nerve syndrome. *J. Bone Joint Surg.* 50A:521, 1968.
6. Feindel, W., and Stratford, J. The role of the cubital tunnel in tardy ulnar palsy. *Can. J. Surg.* 1:287, 1958.
7. Goldman, S., et al. Posterior interosseous nerve palsy in the absence of trauma. *Arch. Neurol.* 21:435, 1969.
8. Goodgold, J., Kopell, H. P., and Spielholz, N. I. The tarsal tunnel syndrome. *N. Engl. J. Med.* 273:742, 1965.
9. Haymaker, W., and Woodhall, B. *Peripheral Nerve Injuries—Principles of Diagnosis.* Philadelphia: W. B. Saunders, 1953.
10. Ilfeld, F. W., and Holder, H. G. Winged scapula. Case occurring in soldier from knapsack. *J.A.M.A.* 120:448, 1942.
11. Keck, C. The tarsal tunnel syndrome. *J. Bone Joint Surg.* 44A:180, 1962.
12. Keegan, J. J., and Holyoke, E. A. Meralgia paresthetica. *J. Neurosurg.* 19:341, 1962.
13. Kopell, H. P., and Thompson, W. A. L. *Peripheral Entrapment Neuropathies.* Baltimore: Williams & Wilkins, 1963.
14. Lambert, E. H. The accessory deep peroneal nerve: A common variation in innervation of the extensor digitorum brevis. *Neurol. (Minn.)* 19:1169, 1969.
15. Mannerfeldt, L. Studies on the hand in ulnar nerve paralysis. A clinical experimental investigation in normal and anomalous innervations. *Acta Orthop. Scand.* (Suppl.) 87:23, 1966.
16. Medical Research Council. *Aids to the Examination of the Peripheral Nervous System.* London: Her Majesty's Stationery Office, 1976.
17. Morris, H. H., and Peters, B. H. Pronator syndrome: Clinical and electrophysiological features in seven cases. *J. Neurol. Neurosurg. Psychiatry* 39:461, 1976.
18. Mumenthaler, M. Topographical Diagnosis of Peripheral Nerve Lesions. In Vinken, P. J., and Bruyn, G. W. (Eds.), *Handbook of Clinical Neurology.* Amsterdam: North-Holland Publishing Company, 1969. Pp. 15–51.
19. Nakano, K. K., Lundergan, C., and Okihiro, M. M. Anterior interosseous nerve (AIN) syndromes: Diagnostic methods and alternative therapies. *Arch. Neurol.* 34:477, 1977.
20. Riche, P. Le nerf cubital et les muscles de l'eminence thenar. *Bull. Mem. Soc. Anat. Paris* 5:251, 1897.

21. Rosenblum, J., Schwarz, G., and Bendler, E. Femoral neuropathy—A neurological complication of hysterectomy. *J.A.M.A.* 195:115, 1966.
22. Roth, G., Ludy, J. P., and Egloff-Baer, S. Isolated proximal median neuropathy. *Muscle Nerve* 5:247, 1982.
23. Rowntree, T. Anomalous innervation of the hand muscles. *J. Bone Joint Surg.* 31B:505, 1949.
24. Spinner, M. The arcade of Frohse and its relationship to posterior interosseous nerve paralysis. *J. Bone Joint Surg.* 50B:809, 1968.
25. Stern, M., Rosner, L., and Blinderman, E. Kiloh-Nevin syndrome. *Clin. Orthop.* 53:95, 1967.
26. Sunderland, S. *Nerves and Nerve Injuries.* London: Churchill Livingstone, 1978.
27. Thompson, W. A. L., and Kopell, H. P. Peripheral entrapment neuropathies of the upper extremity. *N. Engl. J. Med.* 266:1261, 1959.
28. Wilbourn, A. J., and Lambert, E. H. The forearm median-to-ulnar nerve communication: Electrodiagnostic aspects. *Neurology* 26:680, 1976.
29. Witt, C. M. The supracondyloid process of the humerus. *J. Missouri Med. Assoc.* 47:455, 1950.

Chapter 2

THE LOCALIZATION OF LESIONS AFFECTING THE CERVICAL, BRACHIAL, AND LUMBOSACRAL PLEXUSES

Paul W. Brazis

Plexopathies are usually more difficult to recognize than lesions of individual peripheral nerves (peripheral neuropathies) or spinal roots (radiculopathies) because of the complex anatomy of the plexuses. Before the clinician can accurately localize a lesion to a specific division of the plexus, he must have mastered not only the anatomic intricacies of that division but also the motor and sensory supply of all peripheral nerve components supplied by the division.

In the present chapter, the anatomy of the cervical, brachial, and lumbosacral plexuses is considered, and the localization of lesions within these plexuses, which depends essentially on analysis of sensory or motor disturbances, is discussed.

THE CERVICAL PLEXUS

Anatomy. The cervical plexus, which is formed by the anterior primary rami of C1 through C4 [5, 8], is situated behind the sternocleidomastoid muscle and in front of the scalenus medius and levator scapulae muscles. This plexus consists of a series of anastomotic loops that are closely related to the spinal accessory (cranial nerve XI) and hypoglossal (cranial nerve XII) nerves. The branches of the cervical plexus may be divided into those that are predominantly sensory and those that are predominantly motor.

The cutaneous branches (Fig. 2-1) and their areas of sensory supply include the following nerves:

1. *The greater occipital nerve* (C2)—skin of the posterior scalp
2. *The lesser occipital nerve* (C2)—skin of the mastoid process and lateral head
3. *The great auricular nerve* (C2-C3)—skin of the lower cheek over the mandible, the lower part of the external ear, and the upper neck below the external ear
4. *The transverse colli (cutaneous cervical nerves)* (C2-C3)—skin on much of the neck, especially the anterior neck
5. *The supraclavicular nerves* (C3-C4)—skin immediately above the clavicle

It should be noted that there is no dorsal root from C1; thus C1 is a purely motor root.

The muscular branches of the cervical plexus (Fig. 2-2) include the following nerves and branches:

1. *The ansa hypoglossi,* which is a loop formed by fibers from the C1 root (descending hypoglossal rami; the C1 root courses downward in com-

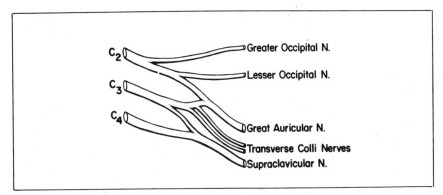

FIG. 2-1. *Sensory branches of the cervical plexus.*

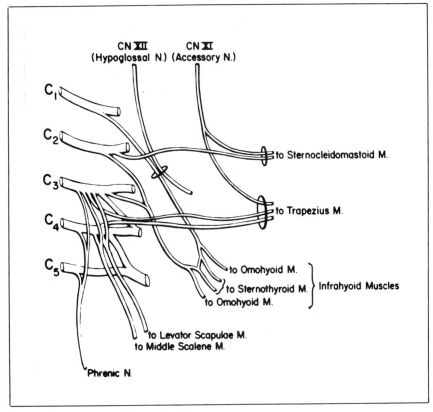

FIG. 2-2. *Motor branches of the cervical plexus.*

42

pany with the hypoglossal nerve proper) joining fibers from the C2 and C3 roots. The fibers of the ansa are distributed to the infrahyoid muscles (sternohyoid, omohyoid, sternothyroid, thyrohyoid, geniohyoid), which aid in head flexion.

2. *The phrenic nerve* (C3–C5), which innervates the diaphragm.
3. *Branches to the middle scalene and levator scapulae muscles* (C3–C4), which are essentially a lateral flexor of the neck and a rotator of the scapula, respectively.
4. *Branches to the accessory nerve* (cranial nerve XI), which supply the sternocleidomastoid (C2) and trapezius (C3–C4) muscles along with the accessory nerve proper.

Lesions of the Cervical Plexus. Injuries to the cervical plexus are infrequent, but any of its branches can be injured by penetrating wounds, surgical injury, or various mass lesions (e.g., enlarged cervical lymph nodes). Involvement of the cutaneous branches results in altered sensation (sensory loss, paresthesias, or pain) in the distribution of these branches (e.g., after a lesion of the great auricular nerve there is loss of sensation over the mandible and lower external ear). When the muscular branches are injured, there is weakness of the infrahyoid and scalene muscles (anterior and lateral head flexion), and the levator scapulae (scapular rotation), and, to some degree, the trapezius (shoulder elevation) and sternocleidomastoid (head rotation and flexion) muscles as well. The muscles affected and the degree of paresis depend on the specific branch of the cervical plexus that is injured.

Injuries to the *phrenic nerve* (C3–C5) deserve special consideration. Paralysis of this nerve results in loss of diaphragmatic movement on the affected side. When unilateral, this paralysis results in little disability at rest, but dyspnea may occur with exertion. On the affected side, the diaphragm fails to descend with inspiration and may paradoxically be drawn upward. When phrenic lesions are bilateral, exertional dyspnea may be prominent, and occasionally severe alveolar hypoventilation and hypercapnia result. Occasionally the phrenic nerve receives an anastomotic branch from the subclavian nerve, in which case a proximal phrenic lesion is associated with no impairment of diaphragmatic action.

THE BRACHIAL PLEXUS

Anatomy. The brachial plexus (Fig. 2-3) is formed from the anterior primary rami of the segments C5, C6, C7, C8, and T1 [8, 10]. The plexus is approximately 15 cm long in the adult and extends from the spinal column to the axilla. It is divided into five major components (in a proxi-

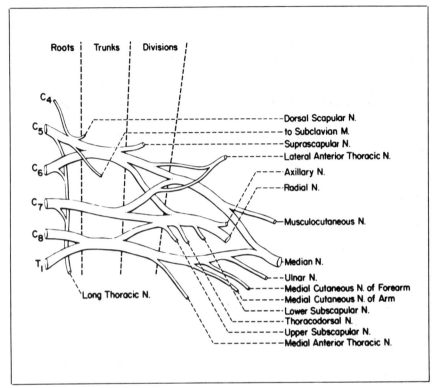

FIG. 2-3. *The brachial plexus.*

mal to distal direction) as follows: roots, trunks, divisions, cords, and branches (the mnemonic *Robert Taylor Drinks Cold Beer* serves as a means of remembering the names and order of these components).

The fifth and sixth cervical roots course downward between the scalenus medius and anterior muscles and unite to form the *upper trunk* of the plexus. The seventh cervical root also inclines downward between the scaleni and at the lateral border of the scalenus anterior emerges as the *middle trunk* of the plexus. The eighth cervical and first thoracic spinal roots unite behind a fascial sheet (Sibson's fascia) and beneath the subclavian artery form the *lower trunk* of the plexus.

The three trunks traverse the supraclavicular fossa protected by the cervical and scalene musculature through most of their course. Lateral to the first rib, where the three trunks are located behind the axillary artery, they separate into *three anterior and three posterior divisions*. The three posterior divisions unite behind the axillary artery to form the posterior cord. The anterior divisions of the upper and middle trunks (C5–C7) unite to form the *lateral cord,* whereas the *medial cord* is formed by the anterior division of the lower trunk (C8–T1). The cords pass through the space formed by the first rib and clavicle *(thoracic outlet)* and then give off the major terminal branches (peripheral nerves).

The major branches of the brachial plexus and the site of origin of these branches are as follows:

BRANCHES ORIGINATING FROM THE SPINAL ROOTS. See Chapter 1 for the distribution of these individual nerves.

THE LONG THORACIC NERVE (C5–C7). This nerve descends vertically behind the plexus to innervate the serratus anterior muscle.

THE NERVE TO THE SUBCLAVIAN MUSCLE (C5–C6). This nerve travels anterior to the plexus to innervate the subclavian muscle.

THE DORSAL SCAPULAR NERVE (C4–C5). This nerve innervates the levator scapulae and rhomboid muscles.

BRANCHES ORIGINATING FROM THE SPINAL ROOTS. See Chapter 1 for the distri-*scapular nerve* (C5–C6) arises from the upper trunk near the latter's origin and innervates the supraspinatus and infraspinatus muscles.

BRANCHES ORIGINATING FROM THE DIVISIONS OF THE BRACHIAL PLEXUS. *The anterior thoracic nerves* (C5–T1, also called the pectoral nerves) consist of the *lateral* anterior thoracic nerve (C5–C7), which arises from the anterior divisions of the upper and middle trunks of the plexus, and the *medial* anterior thoracic nerve (C8–T1), which is a branch of the medial cord of the plexus. They supply the pectoralis major and minor muscles.

BRANCHES ORIGINATING FROM THE CORDS OF THE BRACHIAL PLEXUS. See Chapter 1 for the distribution of these individual nerves. Branches of the lateral cord consist of (1) the *musculocutaneous nerve* (C5–C7), and (2) the *lateral head of the median nerve* (C5–C7). Branches of the medial cord consist of (1) the *medial anterior thoracic nerve* (C8–T1), (2) the *medial cutaneous nerve of the arm* (C8–T1), (3) the *medial cutaneous nerve of the forearm* (C8–T1), (4) the *ulnar nerve* (C7–T1), and (5) *the median head of the median nerve* (C8–T1). Branches of the posterior cord consist of (1) the *subscapular nerve* (C5–C7), (2) the *thoracodorsal nerve* (C5–C8), (3) the *axillary nerve* (C5–C6), and (4) the *radial nerve* (C5–C8).

There may be considerable anatomic variation of the brachial plexus [7]. In the *prefixed plexus* all the components are shifted upward one segment, resulting in a major contribution from the fourth cervical nerve. In the *postfixed plexus* all the components are shifted downward one segment, resulting in little or no contribution to the plexus from the fifth cervical nerve and a distinct contribution from the second thoracic nerve. These "one level" variations in innervation occur in 3 to 5 percent of patients and must be considered in any patient who doesn't fit the usual clinical presentation of a brachial plexopathy.

Lesions of the Brachial Plexus. Brachial plexopathies present with a multiplicity of clinical syndromes [4] that vary with the component of the plexus involved and the situation of the lesion. Trauma is the most frequent cause of damage (causing 50% of all brachial plexopathies) and may occur as a penetrating injury or as a closed injury (traction, compression, or stretch of the plexus). Other causes include serum- and vaccine-induced lesions, heredity, radiation injuries, infections and toxic causes, and mass lesions (e.g., neoplasms).

Plexopathies are usually incomplete and are characterized by muscle paresis and atrophy, loss of muscle stretch reflexes, sensory changes (usually patchy and incomplete), and often shoulder and arm pain (usually accentuated by arm movement). *The most prominent sign of a brachial plexopathy is a clinical deficit that involves more than one spinal or peripheral nerve.*

TOTAL PLEXUS PARALYSIS. This rare syndrome is usually due to severe trauma (usually a fall from a moving vehicle) and consists of several signs.

MOTOR SIGNS. The entire arm is paralyzed and hangs limp at the patient's side. All the arm's musculature may undergo rapid atrophy.

SENSORY SIGNS. There is usually complete anesthesia of the arm distal to a line extending obliquely from the tip of the shoulder down to the medial arm halfway to the elbow.

REFLEX SIGNS. The entire upper extremity is areflexic.

UPPER PLEXUS PARALYSIS (ERB-DUCHENNE TYPE). This lesion results from damage to the fifth and sixth cervical roots or the upper trunk of the brachial plexus. It is a common deficit and is usually due to forceful (traumatic) separation of the head and shoulder but may also be due to pressure on the shoulder (e.g., knapsack paralysis) [3] and idiopathic plexitis ("neuralgic amyotrophy" or Parsonage-Turner syndrome). The upper plexus syndrome consists of the following signs:

MOTOR SIGNS. The muscles supplied by the C5–C6 roots are paralyzed or paretic and atrophic. These include the deltoid, biceps, brachioradialis, and brachialis and occasionally the supraspinatus, infraspinatus, and subscapularis as well. The position of the limb is characteristic;

the limb is internally rotated and adducted, and the forearm is extended and pronated, the palm thus facing out and backward. This is the so-called *policeman's tip* or *porter's tip* position. Shoulder abduction (deltoid and supraspinatus), elbow flexion (biceps, brachioradialis, brachialis), external rotation of the arm (infraspinatus), and forearm supination (biceps) are impaired. Very proximal lesions may also cause weakness of the rhomboids, levator scapulae, serratus anterior, and scalene muscles.

SENSORY SIGNS. Sensation is usually intact, but there may be some sensory loss over the outer surface of the upper arm, especially over the deltoid muscle.

REFLEX SIGNS. The biceps and brachioradialis reflexes are depressed or absent.

MIDDLE PLEXUS PARALYSIS. Lesions of the middle trunk or the corresponding individual anterior primary ramus of the seventh cervical root are rare but occasionally occur on trauma. The seventh cervical fibers to the radial nerve are primarily involved, and thus the extensors of the forearm, hand, and fingers are paretic (including the triceps, anconeus, extensor carpi radialis and ulnaris, extensor digitorum, extensor digiti minimi, extensor pollicis longus and brevis, abductor pollicis longus, and extensor indicis). Forearm flexion is spared because the brachioradialis and brachialis are innervated predominantly by the fifth and sixth cervical segments. The triceps reflex may be depressed or absent, and a sensory defect, although inconsistent and often patchy, may occur over the extensor surface of the forearm and the radial aspect of the dorsum of the hand.

LOWER PLEXUS PARALYSIS (DEJERINE-KLUMPKE TYPE). The lower type of brachial plexopathy (Dejerine-Klumpke type) follows injury to the eighth cervical and first thoracic roots or the lower trunk of the plexus. It is usually the result of trauma, especially arm traction in the abducted position, but is also seen after surgical procedures and is associated with lung tumors (Pancoast tumor) or other mass lesions (e.g., aneurysms of the aortic arch). The lower plexus syndrome consists of the following signs:

MOTOR SIGNS. All of the musculature supplied by the eighth cervical and first thoracic roots are paretic and eventually atrophic. Thus, there will be weakness of wrist and finger flexion and weakness of the intrinsic hand muscles. Often a "claw-hand" deformity is evident.

SENSORY SIGNS. Sensation may be either intact or lost on the medial arm, medial forearm, and ulnar aspect of the hand.

REFLEX SIGNS. The finger flexor reflex (C8–T1) is depressed or absent.

AUTONOMIC SIGNS. When the first thoracic root is injured, the sympathetic fibers, destined for the superior cervical ganglion (and eventually the eye, upper lid, and face), are interrupted. Thus an ipsilateral Horner syndrome (ptosis, miosis, and anhidrosis) results.

LESIONS OF THE CORDS OF THE BRACHIAL PLEXUS

LESIONS OF THE LATERAL CORD. Lateral cord lesions are usually due to surgical or local trauma and result in paresis of the muscles innervated by the musculocutaneous nerve and lateral head of the median nerve. Thus there will be paresis of the biceps, brachialis, and coracobrachialis (which control elbow flexion and forearm supination) due to the musculocutaneous nerve injury as well as paresis of all muscles innervated by the median nerve except the intrinsic hand muscles. As a result, the following muscles are weak: pronator teres (forearm pronation), flexor carpi radialis (radial wrist flexion), palmaris longus (wrist flexion), flexor digitorum superficialis (middle phalangeal flexion of the second through fourth digits), flexor pollicis longus (flexion of the distal phalanges of the thumb), flexor digitorum profundus I and II (flexion of the distal phalanges of the second and third fingers), and pronator quadratus (forearm pronation). The biceps reflex is depressed or absent. Sensory loss may occur on the lateral forearm (the area of distribution of the lateral cutaneous nerve of the forearm, a branch of the musculocutaneous nerve).

LESIONS OF THE MEDIAL CORD. Lesions of the medial cord of the brachial plexus result in weakness of the muscles innervated by the ulnar nerve and medial head of the median nerve (the median-innervated intrinsic hand muscles). The ulnar muscles involved are the flexor carpi ulnaris (ulnar wrist flexion), flexor digitorum III and IV (flexion of the terminal digits of the fourth and fifth fingers), and all the ulnar-innervated small hand muscles. The median muscles involved are the abductor pollicis brevis (abduction of the metacarpal of the thumb), opponens pollicis (opposition of the thumb), superficial head of the plexor pollicis brevis (flexion of the proximal phalanx of the thumb), and the first and second lumbricals. With proximal lesions of the medial cord, the medial anterior thoracic nerve may be injured, resulting in some paresis of the lower sternocostal portion of the pectoralis major muscle and of the pectoralis minor. The finger flexor reflex is decreased or absent. Because the medial cutaneous nerves of the arm and forearm are branches of the medial cord, a sensory loss may be evident on the medial arm and forearm.

LESIONS OF THE POSTERIOR CORD. Lesions of the posterior cord result in disability in the fields of distribution of the subscapular, thoracodorsal, axillary, and radial nerves. Subscapular nerve injury results in paresis of the teres major and subscapularis (internal rotators of the humerus), whereas thoracodorsal nerve injury results in latissimus dorsi paresis. Axillary injury is manifest as deltoid (arm abduction) and teres minor (lateral rotation of the shoulder joint) paresis as well as variable sensory loss in the distribution of the lateral cutaneous nerve of the arm (skin of the lateral arm). Radial injury results in paresis of elbow extension, wrist extension, forearm supination, and finger extension; there is a lesser degree of paresis of elbow flexion. When the radial nerve is involved, the triceps and radial reflexes are decreased or absent, and a variable sensory loss is present on the entire extensor surface of the arm and forearm and on the back of the hand and dorsum of the first four fingers.

BRACHIAL MONONEUROPATHIES. Injuries to individual peripheral nerves arising directly from the plexus may occur and are usually related to closed trauma (e.g., traction and compression injuries) or disease of the vasa nervorum (e.g., diabetic neuropathy). The clinical signs involve motor, reflex, and sensory disturbances in the entire distribution of each nerve involved. These findings are described in Chapter 1.

THORACIC OUTLET SYNDROME (CERVICOBRACHIAL NEUROVASCULAR COMPRESSION SYNDROME). This group of signs and symptoms results from compression of the brachial plexus or the subclavian artery and vein in the space between the first rib and the clavicle (the *thoracic outlet*). There are usually various predisposing compressive factors including a cervical rib, an enlarged seventh cervical transverse process, a hypertrophied anterior scalene muscle *(scalenus anticus syndrome)*, or a fibrous band uniting the seventh cervical transverse process to the first rib or anterior scalene muscle.

The thoracic outlet syndrome [2, 9, 11] may be purely vascular, purely neuropathic, or mixed.

VASCULAR SIGNS AND SYMPTOMS. Because of subclavian artery compression there may be recurrent coldness, cyanosis, and pallor of the hand. Frank gangrene of the digits or Raynaud's phenomenon may occur rarely. A bruit may be present over the supra- or infraclavicular areas of the axilla, especially when the arm is fully abducted. When the arm is fully abducted, the radial pulse is frequently obliterated. (However, pulse obliteration is occasionally seen in normal individuals also.) The subclavian vein may also be compressed, resulting in arm edema, cyanosis, and enlargement of the veins of the arm and chest.

NEUROPATHIC SIGNS AND SYMPTOMS. Usually the lower trunk of the brachial plexus is involved. Pain is the most common sensory symptom and is often referred to the ulnar border of the hand and the medial

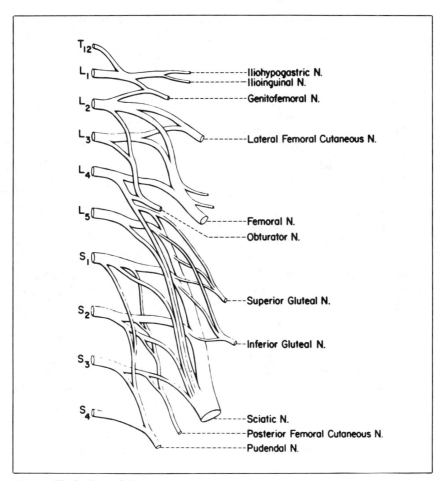

FIG. 2-4. *The lumbosacral plexus.*

forearm and arm. Paresthesias and sensory loss may occur in the same
distribution. The motor and reflex findings are essentially those of a
lower plexus palsy (see Lower Plexus Paralysis, above).

THE LUMBOSACRAL PLEXUS

Anatomy. The lumbosacral plexus (Fig. 2-4) is derived from the anterior
primary rami of the twelfth thoracic through fourth sacral levels and is
situated within the substance of the psoas major muscle [1, 5]. Anomalous derivations of the plexus (prefixed or postfixed) occur in up to 20

percent of normal subjects. The lumbosacral plexus is much simpler than the brachial plexus. This plexus gives off the following nerves (the distribution areas of these nerves are discussed in Chapter 1):

1. The *iliohypogastric nerve* (T12–L1)
2. The *ilioinguinal nerve* (L1)
3. The *genitofemoral nerve* (L1–L2)
4. The *lateral femoral cutaneous nerve* (L2–L3)
5. The *femoral nerve* (L2–L4)
6. The *obturator nerve* (L2–L4)
7. The *superior gluteal nerve* (L4–S1)
8. The *inferior gluteal nerve* (L5–S2)
9. The *sciatic nerve* (L4–S3)
10. The *posterior femoral cutaneous nerve* (S1–S3)
11. The *pudendal nerve* (S1–S4)

Lesions of the Lumbosacral Plexus. Like lesions of the brachial plexus, a lumbosacral plexopathy is recognized by deficits in the distribution of multiple spinal and peripheral nerves in the lower extremity. Among the common causes are neoplasm (lymph nodes, prostate, cervix, rectum), psoas hematoma, trauma, surgery (especially pelvic procedures), and diabetes [1]. A lumbosacral plexus neuropathy may occur with no apparent underlying cause [6]. Most injuries to the lumbosacral plexus involve primarily the lumbar segments, primarily the sacral segments, or individual peripheral nerves. The individual peripheral nerve syndromes are described in Chapter 1.

LESIONS OF THE ENTIRE LUMBOSACRAL PLEXUS. Lesions of the entire plexus are rare and usually are incomplete. They result in paralysis or paresis of the entire lower extremity with hyporeflexia or areflexia and sensory disturbance affecting the entire leg.

LESIONS OF THE LUMBAR SEGMENTS. These lesions also are usually incomplete, and they are most often due to tumor, hemorrhage, or surgical injury. If the entire lumbar plexus is injured, a syndrome results exhibiting the following signs.
MOTOR SIGNS. There are paresis and atrophy, predominantly in the motor distributions of the femoral and obturator nerves. Thus, there will be weakness of thigh flexion (iliopsoas), leg extension (quadriceps), thigh eversion (sartorius), and thigh adduction (adductor muscles).
SENSORY SIGNS. Sensation may be lost in the inguinal region and over the genitalia (iliohypogastric, ilioinguinal, and genitofemoral nerves), on

the lateral, anterior, and medial thigh (innervated by the lateral femoral cutaneous, femoral, and obturator nerves, respectively), and on the medial aspect of the lower leg (innervated by the saphenous nerve, a branch of the femoral nerve).

REFLEX SIGNS. The patellar reflex (femoral nerve) and cremasteric reflex (genitofemoral nerve) may be decreased or absent.

LESIONS OF THE SACRAL PLEXUS. These lesions are frequently incomplete and occur most commonly with neoplasms or surgical trauma. If the entire sacral plexus is injured, the following syndrome results:

MOTOR SIGNS. Lesions of the sacral plexus result in motor disturbances in the field of distribution of the superior gluteal, inferior gluteal, and sciatic nerves. A "flail foot" will result due to paralysis of dorsiflexors and plantar flexors of the foot. There will also be weakness of knee flexion (hamstrings), foot eversion (peronei), foot inversion (tibialis anterior and anterior leg muscles), foot plantar flexion (gastrocnemius and soleus), toe dorsiflexion (extensors of toes), and toe plantar flexion (plantar flexors of toes); all of these muscles are in the sciatic distribution area. Paresis of abduction and internal rotation of the thigh (superior gluteal nerve palsy) and of hip extension (inferior gluteal nerve palsy) will occur.

SENSORY SIGNS. Sensation may be lost in the distribution area of the sciatic nerve (outer leg and dorsum of the foot, sole and inner aspect of the foot) and in the distribution of the posterior femoral cutaneous nerve (posterior thigh and popliteal fossa).

REFLEX SIGNS. The Achilles reflex (ankle jerk) may be decreased or absent due to sciatic nerve involvement.

SPHINCTER SIGNS. Difficulty of bladder or bowel control may result from injury to the pudendal nerve.

REFERENCES

1. Calverley, J. Lumbosacral Plexus Lesions. *In* Dyck, P. J., Thomas, P. K., and Lambert, E. H. (Eds.). *Peripheral Neuropathy*. Philadelphia: W.B. Saunders, 1975.
2. Daube, J. R. Nerve conduction studies in the thoracic outlet syndrome. *Neurology* 25:347, 1975.
3. Daube, J. R. Rucksack paralysis. *J.A.M.A.* 208:2447, 1969.
4. Davis, D., Onofrio, B., and MacCarty, C. Brachial plexus injuries. *Mayo Clin. Proc.* 53:799, 1978.
5. DeJong, R. N. *The Neurologic Examination—Incorporating the Fundamentals of Neuroanatomy and Neurophysiology*. Hagerstown, Md.: Harper & Row, 1979. Pp. 569–575.
6. Evans, B. A., Stevens, J. C., and Dyck, P. J. Lumbosacral plexus neuropathy. *Neurology* 31:1327, 1981.

7. Harris, W. True form of brachial plexus and its motor distribution. *J. Anat. Physiol.* 38:399, 1904.
8. Haymaker, W., and Woodhall, B. *Peripheral Nerve Injuries—Principles of Diagnosis.* Philadelphia: W.B. Saunders, 1953.
9. Kremer, R. M., and Ahlquist, R. E. Thoracic outlet compression syndrome. *Am. J. Surg.* 130:612, 1975.
10. Tsairis, P. Brachial Plexus Neuropathies. *In* Dyck, P. J., Thomas, P. K., and Lambert, E. H. (Eds.). *Peripheral Neuropathy.* Philadelphia: W.B. Saunders, 1975.
11. Urschel, H. C., et al. Objective diagnosis (ulnar nerve conduction velocity) and current therapy of the thoracic outlet syndrome. *Ann. Thorac. Surg.* 12:608, 1971.

Chapter 3

THE LOCALIZATION OF SPINAL NERVE AND ROOT LESIONS

Paul W. Brazis

ANATOMY OF THE SPINAL NERVES AND ROOTS

The afferent (sensory) fibers from the peripheral nervous system enter the spinal cord in the *dorsal roots* and have their perikarya in the *dorsal spinal root ganglia*. The dorsal roots enter the cord in the dorsolateral sulcus. The efferent (motor) fibers arise from the motor neurons located in the ventral horns of the spinal cord and exit from the cord as the *ventral roots*. The ventral and dorsal roots unite to form the *mixed spinal nerve*, which then travels through the intervertebral foramen. After emerging from the foramen, the spinal nerve divides into anterior and posterior primary rami. The smaller *posterior primary rami* supply the skin on the dorsal part of the trunk with sensory fibers and also send motor fibers to the longitudinal muscles of the axial skeleton. The *anterior primary rami* supply the limbs (see Chap. 2), nonaxial skeletal muscles, and skin of the lateral and anterior trunk and neck (by way of the *lateral cutaneous and anterior cutaneous branches*, respectively). The anterior primary rami also communicate with the sympathetic ganglia through *white and gray rami communicantes*.

PRINCIPLES OF SPINAL NERVE AND ROOT LOCALIZATION

The identification of spinal nerve lesions requires a precise knowledge of each group of muscles supplied by a single anterior spinal root *(myotome)* and each cutaneous area supplied by a single posterior spinal root *(dermatome)*. Differentiation from peripheral nerve or plexus lesions thus depends on the *segmental* character of sensory and motor signs and symptoms [15].

Sensory Symptoms. Irritative lesions of a dorsal root result in *radicular pain* or *root pain,* which has a characteristic lancinating or burning quality. This pain is referred to a specific dermatome and is characteristically accentuated or precipitated by maneuvers that cause increased intraspinal pressure or stretching of the dorsal nerve root (e.g., coughing, sneezing, Valsalva maneuver, or spine movements). Pain is often the first manifestation of a sensory radiculopathy and may be associated with paresthesias or dysesthesias in the area involved.

Destructive dorsal root lesions result in hypesthesia or anesthesia that is confined to the specific dermatome involved. Because of the overlap of cutaneous supply by adjacent nerve roots, sectioning of a single dorsal root results in little or no sensory loss. Therefore, the absence of sensory loss does not exclude the possibility of a lesion affecting a single dorsal root. When multiple dorsal root lesions are present, sensory loss is evident, the area of analgesia being larger than the area of anesthesia to light touch.

Motor Signs. Ventral root lesions result in weakness and atrophy in the myotomal distribution of the affected root. Fasciculations are often evident in the affected muscle.

Reflex Signs. Lesions of the dorsal or ventral root may interrupt the afferent or efferent arc, respectively, of a specific muscle stretch reflex. Therefore, with ventral or dorsal lesions, hypo- or areflexia occurs in the muscle subserved by the affected spinal root.

The spinal roots may be injured by direct (e.g., missile or penetrating wounds) or indirect (e.g., spinal traction) trauma and are frequently compressed by lesions in and about the intervertebral foramina (e.g., disc disease, a hypertrophied ligamentum flavum, or primary or metastatic tumors of the vertebrae or spinal nerves). Certain generalized peripheral nervous system diseases have a predilection for the spinal roots (e.g., Guillain-Barré syndrome).

THE LOCALIZATION OF NERVE ROOT SYNDROMES

Lesions Affecting the Cervical Roots. Lesions affecting the spinal nerves and roots [4, 6] give rise to motor and sensory segmental defects and characteristic disturbances in muscle stretch reflexes. Each cervical segment will now be considered in more detail. The individual spinal nerve root syndromes discussed are theoretical because in clinical practice one is usually confronted with lesions that affect multiple segments.

LESIONS AFFECTING C1. Because there is no dorsal root from C1, lesions of this root result in purely motor symptoms. This root supplies muscles that support the head, fix the neck, assist in neck flexion and extension, and tilt the head to one side. These include the longus capiti, rectus capiti, obliquis capiti, longissimus capitis and cervicis, multifidi, intertransversarii, rotatores, semispinalis, and infrahyoid muscles. C1 lesions usually result in minor motor difficulties.

LESIONS AFFECTING C2. Sensory symptoms and signs due to C2 lesions are localized to the scalp posterior to the interaural line (the C2 dermatome). The motor supply of this segment involves the same muscles responsible for head and neck movements as those innervated by segment C1. In addition, the C2 nerve helps to supply the sternocleidomastoid muscle (head rotation and flexion), which is predominantly innervated by the spinal accessory nerve (cranial nerve XI).

LESIONS AFFECTING C3. Sensory disturbances occur on the lower occiput, the angle of the jaw, and the upper neck. Paresis may occur in the scalene and levator scapulae muscles (lateral neck flexion and scapular rotation, respectively), in muscles of the neck (including the infrahyoids, semispinalis capitis and cervicis, longissimus capitis and cervicis, intertransversarii, rotatores, multifidi), and in the trapezius (shoulder elevation), this last muscle being predominantly innervated by the spinal accessory nerve (cranial nerve XI). Diaphragmatic paresis may also result because the phrenic nerve receives some of its fibers from the C3 segment.

LESIONS AFFECTING C4. Sensory signs and symptoms occur on the lower neck with C4 lesions. Paresis occurs in the scalene and levator scapulae muscles (lateral neck flexion and scapular rotation, respectively), rhomboid muscles (scapular elevation and adduction), trapezius muscle (shoulder elevation), and some muscles of the neck. Diaphragmatic paresis may also occur because some fibers go to the phrenic nerve.

LESIONS AFFECTING C5. Sensory disturbances occur on the lateral arm with these lesions. Paresis occurs variably in the following muscles: levator scapulae, rhomboids, subclavian, serratus anterior, supraspinatus, infraspinatus, subscapularis, teres major, pectoralis major, teres minor, deltoid, biceps, brachialis, brachioradialis, and extensor carpi radialis brevis (for methods of examination of each of these muscles, see Chapter 1). Diaphragm paresis may occur owing to C5 fibers reaching to the phrenic nerve. The biceps reflex (subserved by segments C5–C6) and the brachioradialis reflex (C5–C6) may be depressed.

LESIONS AFFECTING C6. Sensory signs and symptoms occur on the lateral forearm, lateral hand, and the first and second digits with C6 lesions. Paresis occurs variably in the following muscles: subclavian, serratus anterior, supraspinatus, infraspinatus, teres major, pectoralis major, latissimus dorsi, teres minor, deltoid, brachialis, biceps, coracobrachialis, pronator teres, flexor carpi radialis, triceps, anconeus, brachioradialis, extensor carpi radialis longus, supinator, and extensor carpi radialis brevis (examination of these muscles is described in Chapter 1). The biceps reflex (segments C5–C6), the brachioradialis reflex (segments C5–C6), and, less often, the triceps reflex (C6–C8) may be depressed.

LESIONS AFFECTING C7. Sensory disturbances occur on the third and fourth digits with C7 lesions. Paresis occurs variably in the following muscles: serratus anterior, pectoralis major, coracobrachialis, subscapularis, teres major, latissimus dorsi, pronator teres, flexor carpi radialis, palmaris longus, flexor digitorum superficialis, flexor pollicis longus, flexor digitorum profundus I to IV, pronator quadratus, flexor carpi ulnaris, triceps, anconeus, extensor carpi radialis longus, extensor carpi radialis brevis, supinator, extensor digitorum, extensor digiti minimi, extensor carpi ulnaris, abductor pollicis longus, extensor pollicis longus, extensor pollicis brevis, and extensor indicis (examination of these muscles is covered in Chapter 1). The triceps reflex (C6–C8) may be depressed.

LESIONS AFFECTING C8. With C8 lesions sensory signs and symptoms occur on the medial forearm and hand and on the fifth digit. Paresis occurs variably in the following muscles: pectoralis major and minor, latissimus dorsi, palmaris longus, flexor digitorum superficialis, flexor pollicis longus, flexor digitorum profundus I to IV, pronator quadratus, abductor pollicis brevis, opponens pollicis, flexor pollicis brevis, all lumbricals, flexor carpi ulnaris, palmaris brevis, abductor digiti minimi, opponens digiti minimi, flexor digiti minimi, all interossei, adductor pollicis, triceps, anconeus, extensor digitorum, extensor digiti minimi, extensor carpi ulnaris, abductor pollicis longus, extensor pollicis longus and brevis, and extensor indicis (see Chapter 1 for examination methods of these muscles). The triceps reflex (C6–C8) and the finger flexor reflex (C8–T1) may be depressed. Sympathetic fibers destined for the superior cervical ganglia are interrupted, resulting in an ipsilateral Horner syndrome (ptosis, miosis, and anhidrosis).

There are frequent intradural communicating fibers between neighboring segments of the cervical posterior roots. These connections are most prominent between a specific cervical segment and the next caudal root. A lesion may therefore be falsely localized clinically to a segment one level higher than its actual location.

The theoretical root syndromes above are also related to an "idealized" brachial plexus and do not take into consideration the possibility of a prefixed or postfixed plexus (see Chap. 2).

Lesions Affecting the Thoracic Roots

LESIONS AFFECTING T1. Sensory disturbances occur on the medial arm with T1 lesions. Paresis occurs variably in the following muscles: pectoralis major and minor, flexor digitorum superficialis, palmaris longus, abductor pollicis brevis, opponens pollicis, flexor pollicis brevis, all lumbricals and interossei, flexor carpi ulnaris, palmaris brevis, abductor digiti minimi, opponens digiti minimi, flexor digiti minimi, and abductor pollicis. The finger flexor reflex (C8–T1) may be depressed. Sympathetic fibers destined for the superior cervical ganglia are interrupted, resulting in an ipsilateral Horner syndrome.

LESIONS AFFECTING SEGMENTS T2–T12. Lesions affecting the thoracic roots and spinal nerves are difficult to diagnose because thoracic and abdominal muscles are difficult to evaluate and there are no muscle stretch reflexes subserved by these levels. Therefore, clinical diagnosis relies predominantly on sensory symptoms and signs.

Thoracic nerves supply (by way of the intercostal nerves) the intercostal and abdominal muscles, which function predominantly in elevation and depression of the ribs, contraction of the abdomen, and flexion of the trunk. Thoracic nerve lesions result in intercostal muscle paralysis, which causes retraction of the costal interspace during inspiration and bulging of the interspace during cough or a Valsalva maneuver. Lower thoracic and upper lumbar root lesions may result in excessive protrusion of the abdomen during inspiration. When the abdominal muscles are affected, there may be difficulty in rising from a recumbent position, and if these muscles are paralyzed unilaterally, the umbilicus is pulled toward the normal side during inspiration or head elevation against resistance (while the patient is in the prone position). When there is bilateral upper abdominal muscle paresis above or at the T10 level, this maneuver results in elevation of the umbilicus (Beevor's sign).

Sensory disturbances are often predominantly or solely subjective. The patient complains of severe burning paresthesias or lightninglike pains. These occur in a unilateral or bilateral segmental distribution (radiating around the thorax or abdomen) and are precipitated by any maneuver that causes increased intraspinal pressure or stretching of the dorsal root (coughing, sneezing, Valsalva maneuver, neck flexion, spine movements). There may be sensory loss in the thoracic dermatome involved, but because of the overlapping cutaneous supply by adjacent nerve roots, complete section of a single dorsal root results in little or no sensory loss.

Lesions of the Lumbar and Sacral Roots

LESIONS AFFECTING L1. Sensory signs and symptoms occur mainly in the inguinal region. Lower abdominal paresis (internal oblique, transversus abdominis) may occur but is difficult to demonstrate.

LESIONS AFFECTING L2. Sensory disturbances occur over the anterior thigh. Paresis may be present in the pectineus (thigh adduction, flexion, and eversion), iliopsoas (thigh flexion), sartorius (thigh flexion and eversion), quadriceps (leg extension), and thigh adductors. The patellar reflex (L2–L4) and cremasteric reflex (L2) may be depressed. With upper lumbar root lesions (L2–L4) the bent-knee pulling test is often positive [2]. The examiner pulls the half-prone patient's knee backward while putting forward pressure on the buttock; the test is positive when lumbar radicular pain is elicited.

LESIONS AFFECTING L3. Sensory signs and symptoms occur on the lower anterior thigh. Paresis occurs variably in the pectineus (thigh adduction, flexion, and eversion), iliopsoas (thigh flexion), sartorius (thigh flexion and eversion), quadriceps (leg extension), and thigh adductors. The patellar reflex (L2–L4) may be depressed.

LESIONS AFFECTING L4. Sensory disturbances occur on the knee and on the medial leg. Paresis occurs variably in the iliopsoas (thigh flexion), quadriceps (leg extension), sartorius (thigh flexion and eversion), thigh adductors, gluteus medius, gluteus minimus, and tensor fasciae latae (adduction and internal rotation of thigh), semimembranosus, semitendinosus, and biceps femoris (knee flexion), tibialis posterior (foot plantar flexion and inversion), and tibialis anterior (foot dorsiflexion and inversion). The patellar reflex (L2–L4) may be depressed.

LESIONS AFFECTING L5. Sensory signs and symptoms occur on the lateral leg and dorsomedial foot. Paresis occurs in the gluteus medius, gluteus minimus, and tensor fasciae latae (adduction and internal rotation of thigh), gluteus maximus (hip extension), semimembranosus, semitendinosus, and biceps femoris (knee flexion), adductor magnus (thigh adduction), tibialis posterior (plantar flexion and inversion of foot), tibialis anterior (dorsiflexion and inversion of foot), extensor hallucis longus (extension of great toe and foot dorsiflexion), and extensor digitorum longus (extension of four lateral toes and foot dorsiflexion). Both the patellar (L2–L4) and the Achilles (S1–S2) reflexes are *spared*. The medial hamstring reflex may be depressed.

LESIONS AFFECTING S1. Sensory disturbances occur on the little toe, lateral foot, and most of the sole of the foot. Paresis occurs in the gluteus medius, gluteus minimus, and tensor faciae latae (adduction and internal rotation of thigh), gluteus maximus (hip extension), semimembranosus, semitendinosus, and biceps femoris (knee flexion), adductor magnus (thigh adduction), gastrocnemius and soleus (plantar flexion of foot), flexor hallucis longus (plantar flexion of foot and terminal phalanx of great toe), flexor digitorum longus (plantar flexion of foot and all toes except large toe), all of the small muscles of the foot, extensor hallucis longus (extension of great toe and dorsiflexion of foot), extensor digitorum longus (extension of four lateral toes and dorsiflexion of foot), and extensor digitorum brevis (extension of large toe and three medial toes). Rarely, an S1 radiculopathy may result in unilateral calf enlargement [3]. The Achilles reflex (S1–S2) is depressed. Occasionally bladder or bowel dysfunction occurs.

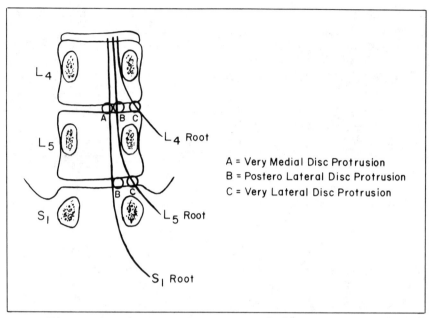

FIG. 3-1. *Disc protrusions: A, very medial disc protrusion; B, posterolateral disc protrusion; C, very lateral disc protrusion.*

LESIONS AFFECTING S2. Sensory disturbances occur on the calf. Paresis may occur in the gluteus maximus (hip extension), flexor hallucis longus (plantar flexion of foot and terminal phalanx of great toe), flexor digitorum longus (plantar flexion of foot and all toes except large toe), and all small foot muscles. The Achilles reflex (S1–S2) is depressed. Occasionally bladder or bowel dysfunction occurs.

LESIONS AFFECTING S3–S5. Sensory disturbances occur on the posterior thigh, buttocks, and perianal region. Bladder and bowel control may be impaired. The external anal sphincter may fail to contract in response to pricking of the skin or mucous membrane of the perianal region (absent *anal wink*).

The Localization of Lumbosacral Disc Disease. Herniation of a lumbar intervertebral disc may result in root compression. Almost all lumbar herniations occur between the fourth and fifth lumbar or the fifth lumbar and first sacral interspaces. Not only the interspace level but also the location of the protruded disc will determine which roots are predominantly affected (Fig. 3-1). For example, an L4–L5 protrusion that occurs posterolaterally will affect the L5 root destined to leave the canal in the L5–S1 foramen. However, a *very lateral* L4–L5 protrusion may affect the L4 root leaving in the L4–L5 interspace, and a *very medial* lesion may affect the S1 root in its downward course. A medial disc may actually affect roots on both sides (bilateral sensorimotor signs and symptoms) or cause a cauda equina syndrome (see Chap. 4).

Similarly, a *very lateral* disc protrusion at L5–S1 will affect the L5 root (which leaves the canal in the L5–S1 interspace), whereas the usual *posterolateral* protrusion will cause symptoms referable predominantly to an S1 distribution.

A thorough knowledge of this intervertebral space–nerve root relationship is necessary in order to localize these nerve root syndromes accurately to the appropriate sites of disc herniation.

REFERENCES

1. Bradley, W. G. Diseases of the Spinal Roots. *In* Dyck, P. J., Thomas, P. K., and Lambert, E. H. (Eds.). *Peripheral Neuropathy.* Philadelphia: W. B. Saunders, 1975.
2. Jabre, J. F., and Bryan, R. W. Bent-knee pulling in the diagnosis of upper lumbar root lesions. *Arch. Neurol.* 39:669, 1982.
3. Mielke, U., et al. Unilateral calf enlargement following S1 radiculopathy. *Muscle Nerve* 5:434, 1982.
4. Spurling, R. G., and Scoville, W. B. Lateral rupture of the cervical intervertebral discs. *Surg. Gynecol. Obstet.* 78:350, 1944.
5. Tonzula, R. F., et al. Usefulness of electrophysiological studies in the diagnosis of lumbosacral root disease. *Ann. Neurol.* 9:305, 1981.
6. Yoss, R. E., et al. Significance of symptoms and signs in localization of involved root in cervical disc protrusion. *Neurology* 7:674, 1958.

Chapter 4

THE LOCALIZATION OF LESIONS AFFECTING THE SPINAL CORD

José Biller and Paul W. Brazis

ANATOMY OF THE SPINAL CORD

Gross Anatomy and Relationship to Vertebral Levels. The spinal cord
[8, 11, 13, 30] extends from the level of the cranial border of the atlas,
where it is continuous with the medulla, to the lower border of the first
lumbar vertebra. During early fetal development the spinal cord extends
to the lower end of the sacrum, but at birth it extends only as far as the
upper border of the third lumbar vertebra. The average length of the
spinal cord is 45 cm in the adult male and 42 to 43 cm in the adult female.
The corresponding average length of the spinal column is 70 cm. Cylin-
drical in shape and flattened in a dorsoventral direction, the spinal cord
demonstrates both cervical and lumbar enlargements. The first corresponds to the segmental innervation of the upper extremities and extends from the C5 to T1 spinal levels, whereas the second corresponds
to the innervation of the lower extremities and extends from L3 to S2.
Below the lumbar enlargement the spinal cord narrows, ending as the
conus medullaris. From the conus medullaris a fine pial thread known as
the *filum terminale* passes down to the dorsum of the first coccygeal segment.

Although the spinal cord is a continuous and nonsegmental structure,
the 31 pairs of nerves originating from it give it a segmental appearance.
On that basis, the spinal cord is considered to have 31 segments
analogous to the spinal nerves (8 cervical, 12 thoracic, 5 lumbar, 5 sacral,
and 1 coccygeal). Due to the different growth rates of the spinal cord and
the vertebral column, the more caudal (lumbar and sacral) spinal roots
must travel a considerable distance in the subarachnoid space before
they reach their corresponding intervertebral foramina. This lower
group of roots congregate around the filum terminale in the spinal theca
and are known as the *cauda equina.*

In the cervical region the spinous process of a particular vertebra
matches the level of the corresponding cord segment; in the upper
thoracic region there is a discrepancy of two segments (e.g., the fourth
thoracic spinal segment overlies the sixth thoracic cord segment), and in
the lower thoracic region there is a discrepancy of three segments. The
eleventh thoracic spinous process overlies the third lumbar cord segment, and the twelfth overlies the first sacral cord segment.

The external surface of the spinal cord is marked by a *ventral median
fissure* and a *dorsal median sulcus* (continued by a dorsal median septum),
which divide the cord into two symmetrical halves. In the posterolateral
surface there is a *dorsolateral sulcus* marking the entrance of the dorsal
roots. In the anterolateral surface there is a *ventrolateral sulcus* that is not
as well delineated as the other sulcus because the ventral roots emerge
as a number of separate twigs.

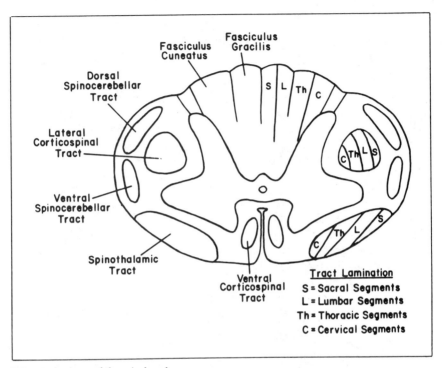

FIG. 4-1. *Anatomy of the spinal cord.*

Cross-Sectional Anatomy of the Spinal Cord. In cross section (Fig. 4-1) the spinal cord consists of the centrally placed gray matter surrounded by white matter. The gray matter is shaped like a modified H with two lateral columns joined by a transverse commissure. Each lateral column has a *dorsal horn* lying dorsolaterally and a *ventral horn* lying ventrolaterally. The central canal of the spinal cord is located in the center of the gray commissure. In addition to these gray columns, there is an *intermediolateral gray column* that extends from spinal segments T1 through L2 and gives rise to preganglionic sympathetic autonomic fibers. There is also an intermediolateral zone of gray matter in the second, third, and fourth sacral segments that is the source of the sacral portion of the parasympathetic outflow. A laminar architecture of nine cell layers or laminae is distinguishable within the gray matter: laminae I through VI (dorsal horn), lamina VII (intermediate zone), and laminae VIII and IX (ventral horn). The *zone of Lissauer* (posterolateral tract of Lissauer) separates the dorsal gray column from the surface of the spinal cord. The portion of gray matter dorsal to the central canal is the *dorsal gray commissure,* and the ventral portion is the *ventral gray commissure.*

Lamina
I	Nucleus posteromarginalis
II	Substantia gelatinosa
III and IV	Nucleus proprius
V	Zone anterior to lamina IV
VI	Zone at base of dorsal horn
VII	Zone intermedia
VIII	Zone in ventral horn (restricted to medial aspect in cervical and lumbar enlargements)
IX	Medial and lateral nuclear columns

Each half of the white matter of the spinal cord is separated into three funiculi by the gray matter and the intramedullary portions of the spinal roots, as follows:

1. The dorsal funiculus: the portion of white matter between the dorsomedian and dorsolateral sulci.
2. The lateral funiculus: the white matter between the dorsolateral and ventrolateral sulci.
3. The ventral funiculus: the white matter between the ventrolateral sulcus and the ventromedian fissure.

There are bands of white matter known as *the dorsal and ventral white commissures* that correlate with the gray commissure. The white matter comprises ascending and descending tracts.

Major Ascending and Descending Tracts of the Spinal Cord

ASCENDING TRACTS. Almost all the sensory afferent input to the spinal cord enters by way of the dorsal roots. The central end of a dorsal root splits into lateral and medial bundles. The finely myelinated or unmyelinated fibers of the lateral bundle bifurcate into short ascending and descending branches within the zone of Lissauer and terminate on neurons of the dorsal horn. The axons of second-order neurons, with cell bodies presumably in laminae VI and VII, decussate over several segments by way of the ventral white commissure; they proceed to the ventrolateral quadrant of the spinal cord and ascend as the *lateral spinothalamic (neospinothalamic) tract* to reach the thalamus (ventral posterolateral nucleus). These fibers convey pain and temperature sensation and have a laminar configuration. As a consequence of this form, those fibers carrying information from cervical regions lie dorsomedially, and those from sacral regions lie ventrolaterally. There seems also to be a segregation between pain and temperature fibers, with fibers carrying temperature information located dorsolaterally to pain fibers.

Pain may also be conducted by way of the *spinoreticulothalamic* (paleospinothalamic) system. Fibers from this system have short axons that synapse in the brainstem reticular formation and terminate in the intralaminar nuclei of the thalamus. The lateral spinothalamic tract conveys information that is perceived as sharp and localized pain, whereas the spinoreticulothalamic system is concerned with poorly localized pain sensation.

Fibers carrying tactile sensibility (light touch) also bifurcate after entering the zone of Lissauer and terminate with interneurons of the dorsal horn. The axons of second-order neurons, whose cell bodies presumably lie in laminae VI and VII, cross over to the opposite side through the ventral white commissure and ascend as the *ventral spinothalamic tract* to reach the ventral posterolateral nucleus of the thalamus. Light touch is also transmitted by way of the *dorsal funiculus — medial lemniscus* pathway.

The heavily myelinated fibers of the medial bundle of the dorsal root pass over the dorsal horn into the dorsal funiculus. After giving rise to collaterals, which terminate largely in laminae III and IV, they ascend in the dorsal funiculus. The fibers from the lowermost part of the body (sacral, lumbar, and lower six thoracic levels) are located more medially and constitute the *fasciculus gracilis*, whereas those coming from the upper part of the body (upper six thoracic and all cervical levels) occupy a more lateral position and constitute the *fasciculus cuneatus*. The fasciculus gracilis ends in the nucleus gracilis of the medulla; the fasciculus cuneatus also reaches the dorsal surface of the medulla and terminates in the nucleus cuneatus. The axons of these two nuclei decussate in the lower medulla and ascend as the medial lemniscus to reach the ventral posterolateral nucleus of the thalamus. These fibers carry information concerning discriminative senses (position sense, vibration sense, weight perception, discriminative touch, pressure touch, two-point discrimination, stereognosis, and shape and movement awareness). Other ascending tracts include the *dorsal spinocerebellar* and *ventral spinocerebellar tracts*, which transmit unconscious proprioceptive information from the lower limbs and inferior half of the body to the cerebellum, and the *cuneocerebellar* and *rostrocerebellar* tracts, which convey similar information from the upper limbs and rostral half of the body.

DESCENDING TRACTS. There are five descending systems that exert tonic effects on the alpha and gamma motor neurons; these systems are thus important in postural control of the limbs. Two of these systems (the *ves-*

tibulospinal tract and the *medial reticulospinal tract*) tend to facilitate the alpha and gamma motor neurons of antigravity muscles, and three (the *corticospinal tract, corticorubrospinal tract,* and *lateral reticulospinal tract*) inhibit the antigravity muscles and facilitate the antagonists.

CORTICOSPINAL TRACT. The fibers of the corticospinal tract originate in areas 4 and 6 (70%) and areas 1, 2, and 3 and the parietooccipitotemporal cortex (30%) of the contralateral hemisphere. These fibers descend through the corona radiata, the posterior limb of the internal capsule, and the ventral portion of the mesencephalon and pons down to the ventral portion of the medulla, where they form two large pyramids. When they reach the caudal portion of the medulla, approximately 90 percent of the 1 million fibers of each pyramid cross over in an interdigitate fashion to descend in a massive tract in the lateral funiculus of the spinal cord known as the *lateral corticospinal tract.* The fibers in the lateral corticospinal tract extend all the way through the spinal cord and terminate in laminae IV through VII and IX.

The other 10 percent of the fibers that do not decussate descend in the ipsilateral ventral funiculus as the *ventral corticospinal tract,* which terminates (after crossing in the ventral white commissure) in lamina VIII of the cervical and upper thoracic regions.

CORTICORUBROSPINAL TRACT. Cells in cortical areas 4, 6, and 1, 2, and 3 project to the ipsilateral red nucleus. The axons of some of these rubral cells decussate and descend through the brainstem tegmentum and lateral funiculus of the spinal cord as the *rubrospinal tract.*

LATERAL RETICULOSPINAL TRACT. This tract originates in the medial medullary reticular formation, chiefly on the ipsilateral side, and descends in the ventrolateral funiculus.

VESTIBULOSPINAL TRACT. Fibers originating in the lateral vestibular nucleus extend through the entire length of the spinal cord in the anterior region of the lateral funiculus. Fibers from the medial vestibular nucleus extend through the cervical and upper thoracic levels in the ventral funiculus.

MEDIAL RETICULOSPINAL TRACT. This pathway originates in the pontine and lateral medullary reticular formations and descends largely uncrossed in the ventral funiculus of the spinal cord.

Arterial Supply to the Spinal Cord. The vascular supply of the spinal cord (Fig. 4-2) can be divided into extraspinal and intraspinal systems [18, 21, 23, 26, 40, 46].

EXTRASPINAL SYSTEM (EXTRAMEDULLARY ARTERIES). The lateral spinal arteries present in early development give rise to radicular arteries, radiculopial

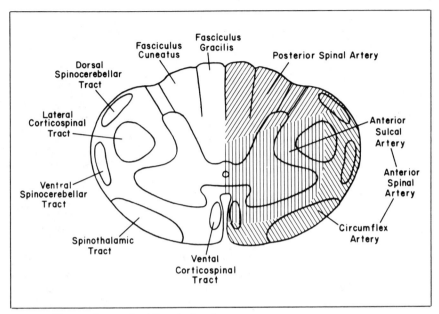

FIG. 4-2. *The vascular supply of the spinal cord.*

arteries, and radiculomedullary arteries. The latter, by way of the anterior and posterior spinal arteries, are responsible for most of the blood supply to the spinal cord. The radiculomedullary arteries are only present at certain segmental levels. Approximately 6 to 10 of them join the anterior spinal artery, and 10 to 23 join the posterior spinal arteries. The *anterior spinal artery* arises from the anastomosis of two branches from the vertebral artery, extends from the level of the olivary nucleus to the tip of the conus medullaris, and supplies the anterior two-thirds of the cord. The *posterior spinal arteries* are paired branches of the intracranial vertebral artery or posterior inferior cerebellar artery. The posterior spinal arteries also extend the length of the cord and supply its posterior third. At the conus medullaris, the anterior and posterior spinal arteries are joined by the anastomosing ansa of the conus. Anastomotic radicular arteries, most of them branches of the aorta, feed both arterial systems at various levels.

Three main functional regions in the vertical axis of the spinal cord have been distinguished according to their unequal blood supply:

1. The *upper or cervicothoracic region*, richly vascularized, embraces the cervical and first two thoracic cord segments. The first four cervical

segments are supplied by the anterior spinal artery and have a limited radiculomedullary supply or none. The lower four cervical and the first two thoracic segments receive their supply by two to four large radicular arteries arising from the vertebral and the ascending and deep cervical arteries. The most important of these radicular arteries is named the *artery of the cervical enlargement;* it enters the cord with the seventh and eighth cervical root. There are a variable number of radiculomedullary vessels feeding the posterior spinal arteries, and they predominate in the cervical enlargement.

2. The *intermediate or midthoracic region,* poorly vascularized, is supplied by branches of the intercostal arteries and includes the third through the eighth thoracic segments. It receives a single radiculomedullary artery, which enters with the sixth, seventh, or eighth thoracic roots. There are two to three segmental feeders to the posterior spinal arteries.

3. The *lower or thoracolumbosacral region* enjoys a rich vascularization and is nourished by radiculomedullary branches of the intercostal and lumbar arteries. The most important source of supply to the anterior circulation depends on the large *anterior radicular artery of Adamkiewicz (artery of the lumbar enlargement)* that enters most frequently (75%) from the left side with the ninth, tenth, eleventh, or twelfth thoracic or first two lumbar roots. Numerous posterior radicular arteries are also present in this region.

INTRASPINAL SYSTEM (INTRAMEDULLARY ARTERIES). Branches of the anterior and posterior spinal arteries form a perimedullary circuitry around the cord. Branches arise from this plexus to supply a substantial amount of white matter and the dorsal horns of the gray matter. The arterial supply of the gray matter is richer than that of the white matter. The largest branches of the anterior spinal artery (sulcocommissural arteries) enter the ventral median fissure and supply the gray matter, except for the dorsal horns and the innermost surface of the white matter. The dorsal horns and funiculi are supplied by the paired posterior spinal arteries, the posterior medullary feeders, and the perforating pial branches.

LESIONS OF THE SPINAL CORD

Complete Spinal Cord Transection (Transverse Myelopathy). With complete cord transection (Fig. 4-3), all ascending tracts from below the level of the lesion and all descending tracts from above the level of the lesion are interrupted [2, 4, 15, 17, 19, 20, 27, 33, 35]. Therefore, all motor and sensory function below the level of spinal cord damage is disturbed. More often, the section is incomplete and irregular, and the findings reflect the extent of the damage.

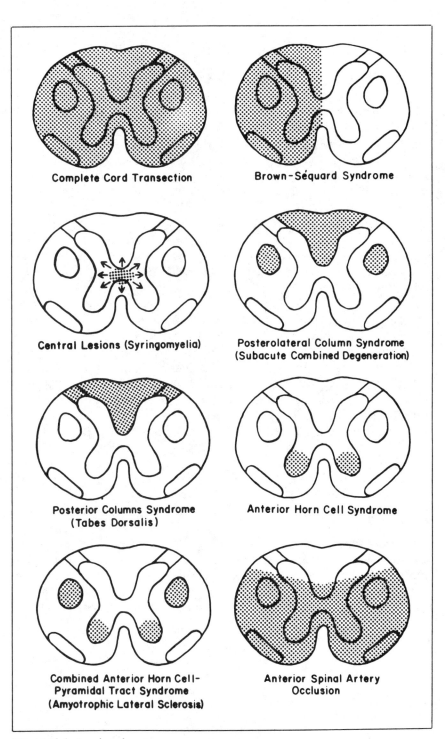

FIG. 4-3. *Spinal cord syndromes.*

SENSORY DISTURBANCES. All sensory modalities (soft touch, position sense, vibration, temperature, and pain) are impaired below the level of the lesion. Radicular pain or segmental paresthesias may occur at the level of the lesion and may be of localizing value for the appropriate spinal level. Localized vertebral pain (over the vertebral spinous process), which is accentuated by palpation or vertebral percussion, may occur with destructive lesions (especially infections and tumors) and may also be of localizing value.

MOTOR DISTURBANCES. Paraplegia (loss of lower limb motor function) or tetraplegia (loss of motor function in all four extremities) occurs below the level of the lesion owing to interruption of the descending corticospinal tracts. Initially, especially with acute lesions, the paralysis is flaccid and areflexic because of spinal shock. Eventually, hypertonic, hyperreflexic paraplegia or tetraplegia occurs with bilateral extensor toe signs, loss of superficial abdominal reflexes, and extensor and flexor spasms. Extension at the hip and knee tends to occur with incomplete or high spinal cord lesions, whereas complete and lower lesions of the spinal cord result in flexion at the hip and the knee.

At the level of the lesion there are lower motor neuron signs (paresis, atrophy, fasciculations, and areflexia) in a segmental distribution due to damage to the anterior horn cells or their ventral roots. These lower motor neuron signs, which in thoracic lesions may be quite subtle, localize the lesion to a specific spinal cord level.

AUTONOMIC DISTURBANCES. Atonic and later, spastic rectal and bladder sphincter dysfunction occurs with lesions at any spinal level. Anhidrosis, trophic skin changes, impaired temperature control, and vasomotor instability occur below the level of the lesion. Sexual dysfunction (especially impotence) also may occur.

Transverse myelopathy of acute onset is often due to traumatic spine injuries, multiple sclerosis, or vascular disorders. Other causes include spinal epidural hematoma or abscess, herniated intervertebral disc disease, tumor, anoxia, and para-infectious or postvaccinal syndromes.

Hemisection of the Spinal Cord (Brown-Séquard Syndrome). Hemisection of the spinal cord results in a characteristic syndrome (the Brown-Séquard syndrome, Fig. 4-3) [10, 14], which consists of:

LOSS OF PAIN AND TEMPERATURE SENSATION CONTRALATERAL TO THE HEMISECTION (DUE TO INTERRUPTION OF THE CROSSED SPINOTHALAMIC TRACT). This sensory level is usually one or two segments below the level of the lesion.

IPSILATERAL LOSS OF PROPRIOCEPTIVE FUNCTION BELOW THE LEVEL OF THE LESION DUE TO INTERRUPTION OF ASCENDING FIBERS IN THE POSTERIOR COLUMNS. Tactile sensation may be normal or minimally decreased. This vibratory and position sense loss may be related more to interruption of the dorsal spinocerebellar tract than to damage of the posterior columns per se [36].

IPSILATERAL SPASTIC WEAKNESS DUE TO INTERRUPTION OF THE DESCENDING CORTICOSPINAL TRACT.

SEGMENTAL LOWER MOTOR NEURON AND SENSORY SIGNS AT THE LEVEL OF THE LESION DUE TO DAMAGE OF THE ROOTS AND ANTERIOR HORN CELLS AT THIS LEVEL. The Brown-Séquard syndrome is characteristically produced by extramedullary lesions.

Lesions Affecting the Spinal Cord Centrally. This syndrome is best exemplified by syringomyelia [3] and intramedullary cord tumors. Cord damage starts centrally and spreads centrifugally to involve other cord structures. Characteristically, the decussating fibers of the spinothalamic tract conveying pain and temperature sensation are compromised initially. This results in thermoanesthesia and analgesia in a "vestlike" or "suspended" bilateral distribution with preservation of soft touch sensation and proprioception *(dissociation of sensory loss)*. With forward extension of the disease process, the anterior horn cells are compromised at the level of the lesion, resulting in segmental neurogenic atrophy, paresis, and areflexia. Lateral extension results in an ipsilateral Horner's syndrome (due to involvement of the ciliospinal center of Budge with C8–T2 lesions), scoliosis (due to involvement of the dorsomedian and ventromedian motor nuclei supplying the paraspinal muscles), and eventually, spastic paralysis below the level of the lesion (due to corticospinal tract involvement). Dorsal extension disrupts dorsal column function (ipsilateral position sense and vibratory loss), and with extreme ventrolateral extension the spinothalamic tract may be affected, producing thermoanesthesia and analgesia below the spinal level of the lesion. Because of the lamination of the spinothalamic tract (cervical sensation dorsomedial and sacral sensation ventrolateral), sacral sensation is spared *(sacral sparing)* by intraparenchymal lesions.

An *acute central cord syndrome* may occur, especially after hyperextension injuries of the neck [38]. These patients become quadriplegic after cervical trauma but regain strength in the legs in a matter of hours or even minutes. However, severe motor impairment in the arms remains ("man in a barrel syndrome"). This syndrome is probably due to damage to the gray matter at the cervical spinal cord enlargement.

Posterolateral Column Disease. The posterior and lateral columns may be selectively damaged in subacute combined degeneration of the spinal cord due to vitamin B_{12} deficiency [1, 25] or to extrinsic cord compression (e.g., cervical spondylosis) [7, 45]. The former usually shows signs of dorsal column dysfunction, including impaired vibration, position, and discriminative tactile sensations, especially those affecting both lower extremities. Pain and temperature sensations are intact because the spinothalamic tracts are not damaged. Bilateral corticospinal tract dysfunction is superimposed and results in spastic paraparesis with extensor toe signs. The muscle stretch reflexes may be hypoactive because vitamin B_{12} deficiency causes peripheral neuropathy as well.

Posterior Column Disease. The posterior columns are selectively damaged by tabes dorsalis (neurosyphilis). This posterior column damage results in impaired vibration and position sense and decreased tactile localization. Due to proprioceptive interruption, the gait is ataxic, and "stomping" or "double-tapping" is characteristic. The gait disorder is much more pronounced when the patient is in the dark or closes his eyes because visual cues can no longer be incorporated in maintaining balance (unlike cerebellar gait ataxia). Often the patient falls forward when the eyes are closed, as in washing the face (positive "sink" sign).

With demyelination of the posterior columns in the cervical region, neck flexion may elicit a characteristic subjective sensation of electrical discharge that spreads inferiorly throughout the spine and lower extremities *(Lhermitte's sign).*

Anterior Horn Cell Syndromes. Certain disease processes selectively damage the anterior horn cells of the spinal cord [9, 31, 37, 43]. The cranial motor nuclei may also be involved. This diffuse anterior horn cell involvement is exemplified by the spinal muscular atrophies (i.e., infantile spinal muscular atrophy of Werdnig-Hoffman, intermediate spinal muscular atrophy or type II spinal muscular atrophy, juvenile spinal muscular atrophy or Kugelberg-Welander disease, and progressive spinal muscular atrophy in motor neuron disease).

When there is diffuse anterior horn cell damage, diffuse weakness, atrophy, and fasciculations are noted in the muscles of the trunk and extremities. Muscle tone is usually reduced but may be normal, and muscle stretch reflexes may be depressed or absent. Sensory changes are absent because the sensory tracts are unaffected.

Combined Anterior Horn Cell and Pyramidal Tract Disease. This syndrome characterizes amyotrophic lateral sclerosis (motor neuron disease), in which degenerative changes occur in the anterior horn cells of the spinal cord (and in the motor nuclei of the brainstem) and in the corticospinal tracts. Diffuse lower motor neuron signs (progressive muscular atrophy, paresis, and fasciculations) are superimposed on the signs and symptoms of upper motor neuron dysfunction (paresis, spasticity, and extensor plantar responses). The muscle stretch reflexes may be depressed (due to lower motor neuron lesions) but are often exaggerated, especially in the lower extremities, due to concomitant corticospinal tract compromise. Sensory changes are absent, abdominal superficial reflexes are characteristically preserved, and the sphincters are spared. Bulbar or pseudobulbar impairment is often superimposed, resulting in explosive dysarthria, emotional incontinence, tongue spasticity or atrophy-paresis, and dysphagia.

Vascular Syndromes of the Spinal Cord. The most important ischemic myelopathy results from involvement of the anterior spinal artery, which supplies the anterior funiculi, anterior horns, base of the dorsal horns, periependymal area, and anteromedial aspects of the lateral funiculi [16, 22, 42]. This syndrome is usually abrupt in onset and is often associated with radicular or "girdle" pain. Loss of motor function (e.g., flaccid tetraplegia or paraplegia) occurs within minutes or hours below the level of the lesion (bilateral corticospinal tract damage) and is associated with impaired bowel and bladder control and thermoanesthesia and analgesia below the level of the lesion (compromise of the spinothalamic tracts bilaterally). Position sense, vibration, and light touch remain intact owing to preservation of the dorsal columns (supplied by the posterior spinal arteries). Spinal cord infarction usually occurs in "watersheds" or border zones where the major arterial systems supplying the spinal cord anastomose at their most distal branches. These border zones include the T1 to T4 segments and the L1 segment.

Initially described with syphilitic arteritis, spinal cord infarction now usually results from aortic dissection, arteriosclerosis, fracture-dislocation of the spine, vasculitis, or aortography. In a substantial number of cases no cause is found.

Extramedullary Cord Lesions and Their Differentiation from Intramedullary Cord Lesions. It is important to determine whether a lesion lies outside the cord (extramedullary) or within the cord (intramedullary) and whether an extramedullary lesion is intradural or extradural. Although the clinical distinction between intramedullary and extramedullary lesions is never absolute, certain clinical guidelines are helpful (Table 4-1) [12, 14, 20, 34].

TABLE 4-1. *Clinical Guidelines to Differentiate Intramedullary and Extramedullary Tumors*

Symptoms and Signs	Intramedullary Tumor	Extramedullary Tumor
Radicular pain	Unusual	Common, may occur early
Vertebral pain	Unusual	Common
Funicular pain	Common	Less common
Upper motor neuron signs	Yes, late	Yes, early
Lower motor neuron signs	Prominent and diffuse	Unusual, if present, segmental distribution
Paresthesias	Descending progression	Ascending progression
Sphincter abnormalities	Early with caudal lesions (conus–cauda equina)	Late
Trophic changes	Common	Unusual

PAIN. In 1923, Oppenheim [32] distinguished three clinical stages of spinal cord compression: (1) a stage of radicular pain and segmental motor and sensory disruption, (2) a stage of incomplete transection (i.e., Brown-Séquard syndrome), and (3) a stage of complete cord transection. Pain is an important early sign of cord compression and may be classified as one of three types: root (radicular) pain, vertebral pain, and funicular (central) pain.

1. *Root pain* is usually described as a unilateral, lancinating, dermatomal pain that is exacerbated by cough, sneeze, or Valsalva maneuver. Radicular pain is common with extradural growths and is unusual with intramedullary lesions. An example of an extramedullary tumor causing radicular pain is the neurilemmoma (usually an intradural-extramedullary lesion). With such lesions root pain predominates and may be the exclusive symptom before dermatomal hypoesthesia and segmental paresis, amyotrophy, and fasciculations occur.
2. *Vertebral pain,* either spontaneous or induced by vertebral palpation or percussion, is common with neoplastic or inflammatory extradural lesions and is uncommon with intramedullary or intradural-extramedullary lesions.
3. *Funicular (central) pain* is common with intramedullary lesions and is very unusual with extradural lesions. It is characterized by deep, ill-defined painful dysesthesias that are usually distant from the affected cord level (and thus of poor localizing value) and are probably related to dysfunction of the spinothalamic tract or posterior columns.

DISTURBANCES OF MOTOR FUNCTION. Motor dysfunction may be secondary to compromise of the lower motor neuron, upper motor neuron, or both. Lesions compressing the corticospinal tract gradually and chronically result in spasticity, whereas acute lesions result in flaccid paresis.

Upper motor neuron signs may occur with intramedullary or extramedullary cord lesions but tend to occur late in the former and early in the latter. The coexistence of upper and lower motor neuron signs suggests an intramedullary lesion but does not exclude an intradural-extramedullary process.

SENSORY DISTURBANCES. Paresthesias may follow a radicular or funicular distribution. Subjective sensory complaints may or may not be associated with objective sensory loss. For example, in the case of monoradicular involvement by a lesion, the patient may have subjective sensory dermatomal complaints, but, because of dermatomal overlap, there is no objective sensory loss. A descending progression of paresthesias suggests an intramedullary lesion, whereas an ascending progression of paresthesias suggests an extramedullary lesion.

A *sensory level* to pain and temperature must be sought in all cases of suspected spinal cord disease. A sensory level is, however, not of great significance in distinguishing intramedullary from extramedullary lesions. A Brown Séquard syndrome is more common with extramedullary lesions but is not unusual with intramedullary lesions.

Dissociated sensory loss and sacral sparing (due to the somatotopic organization of the spinothalamic tract) are characteristic of intramedullary cord involvement. Also, with intramedullary lesions vibratory sensation is usually more impaired than position sense.

DISTURBANCES OF SPHINCTER FUNCTION. Early loss of sphincter control with associated saddle anesthesia is common with tumors arising in the conus medullaris (intramedullary) and with tumors affecting the cauda equina (extramedullary). Lesions at higher spinal levels (intramedullary or extramedullary) usually are associated with disturbances of sphincter function only late in the clinical course.

AUTONOMIC MANIFESTATIONS. Ocular sympathetic palsy (Horner syndrome) can be associated with either extramedullary or intramedullary tumors. In the series of Webb et al. [44], it was most common with extramedullary tumors. Other autonomic manifestations, such as vasomotor and sudomotor abnormalities, are of no clinical value in distinguishing intramedullary from extramedullary lesions.

LOCALIZATION OF SPINAL CORD LESIONS AT DIFFERENT LEVELS

Foramen Magnum Syndrome and Lesions of the Upper Cervical Cord.
The neurologic findings with lesions of the foramen magnum consist of a complex array of sensory, motor, and neuroophthalmologic findings [41]. Suboccipital pain in the distribution of the greater occipital nerve (C2) and neck stiffness occur early. Subjective occipital paresthesias and, rarely, objective sensory findings indicative of posterior column dysfunction or a "syringomyelic type" of sensory dissociation may occur. Numbness and tingling of the fingertips are common. In addition to high cervical cord compression findings (spastic tetraparesis, long tract sensory findings, bladder disturbance), lower cranial nerve palsies (cranial nerves IX–XII) may occur by extension of the pathologic process to the medulla. Lesions of the foramen magnum may also be associated with nystagmus, especially downbeat nystagmus, papilledema (secondary to cerebrospinal fluid circulation obstruction), and cerebellar ataxia.

The pyramidal tract decussates at the medullocervical junction with the arm fibers crossing before the leg fibers (somatotopic lamination). Therefore, a lesion that affects the lateral pyramidal decussation can theoretically produce the unusual combination of contralateral upper extremity paresis associated with ipsilateral lower extremity paresis *(hemiplegia cruciata).*

Compressive lesions of the upper cervical cord (C1–C4 segments) [29, 39] may compromise cranial nerve XI (C1–C5 medullary segments), which innervates the sternocleidomastoid muscle and the upper portion of the trapezius muscle. In addition to sensory loss in the distribution of the level affected, the associated dysfunction of cranial nerve XI results in anomalous head position, inadequate contraction and atrophy of the sternocleidomastoid muscle, and inability to elevate the shoulder toward the ipsilateral ear. Furthermore, diaphragmatic paralysis may occur with lesions involving the C3 through C5 medullary segments.

Lesions of the Fifth and Sixth Cervical Segments. Compression of the lower cervical spinal cord causes lower motor neuron signs at the corresponding segmental levels of the upper extremities associated with upper motor neuron signs below the lesion (e.g., spastic paraplegia). Lesions affecting the C5 and C6 segments cause lower motor neuron signs that affect especially the spinati, deltoid, biceps, brachioradialis, brachialis, pectorals, latissimus dorsi, triceps, and extensor carpi radialis muscles, among others. This lower motor neuron paresis of the arm is associated with spastic paraparesis. Diaphragmatic function may be compromised (C5 affection). With C5 segment lesions, the biceps reflex (segments C5–C6) and the brachioradialis reflex (segments C5–C6) are absent or diminished, whereas the triceps reflex (segments C6–C8) and the finger flexor reflex (segments C8–T1) are exaggerated (the latter two are exaggerated owing to corticospinal tract compression at the C5 level). Thus, C5 segmental lesions result in an *inversion of the brachioradialis reflex.* Tapping of the radius elicits exaggerated finger and hand flexion without flexion and supination of the forearm. With C6 segmental lesions, the biceps (segments (C5–C6), brachioradialis (segments C5–C6), and triceps (segments C6–C8) reflexes are depressed or absent, but the finger flexor reflex (segments C8–T1) is exaggerated. With complete C5 segment lesions, sensory loss occurs on the entire body below the neck and anterior shoulder; with C6 sensory lesions, the same sensory loss occurs except that the lateral arm is spared.

Lesions of the Seventh Cervical Segment. With lesions of the C7 segment, diaphragmatic function is normal. Paresis affects especially the flexors and the extensors of the wrists and fingers. The biceps and brachioradialis reflexes (segments C5–C6) are preserved, whereas the finger flexor reflex (segments C8–T1) is exaggerated. A *paradoxical triceps reflex,* consisting of flexion of the forearm following tapping of the olecranon, occurs (weakness of the triceps prevents triceps contraction and elbow extension, while muscles innervated by normal segments above the lesion are allowed to contract). With C7 segment lesions, sensory loss occurs at and below the third and fourth digits (including the medial arm and forearm).

Lesions of the Eighth Cervical and First Thoracic Segments. Lesions at this level result in weakness that affects predominantly the small hand muscles associated with spastic paraparesis. With C8 lesions, the triceps reflex (segments C6–C8) and the finger flexor reflex (segments C8–T1) are decreased or absent; with T1 lesions, the triceps reflex (segment C6–C8) is preserved, but the finger flexor reflex (segments C8–T1) is decreased. With C8–T1 lesions, there may be a unilateral or bilateral Horner syndrome. Sensory loss involves the fifth digit and the medial forearm and arm as well as the rest of the body below the lesion.

Lesions of the Thoracic Segments. Lesions of the thoracic segments are characterized by root pain or paresthesias that mimic intercostal neuralgia. Segmental lower motor neuron involvement is usually difficult to detect clinically in the thoracic musculature. Paraplegia, sensory loss to a thoracic level, and disturbances of bladder, bowel, and sexual function occur. With lesions above T5, there may also be impairment of vasomotor control resulting in syncope developing upon arising (due to marked orthostatic blood pressure changes).

With a cord lesion at the T10 level, upper abdominal muscular function is preserved, whereas the lower abdominal muscles are weak; therefore, when the head is flexed against resistance (patient supine), the intact upper abdominal muscles will pull the umbilicus upward *(Beevor's sign)*.

If a lesion lies above T6, no superficial abdominal reflexes can be elicited. If a lesion is at or below T10, the upper and middle abdominal reflexes are present; if below T12, all abdominal reflexes are present.

Lesions of the First Lumbar Segment. With L1 segmental cord lesions, all muscles of the lower extremities are weak (spastic paraparesis). Lower abdominal paresis (internal oblique, transversus abdominis muscles) may occur but is difficult to demonstrate. The zone of sensory loss includes both lower extremities up to the groin and the back above the buttocks. With chronic lesions, the patellar (segments L2–L4) and ankle jerks (segments S1–S2) are pathologically brisk.

Lesions of the Second Lumbar Segment. There is spastic paraparesis but no weakness of the abdominal muscles. The cremasteric reflex (segment L2) is not elicitable and the patellar jerks (segments L2–L4) may be depressed. The ankle jerks (segments S1–S2) are hyperactive. There is normal sensation on the upper anterior aspect of the thighs.

Lesions of the Third Lumbar Segment. There is some preservation of hip flexion (iliopsoas and sartorius) and leg adduction (adductor longus, pectineus, and gracilis). The patellar jerks (segments L2–L4) are decreased or not elicitable; the ankle jerks are hyperactive. There is normal sensation on the upper anterior aspect of the thighs.

Lesions of the Fourth Lumbar Segment. There is now better hip flexion and leg adduction. Knee flexion and leg extension are better performed, and the patient is now able to stand by stabilizing the knees. The patellar jerks (segments L2–L4) are not elicitable; the ankle jerks (segments S1–S2) are hyperactive. Sensation is normal on the anterior aspect of the thighs and upper and inner aspects of the knees.

Lesions of the Fifth Lumbar Segment. There is normal hip flexion and adduction and leg extension. Owing to the normal strength of the quadriceps femoris muscles, the patient is able to extend the legs against resistance when the extremities are flexed at the hip and knee. The patellar reflexes (segments L2–L4) are present; the ankle jerks (segments S1–S2) are hyperactive. Sensory function is preserved on the anterior aspect of the thighs and the medial aspects of the legs, ankles, and soles.

Lesions of the First and Second Sacral Segments. With lesions of the S1 segment, there is weakness of the triceps surae, flexor digitorum longus, flexor hallucis longus, and small muscles of the foot. The Achilles reflexes (segments S1–S2) are absent, whereas the patellar reflexes (segments L2–L4) are preserved. There is complete sensory loss over the sole, heel, and outer aspect of the foot and ankle. The medial aspects of the calf and posterior thigh and the outer aspect of the "saddle" area are also anesthetic.

The gastrocnemius and soleus muscles are stronger with S2 segmental lesions; however, the flexor digitorum longus, flexor hallucis longus, and small muscles of the foot remain weak, and the Achilles reflexes (segments S1–S2) may be hypoactive. The sensory loss tends to involve the upper part of the dorsal aspect of the calf, the dorsal lateral aspect of the thigh, and the saddle area.

Lesions of the S3–S5 Segments. This involvement is characterized by normal strength in the lower extremities, preservation of muscle stretch reflexes, and absence of the bulbocavernosus and superficial anal reflexes. Anal-scrotal-perineal anesthesia and sphincter disturbances resulting in an autonomic bladder, fecal incontinence, and impaired sexual function (erection and ejaculation) also occur.

Conus Medullaris Lesions. Lesions of the conus medullaris are characterized by early sphincter dysfunction. Disruption of the bladder reflex arc results in an autonomous neurogenic bladder characterized by loss of voluntary initiation of micturition, increased residual urine, and absent vesical sensation. Constipation and impaired erection and ejaculation are commonly present as well. The patient may have a symmetrical saddle anesthesia. Pain is not common but may occur late in the clinical course and involve the thighs and perineum.

Cauda Equina Lesions. Due to compression of the lumbar and sacral roots below the L3 level, cauda equina lesions are characterized by the early occurrence of radicular pain in the distribution of the sacral nerves [28]. This pain may be unilateral or asymmetrical and is characteristically increased by the Valsalva maneuver. Patients develop flaccid, hypotonic paralysis that affects the glutei, posterior thigh muscles, and anterolateral muscles of the leg and foot, resulting in a true peripheral type of paraplegia. Sensory testing usually reveals an asymmetrical type of saddle anesthesia involving the anal, perineal, and genital regions and extending to the dorsal aspect of the thigh, the anterolateral aspect of the leg, and the outer aspect of the foot. The Achilles reflexes (segments S1–S2) are absent, and the patellar reflexes (segments L2–L4) are variable in their response. Sphincter changes are similar to those noted with conus medullaris lesions but tend to occur late in the clinical course.

Although much has been written about the clinical differentiation between lesions of the conus medullaris and the cauda equina, this distinction is often exceedingly difficult to make and is of little practical value. It can be concluded that lesions of the conus medullaris result in early sphincter compromise, leg pain, and symmetrical sensory manifestations, whereas cauda equina lesions are associated with early pain, late sphincter manifestations, and usually asymmetrical sensory findings.

Neurogenic Bladder with Spinal Cord Lesions. The classification of the neurogenic bladder is complex and requires adequate neuroanatomic and urodynamic knowledge [5, 6, 24]. The storage and evacuation of urine depend ultimately on a spinal reflex arc. However, supraspinal input is needed to preserve continence and to postpone bladder emptying in appropriate circumstances. The afferent arc of this relatively simple reflex arises from the distention of bladder stretch receptors, located in the bladder wall, and travels through the parasympathetic nerves to the S2–S4 segments of the spinal cord. The efferent (parasympathetic) arc travels through the pelvic nerves to the detrusor muscle. Most afferent fibers do not end in the sacral levels of the spinal cord but ascend to synapse in the pontomesencephalic micturition center; others travel further rostrally to the cortical and subcortical bladder centers. From the pontomesencephalic micturition center, efferents descend by way of the reticulospinal tracts to the detrusor nuclei in the sacral gray matter (S2–S4); efferents from the cortical and subcortical centers descend by way of the pyramidal tracts to the pudendal nuclei in the sacral spinal cord (S2–S4).

Two major types of neurogenic bladder follow spinal cord lesions:

1. *The reflex neurogenic bladder.* This type of bladder occurs with lesions above the level of the sacral vesical center and below the level of the pontomesencephalic micturition center. Patients usually present with urinary frequency, incontinence, and inability to initiate micturition voluntarily. Residual urine is increased. The bulbocavernosus and superficial anal reflexes are preserved. With lesions above the splanchnic outflow, bladder fullness may induce a "mass reflex" with headache, paroxysmal hypertension, diaphoresis, and bradycardia.
2. *The autonomous neurogenic bladder.* This type of bladder dysfunction occurs with complete lesions below the T12 segment that involve the conus medullaris and the cauda equina. This is also the type of neurogenic bladder that occurs initially with spinal shock. The patient

presents with urinary retention, inability to initiate micturition, and incontinence. There is no voluntary initiation of micturition, and residual urine is usually increased. There is associated saddle anesthesia with absence of the bulbocavernosus and superficial anal reflexes.

Other types of neurogenic bladders include the *sensory paralytic bladder* secondary to interruption of the afferent sensory fibers and the so-called *motor paralytic bladder* secondary to lesions affecting the anterior horn cells, anterior roots, or peripheral nerves.

REFERENCES

1. Adams, R. D., and Kubik, C. S. Subacute degeneration of the brain in pernicious anemia. *New Engl. J. Med.* 231:1, 1944.
2. Altrocchi, P. H. Acute transverse myelopathy. *Arch. Neurol.* 9:111, 1963.
3. Barnett, H. J. M., Foster, J. B., and Hudgson, P. *Syringomyelia.* Vol. 1, Major Problems in Neurology. Philadelphia: W. B. Saunders, 1973.
4. Bastian, H. C. On the symptomatology of total transverse lesions of the spinal cord with special reference to the condition of various reflexes. *Med. Clin. Trans.* 73:151, 1980.
5. Bors, E., and Comarr, A. E. *Neurological Urology.* Baltimore: University Park Press, 1971. Pp. 138–173.
6. Bradley, W. E., et al. Neurology of micturition. *J. Urol.* 115:481, 1976.
7. Bradshaw, P. Some aspects of cervical spondylosis. *Q. J. Med.* 26:177, 1953.
8. Brodal, A. *Neurologic Anatomy In Relation to Clinical Medicine* (2nd ed.). New York: Oxford University Press, 1969. Pp. 151–254.
9. Brooke, M. H. *A Clinician's View of Neuromuscular Disease.* Baltimore: Williams & Wilkins, 1977.
10. Brown-Séquard, C. E. De la transmission croisée des impressions sensitives par la moelle épiniere. *C. R. Soc. Biol. (Paris)* 2:70, 1850.
11. Carpenter, M. B. *Core Text of Neuroanatomy* (2nd ed.). Baltimore: Williams & Wilkins, 1978. Pp. 44–85.
12. Chade, H. O. Metastatic Tumours of the Spine and Spinal Cord. *In* Vinken, P. J., and Bruyn, G. W. (Eds.). *Handbook of Clinical Neurology.* Amsterdam: North-Holland, 1976. Pp. 415–433.
13. Daube, J. R., et al. *Medical Neurosciences. An Approach to Anatomy, Pathology, and Physiology by Systems and Levels.* Boston: Little, Brown, 1978. Pp. 296–322.
14. De Jong, R. N. *The Neurologic Examination Incorporating the Fundamentals of Neuroanatomy and Neurophysiology* (4th ed.). Hagerstown, Md.: Harper & Row, 1979.
15. DeMyer, W. Anatomy and Clinical Neurology of the Spinal Cord. *In* Baker, A. B., and Baker, L. H. (Eds.). *Clinical Neurology.* Hagerstown, Md.: Harper & Row, 1977.
16. Garland, H., Greenberg, J., and Harriman, D. G. F. Infarction of the spinal cord. *Brain* 89:645, 1966.
17. Gilbert, R. W., Kim, J. H., and Posner, J. B. Epidural cord compression from metastatic tumor: Diagnosis and treatment. *Ann. Neurol.* 3:40, 1978.
18. Gillilan, L. A. The arterial blood supply of the human spinal cord. *J. Comp. Neurol.* 110:75, 1958.

19. Greenfield, J. D., and Turner, J. W. A. Acute and subacute necrotic myelitis. *Brain* 62:227, 1939.
20. Guttmann, L. Clinical Symptomology of Spinal Cord Lesions. *In* Vinken, P. J., and Bruyn, G. W. (Eds.). *Handbook of Clinical Neurology.* Amsterdam: North-Holland, 1969. Pp. 178–216.
21. Hassler, O. Blood supply of the spinal cord. A microangiographic study. *Arch. Neurol.* 15:302, 1966.
22. Henson, R. A., and Parsons, M. Ischaemic lesions of the spinal cord: An illustrated review. *Q. J. Med.* 36:205, 1967.
23. Herren, R. Y., and Alexander, L. Sulcal and intrinsic blood vessels of the human spinal cord. *Arch. Neurol. Psychiat.* 4:678, 1939.
24. Herwig, K. R. The history and physical examination in neurogenic bladder disease. *Urol. Clin. North Am.* 1(1):29, 1974.
25. Hughes, J. T. *Pathology of the Spinal Cord* (2nd ed.). Philadelphia: W.B. Saunders, 1978.
26. Lazorthes, G., et. al. Recherches sur la vascularization artérielle de la moelle: Applications á la pathologie medullaire. *Bull. Acad. Nat. Med.* 141:464, 1957.
27. Lipton, L. H., and Teasdall, R. D. Acute transverse myelopathy in adults. *Arch. Neurol.* 28:252, 1973.
28. Livingston, K. E., and Perrin, R. G. The neurosurgical management of spinal metastases causing cord and cauda equina compression. *J. Neurosurg.* 49:839, 1978.
29. Nakano, K. K., et. al. The cervical myelopathy associated with rheumatoid arthritis: Analysis of 32 patients with 2 postmortem cases. *Ann. Neurol.* 3:144, 1978.
30. Noback, C. R., and Demarest, R. J. *The Human Nervous System: Basic Principles of Neurobiology* (3rd ed.). New York: McGraw-Hill, 1981. Pp. 150–215.
31. Norris, F. H., and Kurland, L. T. (Eds.). *Motor Neuron Disease.* New York: Grune & Stratton, 1969.
32. Oppenheim, H. *Lehrbuch der Nerrenkrankheiten für Ärzte und Studierende,* Vol. 1–7. Auflage, Berlin: S. Karger, 1923.
33. Paine, R. S., and Byers, R. K. Transverse myelopathy in childhood. *Arch. Dis. Child.* 85:151, 1953.
34. Rodriguez, M., and Dinapoli, R. P. Spinal cord compression – with special reference to metastatic epidural tumors. *Mayo Clin. Proc.* 55:442, 1980.
35. Ropper, A. H., and Poskanzer, D. C. The prognosis of acute and subacute transverse myelopathy based on early signs and symptoms. *Ann. Neurol.* 4:51, 1978.
36. Ross, E. D., Kirkpatrick, J. B., and Lastimosa, A. C. B. Position and vibration sensations: Functions of the dorsal spinocerebellar tracts? *Ann. Neurol.* 5:171, 1979.
37. Rowland, L. P., and Layzer, R. B. Muscular Dystrophies, Atrophies, and Related Diseases. *In* Baker, A. B., and Baker, L. H. (Eds.). *Clinical Neurology.* Hagerstown, Md.: Harper & Row, 1973.
38. Schneider, R. C., Cherry, G., and Patrick, H. The syndrome of acute central cervical cord injury: With special reference to mechanisms involved in hyperextension injuries of the cervical spine. *J. Neurosurg.* 11:546, 1954.
39. Strang, R. R. Metastatic tumour of the cervical spinal cord. *Med. J. Aust.* 1:205, 1962.
40. Suh, T. H., and Alexander, L. Vascular system of the human spinal cord. *Arch. Neurol. Psychiat.* 41:4, 1939.

41. Symonds, C. P., and Meadows, S. P. Compression of the spinal cord in the neighborhood of the foramen magnum. *Brain* 60:52, 1937.
42. Toole, J. F. Some Vascular Disorders Affecting the Spinal Cord. Current Concepts of Cerebrovascular Disease. *Stroke* 4(3):11, 1969.
43. Walton, J. N. (Ed.). *Disorders of Voluntary Muscle.* Edinburgh: Churchill Livingstone, 1974.
44. Webb, J. H., Craig, W. M., and Kernohan, J. W. Intraspinal neoplasms in the cervical region. *J. Neurosurg.* 10:360, 1953.
45. Wilkinson, M. *Cervical Spondylosis* (2nd. ed.). Philadelphia: W.B. Saunders, 1978.
46. Yoss, R. E. Vascular supply of the spinal cord: The production of vascular syndromes. *Univ. Mich. Med. Bull.* 16(11):33, 1950.

Chapter 5

THE LOCALIZATION OF LESIONS AFFECTING CRANIAL NERVE I (THE OLFACTORY NERVE)

Paul W. Brazis

ANATOMY OF THE OLFACTORY PATHWAYS

Although the olfactory system is not of major importance in neurologic diagnosis, certain clinical information useful in neuroanatomic localization may be attained by investigating the sense of smell. This investigation requires a basic knowledge of the anatomy of the olfactory pathways [2], especially their relationship to the surrounding neural structures (e.g., frontal lobes).

The olfactory receptors, the sensory cells of the olfactory epithelium, are located on the superior-posterior nasal septum and the lateral wall of the nasal cavity. These ciliated cells give off central processes that form small bundles (approximately 20 in number). These bundles, the filaments of the *olfactory nerve*, penetrate the cribriform plate of the ethmoid bone and enter the *olfactory bulb*. Here the olfactory afferent fibers synapse with the dendrites of the second-order neurons called the *mitral* and *tufted cells*. At the points of synapse, conglomerates of fibers called the *olfactory glomeruli* are formed. The axons of the mitral and tufted cells leave the olfactory bulb and course posteriorly, as the *olfactory tract*, in the olfactory sulcus on the orbital surfaces of the frontal lobe. The olfactory tract divides into a *median* and a *lateral olfactory stria* on either side of the anterior perforate substance (the triangular area formed by the two striae is called the *olfactory trigone*). Some of these strial fibers decussate in the *anterior commissure* and join fibers from the opposite olfactory pathways, terminating in the contralateral cerebral hemisphere. Other strial fibers, especially those of the lateral stria, supply the ipsilateral *piriform lobe* of the cerebral (temporal) cortex (the *primary olfactory cortex*) and terminate in the amygdaloid nucleus, septal nuclei, and hypothalamus.

Although relatively quantitative methods [1, 3, 5, 6] are available to test olfaction (e.g., tests of the minimal perceptible odor or measurements of olfactory fatigue), the sense of smell is usually tested by asking the patient to sniff various nonirritating substances (each nostril is tested separately) and then attempt to identify the odor (*perception* of the smell is of more value than *identification* of the specific substance). Irritating substances (e.g., ammonia) are to be avoided because they stimulate the trigeminal nerve fibers in the nasal mucosa as well as the olfactory fibers.

LOCALIZATION OF LESIONS AFFECTING THE OLFACTORY NERVE

Lesions Causing Anosmia. Anosmia (loss of smell) may or may not be apparent to the patient. He may have some difficulty in tasting various flavors because identification of tasted substances depends in part on the olfactory system.

Local nasal disease (e.g., allergic rhinitis) must first be sought as the cause of anosmia, especially if the olfactory difficulty is bilateral. After local nasal disease has been ruled out, anosmia, especially unilateral anosmia, should raise suspicion of a lesion affecting the olfactory nerve filaments, bulb, tract, or stria. Because the cortical representation for smell in the piriform cortex is bilateral, a unilateral lesion distal to the decussation of the olfactory fibers causes no olfactory impairment.

Head injury [7, 9] is probably the most common cause of disruption of the olfactory fibers prior to their decussation. The olfactory nerve proper (olfactory filaments) may be torn by fractures involving the cribriform plate of the ethmoid bone, but closed head injury without fracture may also disrupt the olfactory pathways unilaterally or bilaterally.

The olfactory bulb and tract are frequently affected by tumors of the olfactory groove (especially meningiomas), which may cause the *Foster-Kennedy syndrome* (see next paragraph). Tumors of the sphenoid or frontal bone (e.g., osteomas), pituitary tumors with suprasellar extension, and aneurysms of the circle of Willis may also compress the olfactory bulb or tract. Any diffuse meningeal process (e.g., meningitis) may involve the olfactory pathways. The anatomic relationship of the frontal lobe to the olfactory bulb and tract is especially important. Mass lesions of the frontal lobe (e.g., glioma or abscess) will often exert pressure on the olfactory system and lead to anosmia even before clear-cut frontal lobe signs and symptoms are noted. Therefore, in any patient with personality changes or subtle signs of frontal lobe involvement, olfaction should be carefully tested.

The Foster-Kennedy Syndrome. This syndrome is occasionally noted with olfactory groove or sphenoid ridge masses (especially meningiomas) or space-occupying lesions of the frontal lobe. The syndrome consists of three signs:

1. *Ipsilateral anosmia* due to direct pressure on the olfactory bulb or tract
2. *Ipsilateral optic atrophy* due to direct injury of the ipsilateral optic nerve
3. *Contralateral papilledema* due to raised intracranial pressure secondary to the mass lesion

A *pseudo Foster-Kennedy syndrome* may be rarely noted when increased intracranial pressure of any cause occurs in a patient who has previous unilateral optic atrophy. Because the atrophic disc cannot become swollen, only the previously normal fundus will demonstrate papilledema. Olfactory nerve involvement will vary depending on the etiology of the increased intracranial pressure, but increased intracranial pressure per se may impair olfaction without any evidence of local olfactory pathway damage. A pseudo Foster-Kennedy syndrome is most often due to ischemic optic neuropathy or optic neuritis in which optic disc edema on one side is associated with optic disc atrophy on the other side [8].

Lesions Causing Parosmia and Cacosmia. Parosmia (perversion of smell) and *cacosmia* (unpleasant odors) [4] are rare phenomena that are usually seen after a head injury or with psychiatric diseases (e.g., depression). Various scents are interpreted as "abnormal" and often unpleasant. Occasionally these unpleasant odors may persist or occur spontaneously as an olfactory hallucination. It is not clear whether these phenomena are of cortical origin (due to primary olfactory cortex injury) and thus possibly ictal in nature or are due to direct irritation of the olfactory pathways.

REFERENCES

1. Bosanyi, S. J., and Blanchard, C. L. Psychogalvanic skin response olfactometry. *Ann. Otol. (St. Louis)* 71:213, 1962.
2. Brodal, A. *Neurological Anatomy in Relation to Clinical Medicine* (3rd ed.). New York: Oxford University Press, 1981.
3. Caruso, V., Hagan, J., and Manning, H. Quantitative olfactometry in measurement of posttraumatic hyposmia. *Arch. Otolaryngol.* 90:500, 1968.
4. DeJong, R. N. *The Neurologic Examination—Incorporating the Fundamentals of Neuroanatomy and Neurophysiology* (4th ed.). Hagerstown, Md.: Harper & Row, 1979. Pp. 83–88.
5. Elsberg, C. A., and Levy, I. The sense of smell. I. A new and simple method of quantitative olfactometry. *Bull. Neurol. Inst. N.Y.* 4:5, 1935.
6. Fordyce, I. D. Olfaction tests. *Br. J. Ind. Med.* 18:213, 1961.
7. Leigh, A. D. Defects of smell after head injury. *Lancet* 1:35, 1943.
8. Schatz, N. J., and Smith, J. L. Non-tumor causes of the Foster Kennedy syndrome. *J. Neurosurg.* 40:245, 1948.
9. Sumner, D. Post-traumatic anosmia. *Brain* 87:107, 1964.

Chapter 6

THE LOCALIZATION OF LESIONS
AFFECTING THE VISUAL PATHWAYS

Joseph C. Masdeu

ANATOMY OF THE VISUAL SYSTEM

The Retina. The retina extends anteroposteriorly from the ora serrata to the optic disc, which corresponds to the attachment of the optic nerve, slightly nasal to the posterior pole of the eyeball. Approximately at the posterior pole of the globe is the macula, a circular area of the retina that appears yellow when viewed with the ophthalmoscope. Each retina can be divided into four quadrants by a vertical and a horizontal meridian intersecting at the macula (Fig. 6-1). The horizontal meridian separates the retina into superior and inferior portions. The vertical meridian separates the nasal (medial) retina from the temporal (lateral) retina.

The first neuronal elements in the visual system are located deep in the retina, separated from the choroid by the retinal pigment epithelium. These elements, the *rods* and *cones*, contain pigments that, reacting to visible light, produce electrical activity. This activity is conveyed to the more superficially located ganglion cells by short *bipolar cells* and by horizontally disposed *amacrine cells* (Fig. 6-2). The *ganglion cells* send their axons to the lateral geniculate body or to the superior colliculus.

The photoreceptors, rods and cones, are oriented toward the pupillary opening rather than toward the center of the globe. The pigment of the rods is a glycoprotein called rhodopsin, which reacts to light within the visible wavelength, from 400 to 800 nm. The approximately 100 million rods are unevenly distributed throughout the retina. They become more tightly packed in the fundus of the globe but are absent from the optic disc (blind spot) and from the macula.

Three different types of cones react maximally to red, green, or blue light. The retina contains about 7 million cones, 100,000 of which are concentrated in the macular region. In the center of the macula there is a small region (the foveola, measuring 0.35 mm across), which is devoid of vessels and neural elements other than the tightly packed cones. Visual discrimination is greatest here, where light can reach the photoreceptors while avoiding the layers present in the rest of the retina.

An estimated 1.2 ganglion cells populate the inner aspect of the retina. Their receptive fields become smaller in the region of the posterior pole of the globe, where ganglion cells are much more numerous than in the periphery and the cones have one-to-one connections with their own ganglion cells. By contrast, in the periphery there is an extensive overlapping among receptive fields. This anatomic arrangement may explain the relative sparing of peripheral vision with lesions that affect the ganglion cells preferentially.

At least two types of ganglion cells have been identified. "X" cells, concentrated in the fundus, provide fine spatial discrimination and send their axons to the lateral geniculate body. "Y" cells mediate analysis of

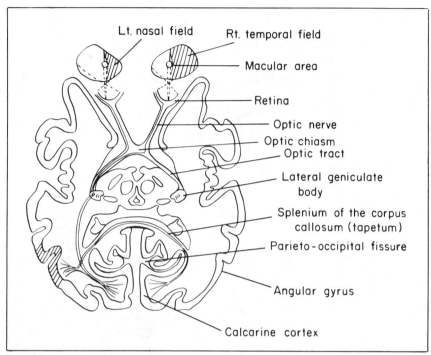

Lt. nasal field

Rt. temporal field

Macular area

Retina

Optic nerve

Optic chiasm

Optic tract

Lateral geniculate body

Splenium of the corpus callosum (tapetum)

Parieto-occipital fissure

Angular gyrus

Calcarine cortex

FIG. 6-1. *Schematic horizontal section at the level of the lateral geniculate bodies, depicting the optic pathways. Right hemifield has been shaded, and fibers from the corresponding retina have been traced.*

movement and the initiation of visual fixation reflexes. Many of them synapse in the superior colliculi.

The axons of the ganglion cells constitute the innermost layer of the retina, which is separated from the vitreous by a thin basement membrane. The position of the axons in the nerve fiber layer depends on their origin in the retina. As the axons converge toward the optic disc, the ganglion cells closer to the disc send their axons through the whole thickness of the nerve fiber layer. Thus, the more peripherally generated axons are deeper in this layer, whereas the ones originating centripetally rest nearer to the vitreous (Fig. 6-2).

Nerve fibers nasal to the optic disc and those originating in the nasal side of the macula (papillomacular bundle) take a straight course as they converge into the optic disc (Fig. 6-3). The remaining fibers arch around the papillomacular bundle, adopting a disposition that bears on the visual field defects that are secondary to retinal and optic nerve lesions. Fibers from the superior half of the temporal aspect of the macula arch

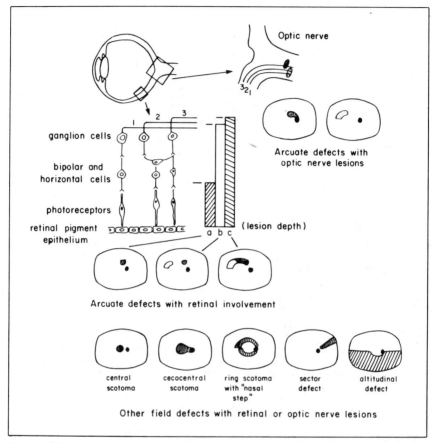

FIG. 6-2. *Diagrammatic representation of the retinal layers, disposition of fibers in the nerve fiber layer and optic nerve, and visual field defects caused by retinal or optic nerve lesions. The vertical bars (a, b, c) represent partial (a) to complete (c) retinal lesions; the corresponding field defects are depicted underneath. Retinal lesions affecting the fiber layer have an arcuate shape with the base located peripherally and, in temporal retinal lesions, in the horizontal meridian. Compare with Figure 6-3.*

superiorly and then down toward the disc. Fibers from the inferior half of the temporal aspect of the macula arch inferiorly and then ascend to reach the disc. Fibers from the temporal retina, particularly those closer to the horizontal meridian, follow a similar course. Thus, between the nerve fibers from the superior temporal retina and those from the inferior temporal retina a raphe is formed, located in the horizontal meridian (Fig. 6-3).

The axons of the ganglion cells on the temporal side of a vertical line

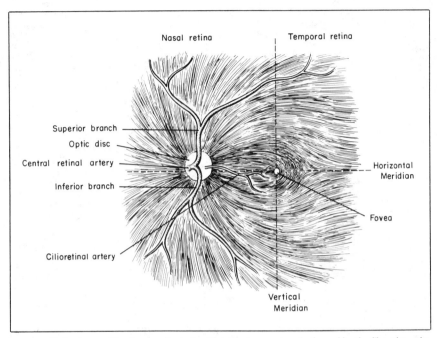

FIG. 6-3. *Retinal nerve fiber layer and arteries. Note the temporal raphe formed by the fibers from the superior and inferior retina.*

drawn through the fovea project to the ipsilateral lateral geniculate body, whereas the ones from the nasal side cross at the optic chiasm (Fig. 6-1). However, this separation is not sharp. The neurons subserving the macular region and a vertical strip of about 1 degree, centered in the fovea, project to either lateral geniculate body.

The Optic Nerves and Optic Chiasm. Each optic nerve is about 50 mm long and has four portions from the globe to the chiasm (Fig. 6-4):

1. *Intraocular Portion.* In this portion, also called the optic nerve head (1 mm in length), the axons become myelinated (central type of myelin). The funduscopic appearance of the optic nerve depends on the angle of the nerve head to the eye. When the angle between the nerve and the sclera is less than 90 degrees, a rim of choroid or sclera may be seen on the flat temporal side of the disc, whereas the nasal edge will appear elevated.
2. *Intraorbital Portion.* This section (25 mm in length) is shaped like an elongated S to allow mobility within the orbit. Here the optic nerve is

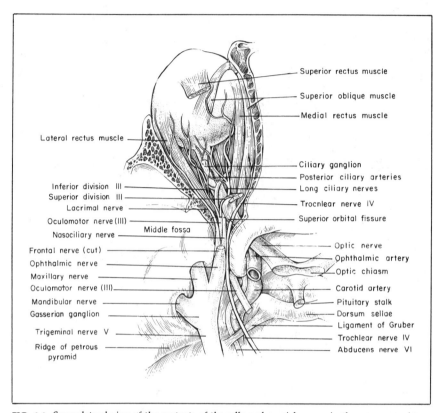

FIG. 6-4. *Superolateral view of the contents of the sella and cranial nerves in the cavernous sinus.*

surrounded by fat contained in the cone formed by the ocular muscles. The apex of this cone (which is open to the optic foramen and to the superior orbital fissure) is directed posteriorly and slightly displaced nasosuperiorly in the orbit (Fig. 6-4). In addition to the ophthalmic artery, the ciliary ganglion and nerves and the nerves to the extraocular muscles are here in close relation to the optic nerve.

3. *Intracanalicular Portion.* This portion (approximately 9 mm in length) is the part of the nerve that travels the optic canal. Each optic canal is oriented posterosuperomedially, at an angle that approximates 45 degrees to the sagittal and horizontal planes. The ophthalmic artery and some filaments of the sympathetic carotid plexus accompany the optic nerve within the optic canal.

4. *Intracranial Portion.* This part (approximately 4–16 mm in length, depending on the position of the chiasm) stretches between the proximal

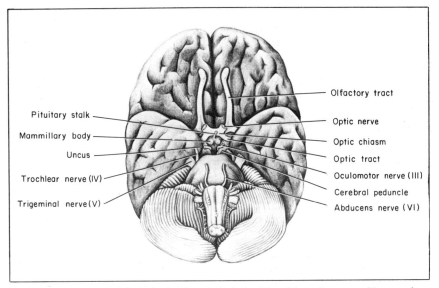

FIG. 6-5. *Inferior aspect of the brain showing some relationships of the optic nerves, chiasm, and optic tracts.*

opening of the optic canal and the chiasm (Fig. 6-4). Each optic nerve lies above the respective carotid artery as this vessel exits from the cavernous sinus and gives off the ophthalmic artery. Inferomedially, the optic nerve lies over the bony roof of the sphenoid sinus, which can be quite thin, and over the contents of the sella turcica when the chiasm is posteriorly placed. Superior to each optic nerve is the horizontal portion of the anterior cerebral artery, which is overlaid by the gyrus rectus of the frontal lobe, the olfactory tract, and the anterior perforated substance (Fig. 6-5). The anterior communicating artery is superior to the optic nerves or to the optic chiasm.

Proximal to the angled optic canal, the optic nerves maintain a 45-degree angle to the horizontal plane, and the chiasm is similarly tilted over the sella turcica, with the suprasellar cistern lying between them. The relation between the chiasm and the sella varies among different individuals. In brachycephalic heads the chiasm tends to be more anterior and dorsal than in dolichocephalic heads. Autopsy studies have shown that in about 5 percent of individuals the chiasm overlies the anterior margin of the sella *(prefixed chiasm)*; in 12 percent it lies over the diaphragma sellae; in 79 percent it is above the dorsum sellae; and in 4 percent it projects behind the dorsum sellae *(retrofixed chiasm)*. The chiasm is located below the suprachiasmatic recess of the third ventricle in close

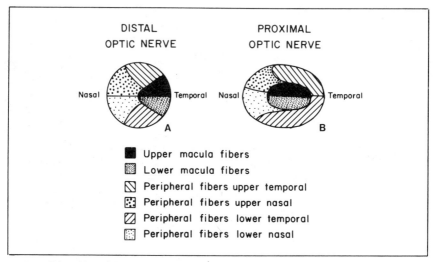

FIG. 6-6. *Disposition of the ganglion cell axons in a cross section of the optic nerve. (A) Distal portion, near the globe. (B) Proximal portion, where the macular fibers have shifted to the core of the nerve.*

proximity to the hypothalamus. Above the chiasm are the lamina terminalis and the anterior commissure. Immediately posterior to it, the pituitary stalk runs an anteroinferior course. From the posterolateral corners of the chiasm arise the optic tracts (Fig. 6-5).

Nerve fibers in the optic nerve follow a topical arrangement similar to that found in the retina (Fig. 6-6). Superior retinal fibers run superiorly in the optic nerve, inferior fibers are below, and those from the temporal and nasal retina run in the corresponding parts of the optic nerve. In the distal portion of the nerve, near the globe, the macular fibers occupy a wedge-shaped sector just temporal to the central vessels (Fig. 6-6). More proximally, they shift toward the core of the nerve.

At the chiasm, about half of the fibers (those originating in ganglion cells of the nasal retina) cross to reach the contralateral optic tract (Fig. 6-1). Fibers from the inferior part of the nasal retina are ventral in the chiasm and loop into the proximal portion of the contralateral optic nerve *(Wilbrand's knee)* before reaching the lateral aspect of the optic tract (Fig. 6-7). Those from the superior nasal retina remain dorsal in the chiasm and become medial in the optic tract.

Uncrossed fibers, originating from the temporal retina, maintain their dorsal or ventral position in the chiasm. The macular fibers, which constitute a large proportion of the total number of chiasmatic fibers, are

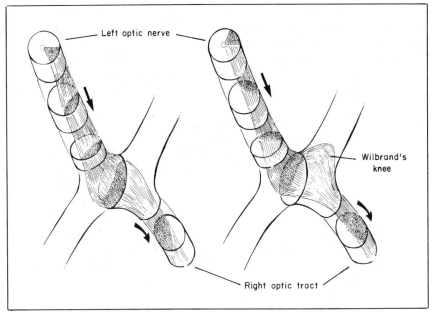

FIG. 6-7. *Crossing of nasal fibers in the optic chiasm. Fibers from the inferior retina make a forward loop into the opposite optic nerve (Wilbrand's knee). (Modified from W. F. Hoyt, O. Luis.* Arch. Ophthalmol. *68:94, 1962.)*

also crossed and uncrossed. However, the separation between temporal and nasal ganglion cells is not sharp. Both nasal and temporal sides of the macula originate crossed and uncrossed fibers. In the optic tract, the macular fibers occupy a dorsal position.

The Optic Tracts and Lateral Geniculate Bodies. The *optic tracts* extend from the dorsolateral corners of the chiasm to the lateral geniculate bodies. From the chiasm the tracts run posterolaterally, limiting a triangular space for the hypothalamus; they then sweep around the cerebral peduncles, and, as soon as they cross them, reach the lateral geniculate bodies in the posterior part of the ventral aspect of the thalami (Fig. 6-1). Several large vessels are located below the optic tracts. The posterior communicating artery crosses their distal portion, in the suprasellar cistern. In the perimesencephalic cistern, the posterior cerebral artery and the basilar vein of Rosenthal are apposed to the tracts. Inferolaterally, the uncus of the temporal lobe covers the proximal portion of each tract (Fig. 6-5).

The *lateral geniculate body*, a thalamic nucleus, provides a relay station for all the axons of the retinal ganglion cells subserving vision. Neurons from the lateral geniculate body project, by way of the optic radiations, to the pericalcarine cortex of the occipital lobe, which is the primary cortical area for vision (Fig. 6-1). The lateral geniculate body is in the roof of the perimesencephalic cistern (cisterna ambiens), just medial to the hippocampal gyrus of the temporal lobe. Anteriorly, the lateral geniculate body receives the optic tract and sends out the ventral optic radiations, which lie in close association with the posterior limb of the internal capsule. Dorsolaterally, the lateral geniculate body is covered by the optic radiations. Dorsomedial to the lateral geniculate body the auditory radiations, originating from the medial geniculate body, pass on their way to the transverse temporal gyrus of Hechsl, where the primary auditory cortex is located. Superomedial to the lateral geniculate body is the pulvinar of the thalamus.

Shaped on midsection like Napoleon's hat, with its concave aspect (hilus) facing inferoposteromedially, the lateral geniculate body has a deep brown color with stripes (striae) of white matter that are visible to the naked eye. The geniculate neurons, as numerous as the fibers in the optic tract, are disposed in six laminae, numbered from I to VI, beginning from the hilus of the nucleus (see Fig. 6-10). Layers I, IV, and VI serve the contralateral eye, whereas II, III, and V are connected with the ipsilateral eye. These six laminae are clearly distinguished in the center of the lateral geniculate body, where the macular region of the retina is represented, but only one or two are present in the peripheral part of the nucleus, which receives axons from ganglion cells in the peripheral retina.

The postchiasmatic shift in the position of the fibers (the superior retinal fibers become superomedial and the inferior fibers become inferolateral [Fig. 6-7]), persists in the synaptic areas of the lateral geniculate body. This shift is straightened out in the optic radiations, where again the superior fibers correspond to the superior retina and those below to the inferior retina. A similar representation is found in the calcarine cortex.

The Optic Radiations. The optic radiations sweep posteriorly around the lateral aspect of the posterior portion of the lateral ventricles (Fig. 6-8), forming the external sagittal stratum, which is separated from the ventricle by the internal sagittal stratum, made up of occipitomesencephalic fibers. Three bundles can be distinguished in the radiations: (1) the upper bundle, originating in the medial part of the lateral geniculate body and corresponding to the superior retina, which courses in the deep parietal white matter and ends in the superior lip of the calcarine fissure; (2) the central bundle, originating from the medial part of the

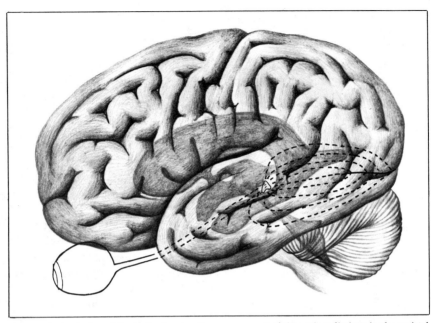

FIG. 6-8. *Lateral view of the brain showing the arrangement of the optic radiations in the parietal and temporal lobes, lateral to the ventricular system.*

nucleus and serving the macular region, which travels the posterotemporal and occipital white matter and ends in the posterior part of the calcarine fissure, on both lips; and (3) the lower bundle, originating from the lateral part of the nucleus and corresponding to the lower retina, which sweeps first anteriorly and then posteriorly around the temporal horn of the lateral ventricle (Fig. 6-8), terminating in the lower lip of the calcarine fissure. As they sweep lateral to the ventricle (Meyer's loop), the lower radiations reach a point located approximately 5 cm behind the tip of the temporal lobe.

In the anterior part of the radiations, fibers corresponding to adjacent retinal units are spatially separated, and the macular fibers, instead of being interposed between fibers from the superior and inferior peripheral retina, run medial to them. Also, fibers from either eye seem to have a similar anterior extent in Meyer's loop, with those from the contralateral eye lying medial to the ones coming from the ipsilateral eye.

The Visual Cortex and Visual Association Areas. Cortical area 17 of Brodmann, located along the superior and inferior lips of the calcarine fissure in the medial aspect of the occipital lobe, receives the axons from neurons of the lateral geniculate body and represents the first link in the cortical processing of visual information (primary visual cortex, see Figs. 19-1, 19-4, and 19-5). The primary visual cortex actually extends farther than the posterior extent of the calcarine fissure, spreading for about 1 cm around the posterolateral aspect of the occipital pole. On cross section of the cortex, a white matter stria (stria Gennari) can be seen with the naked eye. This characteristic feature has won the term *striate cortex* for area 17. The line of Gennari corresponds to a thick band of white matter in layer IV of the cortex, which is devoid at this point of pyramidal cells but is very rich in granular cells. The fascinating discoveries of recent years about the physiology of the visual neurons do not bear on localization of anatomic lesions and will not be reviewed.

Each occipital lobe receives projections from the nasal half of the opposite eye and from the temporal half of the ipsilateral retina. More simply, it receives projections from the two halves of the retinas on the same side as the occipital lobe (Fig. 6-1). This unilateral representation includes the macular region. The superior and inferior retinal projections extend to the superior and inferior lips of the calcarine fissure, respectively. Finally, the macular retina is represented in the posterior pole of the calcarine cortex, while the more peripheral retina is more anteriorly represented [9].

Vascular Supply of the Visual Pathways. The vascular supply of the retina is derived from the ophthalmic artery, which branches from the carotid artery shortly after this vessel exits from the cavernous sinus. At the optic canal, the ophthalmic artery lies below and lateral to the nerve. At a point 5 to 15 mm from the globe, it gives off the central retinal artery, which pierces the optic nerve and courses forward in its core, to divide into a superior and an inferior branch at the optic disc (Fig. 6-3). Second-order nasal and temporal branches supply the inner layers of the retina. From the anatomic arrangement of these vessels it follows that complete occlusion of the central retinal artery results in global retinal ischemia, except when the macular area is supplied by cilioretinal arteries, and occlusion of one of its branches causes superior or inferior retinal ischemia. The consequence of such a lesion will be an inferior or superior altitudinal field defect (Fig. 6-2). Infarction in the territory of the central retinal artery is generally caused by emboli.

In addition to the central retinal artery, the ophthalmic artery gives off several posterior ciliary arteries, which form a rich anastomotic circle on the posterior aspect of the globe near the optic nerve and supply some sectors of the optic disc, the outer layers of the retina, and the choroid. In about half of the population, the region of the macula and the papillomacular bundle receives its vascular supply from one or more cilioretinal arteries, which are branches of the posterior ciliary arteries (Fig. 6-3).

This explains the sparing of central vision that occurs in these people despite central retinal artery occlusion with global retinal ischemia. Unlike ischemia in the territory of the central retinal artery, ischemia in the territory of the posterior ciliary arteries is seldom related to emboli but is usually caused by either arteriosclerotic disease of the larger vessels (acute anterior ischemic optic neuropathy of the elderly) or a vasculitis involving the ophthalmic artery (temporal arteritis). However, field defects resulting from lesions in the territory of the posterior ciliary arteries are also altitudinal, and the differentiation of lesions in either territory rests on the ophthalmoscopic findings. Edema of the retina is obvious in the acute stages of retinal infarction owing to central retinal artery occlusion, but the retina may appear normal or show axonal swellings (cotton-wool spots) in a segmental distribution in the presence of ischemia in the territory of the posterior ciliary arteries.

The proximal part of the optic nerve is supplied by small branches of the ophthalmic artery and, as it approaches the chiasm, by thin vessels from the carotid and anterior cerebral arteries. Similarly, thin vessels arising in the region of the anterior communicating artery supply the dorsal aspect of the chiasm, whereas the inferior aspect receives arterioles from the carotid, posterior communicating, and posterior cerebral arteries. The latter two vessels also supply the optic tract, which in addition is fed by the anterior choroidal artery, a branch of the internal carotid. The lateral geniculate body receives a dual supply, from the anterior choroidal artery laterally and from the lateral posterior choroidal artery medially. The upper (parietal) portion of the optic radiations is supplied by branches of the middle cerebral artery, whereas the lower part receives branches from the posterior cerebral artery. The posterior cerebral artery, particularly its calcarine branch running in the calcarine fissure, supplies the primary visual cortex. Anastomotic branches from the middle cerebral artery (generally the angular or posterior temporal arteries) also play an important role in the vascular supply of the occipital pole, in which the macular region is represented.

LOCALIZATION OF LESIONS IN THE OPTIC PATHWAYS

The long course of the visual pathways along the base of the brain and their relative simplicity render them a very useful tool in lesion localization. An excellent discussion of this subject can be found in Miller's recent monograph [6]. The different techniques of neuroophthalmologic testing are reviewed by Glaser [4]. Detailed, quantitative testing allows:

1. The detection of subtle deficits that may escape detection by bedside maneuvers.

2. Better definition of abnormalities, such as the exact shape of a field defect, which may be important in lesion localization.
3. The quantification of the extent and intensity of a deficit, which are very useful data when judging the evolution of a disease process.

However, detailed testing requires equipment that is unavailable at the bedside and a degree of active cooperation that is often lacking in patients with brain disorders.

Lesions in the visual system may cause impaired visual perception or objective deficits. Impaired visual perception may include (1) poor discrimination of fine details of high contrast (visual acuity), which results in difficulty with tasks such as reading a printed page; (2) impaired color recognition; (3) impaired discrimination of objects that have little contrast with the background (contrast discrimination); (4) visual field defects, the pattern of which is often the most helpful clue to lesion localization. Objectively, retinal changes caused by retinal or more proximal lesions can be seen with the ophthalmoscope, and an impaired pupillary response to light may betray a lesion in the afferent arc of this reflex.

Changes in Visual Perception

VISUAL ACUITY. *Visual acuity*, the capacity for visual discrimination of fine details of high contrast, such as small black letters on a white page, reflects the function of the macular region. It remains unimpaired by unilateral lesions dorsal to the optic chiasm [3]. In practice, visual acuity is most often impaired by changes in the shape of the globe and in the refractory characteristics of the transparent media of the eye. Patients with these refractory defects regain a much better acuity when looking through a pinhole (pinhole test), because this maneuver restricts vision to the central beam of light, which is undisturbed by abnormal ocular distances or transparent media. At the bedside, visual acuity can be tested by asking the patient to read a "near card" with the Snellen optotypes printed on it. The card should be well illuminated and held 14 inches in front of the patient's eyes. For screening purposes, it is well to begin by asking the patient to read the 20/15 line because the visual acuity of most normal adults is better than 20/20 [3].

Once refractory defects have been excluded, it can be accepted that changes in visual acuity are secondary to lesions in the *macular region* or its projection. The macula is the only part of the retina that has a high visual acuity. Virtually all compressive and most noncompressive lesions of the *optic nerve* cause a drop in visual acuity, often even before a field defect can be detected. *Medial chiasmal lesions behave in a similar* manner. *Lateral chiasmal* lesions tend to impair visual acuity in the ipsilateral eye only. From these findings and from the sparing of visual acuity that occurs with retrochiasmatic lesions, Frisen postulated that acuity will remain normal if either the crossing or the noncrossing set of nerve fibers from the fovea remains intact [3]. Both sets of fibers are often affected with medial chiasmal lesions. Unilateral lesions of the *optic tract, lateral geniculate body, visual radiations, orstriate cortex* do not impair visual acuity. When the retrochiasmatic pathways are affected bilaterally, visual acuity fails to the same degree in both eyes.

CONTRAST SENSITIVITY. *Contrast sensitivity* testing may detect more subtle impairments in the function of the macula, optic nerve, and chiasm than visual acuity testing [5]. For instance, visual acuity may become normal after an acute optic neuritis, yet the patient may complain of "dimness" or "fuzzy vision" in that eye. This patient's ability to perceive a series of bars that have very little contrast from the background will probably be abnormal [1]. Impaired contrast sensitivity probably has localizing significance that is similar to that of impaired visual acuity, but it has been studied less thoroughly.

PERCEPTION OF COLOR. *Color perception* is often degraded in areas of the visual fields that correspond to a partial field defect. For instance, a scotoma for blue or for red may be demonstrated when vision for white targets is still good. In confrontation testing of the visual fields, one of the most useful techniques is to ask the patient which one of two identically bright red objects is more red, because a desaturation for red is often caused by lesions of the visual pathways. By contrast, damage to the photoreceptors in the retina often causes a greater impairment in the perception of blue. Impairment of color vision may also be detected by asking the patient to read numbers composed of an assembly of dots of different colors embedded in a background of differently colored dots (Ishihara plates). Color-blind patients cannot perform this task, which reflects mainly macular function. Because optic nerve and chiasmatic lesions often affect the macular fibers, monocular reading of the Ishihara or similar plates is often defective on the side of the lesion. Color vision loss usually parallels visual acuity loss, but in optic neuritis color vision is much worse.

Impairment of color perception also occurs with lesions in the posterior visual pathways. A visual field defect for red may betray the presence of a lesion when the fields for white stimuli are full. Patients with bilateral lesions of the inferomedial occipital region often have color blindness with normal visual acuity [2, 8].

VISUAL FIELDS. The shape and distribution of *visual field* loss closely reflects the site of the lesion (Fig. 6-2 and 6-9). Thus, careful plotting of the visual fields is most helpful in localization of lesions of the visual pathways when examining a cooperative patient. In patients with a markedly reduced attention span or other disturbances in alertness, the gross extent of the visual fields can be estimated from the patient's response to moving objects in the different quadrants. A moving object strongly induces the patient to look at it. However, small field defects are missed with this technique [11]. In cooperative patients, central visual field testing with the tangent (Bjerrum) screen and peripheral testing with a modern perimeter, using stimuli of different colors, provide a detailed map of the visual fields. By convention, in representing the visual fields the field for the left eye is represented to the left of the field for the right eye (Fig. 6-9). Thus, the *nasal retina* of the left eye "sees" the *temporal field* of the left eye. This terminology explains why a chiasmal lesion that destroys the *nasal fibers* from both retinas causes a *bitemporal* hemianopia. Similarly, a macular lesion yields a central defect, whereas a lesion in the nasosuperior retina of the right eye results in a field defect in the temporoinferior portion of the visual field corresponding to the right eye.

TYPES OF VISUAL FIELD DEFECTS. *Hemianopia* is a field defect that encompasses roughly half of the field, with a fairly sharp margin at the vertical or horizontal meridian (Fig. 6-9). Vertical hemianopia may be nasal or temporal. Horizontal or "altitudinal" hemianopia may be superior or inferior. When only one quarter of the field is affected, the resulting deficit is called *quadrantanopia.*

A *central* defect occupies the position of the macula (Fig. 6-2). A *cecocentral* defect affects the area of the macula and of the papillomacular bundle. Other field defects (also called *scotomas* when they are relatively small) are peripheral. *Peripheral* defects in the nasal field tend to have an *arcuate* shape when they are secondary to retinal or optic nerve disease, as they often are. The field defect takes this arcuate shape because of the disposition of the fiber layer in the retina and in the optic nerve (Fig. 6-2). Small, deep retinal lesions result in a discrete defect that is localized to the point of the lesion because the fiber layer remains unaltered. Larger lesions affect the superficial fiber layer and therefore give rise to a fan-shaped arcuate defect, with its tip pointing toward the lesion and its base fanning peripherally toward the nasal horizontal meridian. Similar defects occur with lesions in the optic nerve, but in this case the tip of the defect reaches to the blind spot (Fig. 6-2). Defects in the temporal field lateral to the blind spot have the appearance of a *sector* rather than an arc. The straight course of the retinal fibers of the nasal retina toward the nerve head explains this configuration (Fig. 6-3).

Peripheral field defects may have a *crescent* shape. The most important factor in localizing the lesion is to note whether the field defect is

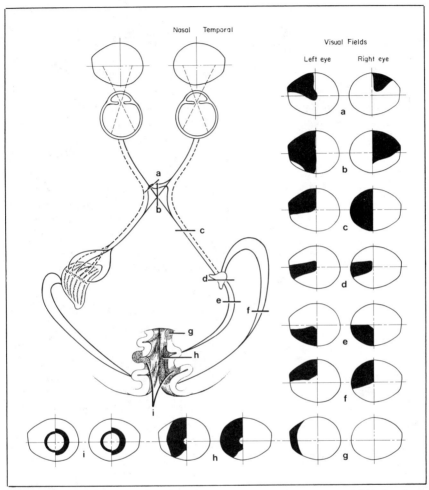

FIG. 6-9. *Visual field defects with chiasmatic and retrochiasmatic lesions. Visual fields from both eyes are usually abnormal. There is greater similarity between the field defects on each eye (congruity) with more posteriorly located lesions.*

monocular, in which case the lesion usually affects the retina or the optic nerve, or *binocular*, in which case the lesion is localized to or beyond the optic chiasm. Obviously, multiple lesions in the visual pathways, which occur frequently with multiple sclerosis and other conditions, may result in bilateral loss even when the anterior optic pathways are involved.

Occasionally the field defect has the appearance of a *ring*, with preserved vision central and peripheral to the scotoma. A unilateral pericentral scotoma indicates macular involvement. Retinitis pigmentosa often results in a large peripheral ring scotoma. Paracentral and arcuate scotomas are characteristic of glaucoma; fusion of superior and inferior arcuate defects gives rise to ring scotomas. These ring-shaped defects have a characteristic *horizontal step* (Fig. 6-2), which distinguishes them from lesions located more proximally in the visual pathways. When only central vision is intact, the visual field is said to be narrowed, and the patient has "funnel vision," not to be confused with tunnel vision, a field defect characteristic of hysteria or malingering. This field defect can easily be mapped on a tangent screen by plotting the fields with the patient sitting 1 meter and 2 meters from the screen. Logically, with an organic field defect, the field projected at 2 meters will be larger than the field plotted at 1 meter (funnel vision). Identical fields are obtained when the constriction of the field is not due to a lesion of the visual system. Bilateral field defects are said to be *homonymous* when they are similarly located in both visual fields. They are *congruous* when there is a point-to-point correspondence of the defect in either field; otherwise, they are called *incongruous* (Fig. 6-9).

Unilateral visual inattention refers to the phenomenon found in some patients with parietooccipital lesions—no field defect is found on unilateral testing, but when stimuli are placed on both right and left hemifields, the patient appears not to see the object on the field opposite the lesion. Unilateral visual inattention is often seen in patients with incomplete homonymous defects and in those recovering from a dense field defect, particularly at the margins of the defect.

Dissociation of the perception of *kinetic* and *static* stimuli (Ridoch's phenomenon) occasionally occurs with occipital lesions, and less often with lesions anywhere in the optic pathways. In this case, the patient can still appreciate moving objects within a dense field defect for static stimuli.

LOCALIZATION OF VISUAL FIELD DEFECTS. *Monocular* scotomas indicate retinal or optic nerve disease. However, in the early stages of a chiasmatic lesion the loss may be restricted to the temporal portion of the central field corresponding to the ipsilateral eye (Fig. 6-9). Also, lesions located in the most anterior extent of the calcarine cortex cause a crescent-shaped defect that is restricted to the temporal field of the contralateral eye (Fig. 6-9). Similarly, an occipital lesion that spares the foremost part of the calcarine cortex will result in a homonymous hemianopia that spares the unpaired temporal crescent (Fig. 6-9).

The pattern of the visual field loss can seldom differentiate retinal from optic nerve disease. However, retinal involvement is generally accompanied by obvious ophthalmoscopic abnormalities.

Bitemporal hemianopia localizes the lesion to the chiasm. Rarely, processes that cause rapidly developing hydrocephalus in children may result in this type of field defect, perhaps through dilation of the optic recess of the third ventricle. Papilledema is usually present in these cases.

A *central* defect in one field with a *superior temporal* defect in the opposite field points to involvement of the anterior angle of the chiasm, with damage of the ipsilateral optic nerve and of the loop made by the fibers from the inferonasal retina of the other eye (Wilbrand's knee; Figs. 6-7 and 6-9). Because of its localizing implications, this type of visual field defect has been termed *junctional scotoma*.

Homonymous hemianopias appear with lesions in the retrochiasmatic pathways. Those affecting the tract and lateral geniculate body tend to be *incongruous*, but the more posteriorly the lesion is located in the optic radiation, the greater the congruity of the defect in either field. Medial occipital lesions cause highly *congruous* homonymous hemianopias (Fig. 6-9). Sparing of central vision *(macular sparing)* is common with occipital lesions.

Superior quadrantic defects may result from lesions in the temporal loop of the optic radiations or in the inferior bank of the calcarine fissure. To cause a quadrantic defect the lesion must be quite extensive; small lesions will result in scotomas. Large medial occipital lesions are seldom restricted to one bank of the calcarine fissure. Thus, quadrantic defects more often point to a lesion of the optic radiations. Involvement of the optic radiations in the depth of the parietal lobe gives rise to an *inferior quadrantic* defect.

Monocular altitudinal defects (Fig. 6-2), which are often accompanied by macular sparing, are characteristic of disease in the distribution of the central retinal artery. Central vision may be spared because the blood supply for the macula often derives from the cilioretinal arteries (Fig. 6-3). *Bilateral altitudinal* defects may result from bilateral ischemic disease of the retinas or optic nerves, but bilateral occipital lesions are more commonly responsible for this type of defect.

Bilateral ring defects may be the consequence of retinal disease, but bilateral occipital involvement may cause a similar field defect (Fig. 6-2). However, in occipital lesions, a vertical step can regularly be identified between the two halves of the ring (Fig. 6-9).

OTHER CHANGES IN VISUAL PERCEPTION. Patients with lesions in the anterior optic pathways usually complain of difficulty in reading and dimming of vision. Altitudinal field defects are often described as a curtain coming down or the sensation of looking over the horizon. Vertical hemianopic defects are often detected when the patient finds himself colliding with objects in the blind field or is unable to see half of the page or the keyboard. However, there are other, less common subjective complaints that also have some localizing value.

Metamorphopsia (objects appearing misshapen) and *micropsia* (objects appearing reduced in size) are due to retinal disease, which causes displacement of the receptor cells. Micropsia is probably related to excessive separation of the photoreceptors by edematous fluid. Distorted perception of the shape and size of objects can also occur with occipital disease. In this case the misperception is often transient because it is linked to the prodroma of migraine or to focal seizures.

Patients with chiasmatic lesions may lose central vision when their eyes converge, because convergence makes the bitemporal defects overlap. This deficit stands in the way of activities such as threading a needle or drawing. Chiasmatic lesions may also cause image displacement in the absence of damage to the oculomotor nerves. Small motor imbalances, which are easily compensated by binocular fixation when the fields are full, are manifest in the presence of a bitemporal defect by horizontal or vertical deviation of the images from either eye *(hemifield slide phenomenon)*.

Objective Findings with Lesions of the Optic Pathways. In addition to neurologic abnormalities, such as oculomotor paresis or hemiparesis, that are due to involvement of neighboring structures, lesions in the optic pathways may betray their presence by changes in the appearance of the retina or by impairment of the afferent arc of the light reflex.

OPHTHALMOSCOPIC APPEARANCE OF THE RETINA. Lesions of the retina and optic nerve may produce identical visual field defects and loss of visual acuity. However, retinal lesions are often apparent on ophthalmoscopic examination. Chronically increased intraocular pressure in glaucoma results in cupping of the optic disc. This finding is evident by the time visual acuity decreases or arcuate scotomas appear.

Many *optic nerve* lesions cause initial swelling of the nerve, appreciable with the ophthalmoscope as papilledema, followed in time by optic atrophy. Thus, when a lesion affects both optic nerves successively, optic atrophy may be seen in the eye involved earlier while the other still has papilledema *(Foster-Kennedy syndrome)*. Foster-Kennedy syndrome due to a tumor generally results from direct compression of the optic nerve on the side of the lesion, while contralateral papilledema is due to increased intracranial pressure. Although classically described with frontal lobe tumors on the side of the optic atrophy, this syndrome occurs more often with bilateral and successive optic neuritis or ischemic optic neuropathy. Lesions in the chiasm, optic tract, or lateral geniculate body may also induce optic atrophy.

Striking optociliary shunt veins, like tiny varices, may appear in the region of the disc in cases of chronic increased pressure in the optic canal or cranial cavity. They represent anastomotic channels between the retina and the choroidal venous system that are enlarged in an effort to bypass the compressed venous channels of the optic nerve.

Because the nerve fiber layer of the retina is composed of axons of ganglion cells on their way to the lateral geniculate body, any lesion between this nucleus and the eye may cause changes in the ophthalmoscopic appearance of the fiber layer. These changes, better appreciated with red-free light, may have one of four basic patterns: slit or rake defects, sector atrophy, diffuse atrophy, or density changes in the nerve fibers themselves [7]. Because the course of the axons through the anterior optic pathways is known, the retinal distribution of these changes may suggest the location of the process. For instance, *chiasmatic* lesions affect the fibers nasal to the optic disc and nasal to the macula (papillomacular bundle; see Figs. 6-2 and 6-3). As a result, sector atrophy occurs at both sides of the disc, and the remaining fibers, somewhat thinned out, adopt the shape of a vertically disposed bow tie, with the knot representing the optic disc. This pattern is present in both eyes when the lesion is in the chiasm but may appear in only one eye, the one contralateral to the lesion, when the lesion is in the optic tract or geniculate body [9].

PUPILLARY LIGHT REFLEX. The fibers that constitute the afferent arc of the pupillary light reflex leave the visual sensory pathway just before the lateral geniculate body, without synapsing in it, to reach the dorsal midbrain. Retinal lesions must be quite large to impair the light reflex, but changes in pupillary responses, particularly the so-called *Marcus-Gunn pupil*, are very helpful in detecting *asymmetrical optic nerve* or *chiasmatic* lesions. This pupillary sign is characterized by a normal bilateral pupillary response when the sound eye is illumined, but pupillary dilatation occurs when the flashlight is quickly switched to the diseased side.

A few patients with *optic tract* involvement have unequal pupils, with the larger pupil on the side of the hemianopia — that is, contralateral to the lesion *(Behr's pupil)*. A more common sign in optic tract disease is an impaired pupillary response when the light is directed into the eye contralateral to the lesion. *Lateral geniculate body* lesions and those in the *geniculocalcarine* segment of the optic sensory pathways leave the pupillary light reflex unimpaired.

This chapter has dealt with the signs and symptoms that are most helpful in localizing a lesion in the optic pathways. These signs are summarized in Table 6-1, which also lists the most likely findings with lesions in each portion of the visual system.

TABLE 6-1. *Signs and Symptoms in Visual Pathways*

	Visual Perception				Objective Evaluation	
	Visual Acuity: Contrast Sensitivity	Color Perception	Visual Field Defects	Other Visual Changes	Pupillary Light Reflex	Ophthalmoscopic Appearance
Retina	Normal, if macula is spared. Decreased, if macula is affected	Blue affected more than red with photoreceptor lesions	Corresponds to retinal damage. Central, cecocentral, or arcuate. Sectorial ring with nasal step. Altitudinal	Micropsia, metamorphopsia	Unimpaired unless lesion is large	Focal or regional retinal changes corresponding to location and degree of visual field defect
Optic nerve	Decreased	Red most affected	Monocular with unilateral lesions. Same shape as retinal lesions		Afferent arc defect. Marcus-Gunn pupillary sign when lesion is asymmetrical	Papilledema followed by optic atrophy. Retinal nerve fiber layer atrophy
Optic chiasm	Decreased in both eyes when the medial part of the chiasm is affected. Decreased in the eye ipsilateral to a lateral chiasmatic lesion	Red most affected	*Anterior angle:* Ipsilateral–temporal or paracentral; contralateral–upper temporal. *Body:* Bitemporal, often only superior or paracentral	Impaired central vision on convergence. Hemifield slide phenomenon with pseudodiplopia	Afferent arc defect. Ipsilateral impairment in lateral chiasmatic lesions	Nerve fiber layer atrophy with a "bow tie" configuration

Optic tract	Normal with unilateral lesions	Red most affected in areas of visual field loss	Contralateral homonymous hemianopia; incongruous	Afferent defect in contralateral eye	Bilateral segmental optic atrophy. Bilateral nerve fiber layer atrophy, nasal retina in contralateral eye, temporal retina in ipsilateral eye
Lateral geniculate body	Normal with unilateral lesions	Red most affected in areas of visual field loss	Contralateral homonymous hemianopia; may be incongruous	Normal	Bilateral segmental optic atrophy. Bilateral nerve fiber layer atrophy, nasal retina in contralateral eye, temporal retina in ipsilateral eye
Optic radiations	Normal with unilateral lesions	Red most affected in areas of visual field loss	Contralateral homonymous hemianopia (total lesion) or quadrantanopia (inferior with parietal lesion; superior with temporal lesion). Macular sparing with purely **quadrantic defects.**	Normal	Normal

TABLE 6-1 (continued)

	Visual Perception				Objective Evaluation	
	Visual Acuity: Contrast Sensitivity	Color Perception	Visual Field Defects	Other Visual Changes	Pupillary Light Reflex	Ophthalmoscopic Appearance
Calcarine cortex	Normal with unilateral lesions; impaired with lesions affecting both occipital poles	Red most affected. Achromatopsia with bilateral inferomedial occipital lesions	Contralateral homonymous hemianopia, congruous. Macular sparing. Involvement or sparing of contralateral unpaired temporal crescent. Ring shape or altitudinal with "vertical step" in bilateral lesions	Kinetic stimuli perceived better than static ones. Unilateral visual inattention with occipitoparietal lesions. Pseudo-diplopia (pallinopsia)	Normal	Normal

REFERENCES

1. Arden, G. B., and Jacobson, J. J. A simple grating test for contrast sensitivity: Preliminary results indicate value in screening for glaucoma. *Invest. Ophthalmol. Vis. Sci.* 17:23, 1978.
2. Damasio, A., et al. Central achromatopsia: Behavioral, anatomic, and physiologic aspects. *Neurology* 30:1064, 1980.
3. Frisen, L. The neurology of visual acuity. *Brain* 103:639, 1980.
4. Glaser, J. S. *Neuro-ophthalmology*. Hagerstown, Md.: Harper & Row, 1978. Pp. 5–24.
5. Kupersmith, M. J., Siegel, I. M., and Carr, R. E. Reduced contrast sensitivity in compressive lesions of the anterior visual pathway. *Neurology* 31:550, 1981.
6. Miller, N. R. *Walsh and Hoyt's Clinical Neuro-Ophthalmology* (4th ed.). Baltimore: Williams & Wilkins, 1982.
7. Newman, N., Tornambe, P. E., and Corbett, J. J. Ophthalmoscopy of the retinal nerve fiber layer. Use in detection of neurologic disease. *Arch. Neurol.* 39:226, 1982.
8. Pearlman, A. L., Birch, J., and Meadows, J. C. Cerebral color blindness: An acquired defect in hue discrimination. *Ann. Neurol.* 5:253, 1979.
9. Savino, P. J., et al. Optic tract syndrome: A review of 21 patients. *Arch. Ophthalmol.* 96:656, 1978.
10. Spector, R. H., et al. Occipital lobe infarctions: Perimetry and computed tomography. *Neurology* 31:1098, 1981.
11. Trobe, J. D., et al. Confrontation visual field techniques in the detection of anterior visual pathway lesions. *Ann. Neurol.* 10:28, 1981.

Chapter 7

THE LOCALIZATION OF LESIONS IN THE OCULOMOTOR SYSTEM

Joseph C. Masdeu

Abnormalities of ocular motility serve as valuable signposts for the localization of lesions of the cerebral hemispheres, brainstem, cranial nerves, or even striated muscle. Ocular symptoms and signs are particularly helpful when examining the patient in coma (see Chap. 21).

In this chapter, the term *ocular motor* refers to cranial nerves III, IV, and VI, collectively, whereas the word *oculomotor* designates specifically cranial nerve III. This follows the convention adopted by Leigh and Zee [20] in their excellent review of ocular motility.

In this chapter we will discuss first the anatomy and localization of lesions of the ocular motor nuclei and nerves and then the control systems that the brain uses to produce precise, smooth, quick, stable, and binocular eye movements. Disturbances of these "supranuclear" mechanisms and their clinical expression will occupy the last pages.

OCULAR MOTOR MUSCLES AND NERVES

Orbital Muscles. Each eye globe is moved by six muscles, four recti (superior, inferior, medial, and lateral) and two oblique (superior and inferior). The action of the medial (eye-in) and lateral (eye-out) recti requires no further comment. The superior rectus elevates the eye (displaces the cornea upward) when the eye is deviated outward (abducted) (Fig. 7-1). Likewise, the inferior rectus depresses the eye only when the globe is abducted. By contrast, when the eye is adducted (turned inward), the superior rectus intorts it (moves it counterclockwise in the case of the left eye), and the inferior rectus extorts it (moves the left eye clockwise). The oblique muscles have a similar but complementary action in moving the eyes in the vertical plane. They move the eyeball in a vertical plane when the eye is adducted and act as rotators when it is abducted. However, unlike the recti, the oblique muscles function as if they were inserted in the anterior part of the orbit and in the posterior part of the globe. Thus, the *superior* oblique *depresses* the eye or twists it inwardly (counterclockwise in the case of the left eye) and the *inferior* oblique *elevates* the eye, or extorts it when abducted (moves the left eye clockwise).

Two muscles, both in the upper eyelid, act together to widen the palpebral fissure. Mueller's muscle receives sympathetic innervation and is responsible for the wide stare that accompanies states of enhanced alertness. However, the levator of the lid, innervated by cranial nerve III, plays the greater role in eyelid opening. Eye closure is effected through cranial nerve VII.

Testing for Diplopia. The commonest subjective complaint elicited by lesions in the ocular motor system is diplopia. This disorder occurs more frequently with lesions of the extraocular muscles or ocular motor

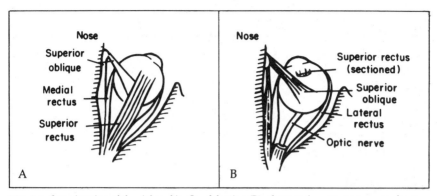

FIG. 7-1. *Superior view of the right orbit. On abduction (B), the superior rectus acts as an elevator, and the superior oblique intorts the eye (brings the upper pole toward the nose). In adduction (A), the superior oblique acts as an elevator and the superior rectus intorts the eye. In (B), the superior rectus has been removed to show the position of the superior oblique.*

nerves than with supranuclear brainstem lesions, which often result in gaze palsies. Diplopia (double vision) results from lack of visual fusion. The perceived object is projected to noncorresponding points of the retina and is therefore seen as two objects. Often, particularly when the defect is mild, the patient sees a blurry rather than a double image.

Diplopia is unilateral when it persists despite covering one eye. Displacements of the lens and retina are often to blame, but occasionally occipital disease is the cause. In the latter case, objects tend to appear doubled or multiplied (polyopsia) on the field opposite the lesion, regardless of the eye that is occluded. A partial homonymous hemianopia may also be present.

Before diplopia testing is undertaken, it is important to ascertain visual acuity in both eyes and to inspect them for lens or retinal displacements. Although somewhat difficult to perform, a forced duction test may be done to determine whether the restriction of eye movement is due to muscle weakness or to mechanical restriction in the movement of the globe. Using topical anesthesia and an ophthalmic forceps, an attempt is made to move the eye passively onto the restricted field of movement. If this attempt succeeds, mechanical restriction is discarded as the cause of the diplopia.

To identify the muscle or nerve involved, subjective and objective tests should be used. Greater difficulty with near vision suggests impairment of the medial rectus muscle, oculomotor nerve, or convergence system. Abducens weakness results in horizontal diplopia when viewing distant objects. Vertical diplopia becomes worse in near vision when an oblique muscle is weak.

SUBJECTIVE TESTING. Although a peripheral nerve or muscle may be so severely affected that the diagnosis can be made by mere inspection of the position of both eye globes in the orbit, often the objective findings are subtle and subjective diplopia testing is most helpful. To ascertain which image belongs to which eye, a red glass may be placed in front of one eye, or each eye may be covered and uncovered alternately. Instead of a red glass, a simple instrument, the Maddox rod, can be used to separate the two images even more conclusively [20]. Two rules are then applied: First, image separation is greatest in the direction of the weak muscle. For instance, a palsy of the left abducens nerve will result in greatest image separation with leftward gaze. Second, in the position of greatest image separation, the image seen more peripherally corresponds to the eye with poorer motility. Paresis of the lateral or medial recti can be easily diagnosed using these rules. Vertical gaze palsies can also be diagnosed in this manner, taking into account the action, described above, of the eight muscles that participate in vertical movement. However, the following steps are often preferable: (1) Determine which eye is higher. If the right eye is higher, the right depressors or the left elevators are weak. (2) Have the patient look to both sides. If the images now appear farther apart on left lateral gaze, either the right superior oblique or the left inferior rectus is weak. (3) Have the patient look up and down toward the side where separation was greater. If this maneuver elicits greater separation on down-gaze, the right superior oblique is the weak muscle. These steps can be supplemented with *Bielchowsky's head-tilt test,* which is usually positive with an oblique muscle palsy. Tilting the head toward the side of a weak superior oblique will increase the separation of the images, which will become single when the head is tilted opposite the side of the weak muscle. Diplopia caused by a right superior oblique palsy will be compensated by a leftward tilt of the head. Thus, a vertical muscle palsy must be suspected in patients with a head tilt. Other unusual head positions, such as turns or inappropriate flexion or extension, may result from an effort to compensate for an ocular motor palsy.

OBJECTIVE TESTING. Objective diplopia testing is used when the patient is uncooperative or when, as sometimes occurs, misalignment of the eyes suggests ocular motor weakness but the patient denies diplopia. This situation occurs more often with longstanding ocular motor weakness or with defects of visual perception. However, it may rarely occur with subacute lesions when the image of the nonfixating eye is suppressed. In this instance, the patient may give a history of transient diplopia.

The *alternate cover test* is performed by having the patient fixate on a

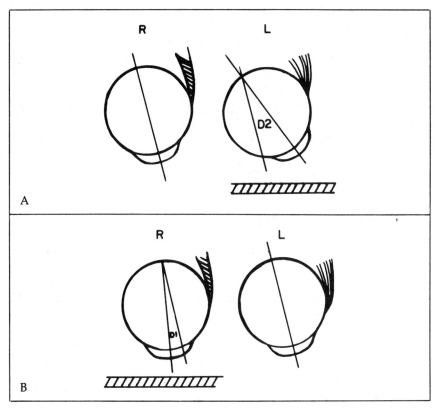

FIG. 7-2. *Alternate cover test in a right medial rectus palsy. (A) When the right (weak) eye fixates, the left is drawn in the direction of gaze (secondary deviation, D2) and is deviated from the orientation to the target (bold line). (B) When the right eye is covered, the left eye is oriented to the target, having covered an angle equal to the amount of the secondary deviation (D2). However, the right eye now drifts toward midposition, deviating (primary deviation, D1) from the orientation to the target.*

target in each of the nine positions of gaze. While in each position, the eyes are watched for angular deviations from the direction of the target as each eye is alternately covered (Fig. 7-2). In a patient with a right third nerve palsy, both eyes will remain parallel on gaze to the right, but on left lateral gaze the uncovered eye will be directed toward the target while the covered eye will be at an angle to it. When the right eye is covered and the left eye fixates, the right eye will deviate outward (exophoria), and when the cover is placed over the left eye, the right eye will move inward and the left eye will move outward. The deviation of the paretic eye, termed *primary deviation,* is smaller than the deviation of the sound eye, called *secondary deviation.* In the example mentioned above of a right third nerve palsy, it is logical that, when the eyes look to the left, the outward deviation of the covered left eye when the right eye fixates is greater than it is when the cover is switched because a strong leftward gaze movement has to compensate for the weakened right medial rectus to allow the right eye to fixate.

Disease of the Ocular Muscles. Disease of isolated extraocular muscles, particularly when it affects the lateral rectus or the superior oblique or causes patterns of weakness that resemble central involvement, may be difficult to differentiate from neurogenic weakness.

Processes that limit the range of motion of the globe by shortening or fibrosis of the muscles, such as old trauma or chronic progressive ophthalmoplegia, can easily be distinguished from neurogenic weakness because forced duction, described above, is normal in neurogenic weakness.

Thyroid ophthalmoplegia is generally preceded by exophthalmos and orbital edema. Upward gaze tends to be impaired initially. Abduction may induce extorsion of the eyeball. This phenomenon is probably related to the frequent myositis that involves the inferior oblique muscle.

Myasthenia gravis should be ruled out in any case of ocular motor weakness without an obvious cause because it can easily mimic neurogenic paresis. In myasthenia gravis the receptor side of the motor endplate of striated muscle has a reduced set of acetylcholine receptors. Characteristically, weakness increases with sustained effort. These patients often have asymmetrical ptosis that becomes more pronounced on sustained up-gaze. During refixations from down to straight ahead, the upper eyelid may bare the sclera transiently (Cogan's eyelid twitch sign).

The diagnosis is made by the marked improvement that is observed shortly after injection of the anticholinesterase agent, edrophonium chloride (Tensilon). The Tensilon test should always be performed in a double-blind fashion, and atropine should be kept readily available. Botulism, like myasthenia gravis, affects the neuromuscular junction and can cause similar eye findings. The myasthenic (Eaton-Lambert) syndrome, due to impaired release of acetylcholine in the motor endplate, seldom causes ophthalmoparesis. Gaze abnormalities due to myasthenia may mimic internuclear ophthalmoplegia or other central lesions and will be discussed later with them.

Ocular Motor Nerves and Localization of Lesions. Three brainstem nuclei contain the lower motor neurons that control the eye muscles: (1) the cranial nerve III (oculomotor) nucleus in the midbrain; (2) the cranial

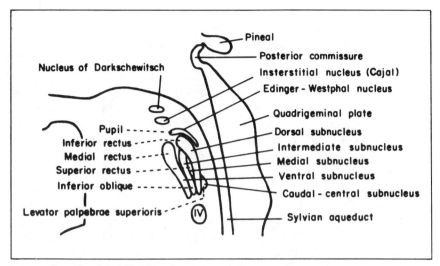

FIG. 7-3. *Lateral aspect of the left oculomotor complex.*

nerve IV (trochlear) nucleus at the level of the midbrain-pontine junction; and (3) the cranial nerve VI (abducens) nucleus in the lower pons. All are paired structures located in the dorsal part of the tegmentum at their respective levels. The sixth nerve innervates the lateral rectus, and the fourth nerve supplies the superior oblique. All of the other muscles are innervated by the third cranial nerve. Muscles innervated by neurons on the same side (ipsilateral innervation) include the lateral (sixth nerve) and medial (third nerve) recti, the inferior rectus (third nerve), and the inferior oblique (third nerve). The superior rectus (third nerve) and inferior oblique (fourth nerve) are innervated by neurons located on the contralateral side. However, the fibers to the superior rectus cross at the level of the nucleus, so that nuclear lesions result in bilateral weakness. Similarly nuclear lesions cause bilateral ptosis because the nuclear group for the levator of the lid is located in the midline [4, 12].

OCULOMOTOR NERVE (CRANIAL NERVE III)

ANATOMY. The third nerve *nuclear complex* extends rostrocaudally for about 5 mm near the midline in the midbrain at the level of the superior colliculus (see Fig. 14-3). It lies ventral to the Sylvian aqueduct, separated from it by the periaqueductal gray matter, and dorsal to the two medial longitudinal fasciculi. One unpaired and four paired rostrocaudal columns can be distinguished in the oculomotor nuclear complex (Fig. 7-3). The unpaired column, shared by the right and left nuclei, is in the most dorsal location and contains the visceral nuclei (Edinger-Westphal nucleus) rostrally and the subnucleus for the levator palpebrae superioris caudally. The Edinger-Westphal nucleus mediates pupillary constriction, which is increased by light and during accommodation. Of the four paired subnuclei, the most medial innervates the superior rectus muscle. This is the only portion of the oculomotor nucleus that sends its axons to the opposite eye. However, the decussation occurs right in the nuclear complex, and the decussating fibers actually traverse the contralateral subnucleus for the superior rectus. Hence, a destruction lesion in one superior rectus subnucleus results in bilateral denervation of the superior recti. Laterally in each oculomotor complex there are three subnuclei (Fig. 7-3): dorsal (inferior rectus), intermediate (inferior oblique), and ventral (medial rectus).

The axons of the oculomotor neurons cross the medial longitudinal fasciculus, decussating fibers of the superior cerebellar peduncle and the red nucleus before exiting on the anterior aspect of the midbrain just medial to the cerebral peduncles. In the *subarachnoid space* each third nerve passes between the superior cerebellar and the posterior cerebral arteries, courses forward near the medial aspect of the temporal uncus, pierces the dura just lateral to the posterior clinoid process, and enters the *cavernous sinus* (see Fig. 6-4). Here, the nerve runs over the trochlear nerve, lying superior to the abducens nerve and medial to the ophthalmic branch of the trigeminal nerve. Once it reaches the *superior orbital fissure*, the oculomotor nerve divides into a superior ramus, which supplies the superior rectus and the levator of the lid, and an inferior ramus, which supplies the medial and inferior recti, the inferior oblique, and the ciliary ganglion.

LOCALIZATION OF LESIONS. Lesions can affect the third nerve in the brainstem (nucleus or fascicular portion), in the subarachnoid space, in the cavernous sinus, at the superior orbital fissure, or in the orbit.

Pure unilateral *nuclear lesions* are very rare. Paresis of an isolated muscle innervated by the oculomotor nerve almost always results from lesions in the orbit or from muscle disease. However, nuclear lesions may give rise to isolated weakness of one of the muscles innervated by the oculomotor nerve, with the exception of the following muscles: superior rectus, levator of the lid, and constrictor of the pupil. These muscles would be affected bilaterally with even small nuclear lesions. More characteristic of nuclear involvement is weakness of all the muscles innervated by the ipsilateral third nerve, contralateral superior rectus weakness, and bilateral incomplete ptosis. Bilateral third nerve palsies with sparing of the lid levators may also be caused by nuclear lesions. Disturbances of alertness are generally prominent in these cases.

Fascicular lesions often accompany nuclear lesions because infarction is a common cause of a nuclear third nerve palsy, and the paramedian branches near the top of the basilar artery often feed both structures. However, pure fascicular lesions cause a peripheral type of oculomotor palsy that is associated both with ipsilateral involvement of all the muscles innervated by it and with sparing of the other eye. Furthermore, involvement of brainstem structures other than the fascicles of the third nerve helps in identifying the extent and location of the lesion. Concomitant damage of the red nucleus will cause contralateral ataxia and outflow tract cerebellar tremor (Claude syndrome). Larger lesions that affect in addition the subthalamic region may produce contralateral choreiform movements (Benedikt syndrome). Lesions that, extending caudally, involve the third nerve and ipsilateral brachium conjunctivum below the decussation cause cerebellar findings ipsilateral to the third nerve palsy (Nothnagel syndrome). A more anterior lesion, affecting the peduncle, gives rise to contralateral hemiparesis (Weber syndrome).

Other common manifestations of lesions in this region include disorders of gaze and convergence, paucity of speech and even mutism, somnolence, and hallucinations (peduncular hallucinosis) [4]. Abduction toward the contralateral side may be impaired [4, 12, 21]. Although displacement and irregularity of the pupils (corectopia) are occasionally found with peripheral third nerve lesions and are often due to focal pathology in the iris, they may also result from midbrain lesions [24].

An isolated third nerve palsy is most often related to an ischemic neuritis or to lesions in its *subarachnoid portion*. Among these, compression by aneurysms in the junction between the posterior cerebral and posterior communicating arteries is common. Elongation by a herniated uncus causes, first, pupillary dilatation, associated with poor response to light but relatively preserved convergence, followed by weakness of the extraocular muscles when the pupil becomes fixed. Ectatic vessels, tumors (particularly meningiomas, metastases, and chordomas), Guillain-Barré syndrome, inflammatory processes of the meninges, or stretching during neurosurgical procedures may also damage the third nerve in its subarachnoid course.

In the *cavernous sinus*, compressive lesions often involve also the other ocular motor nerves and the ophthalmic branch of the trigeminal nerve. However, lesions in the neighborhood of the posterior clinoid process may for some time affect only the third nerve as it pierces the dura (e.g., breast and prostatic carcinoma). Medial lesions in the cavernous sinus, such as a carotid artery aneurysm, may affect only the ocular motor nerves but spare the more laterally located ophthalmic branch of the trigeminal nerve, resulting in painless ophthalmoplegia. On the contrary, lesions that begin laterally, as in some cases of nasopharyngeal carcinoma, present with retroorbital pain first, and only later does ophthalmoparesis supervene. The clinical findings are similar when the process extends to or is primarily located in the *superior orbital fissure*. However, with space-occupying lesions, proptosis is a strong indication of the latter location [10]. When evaluating a patient with an oculomotor palsy for proptosis, it must be remembered that flaccidity of the muscles may result in proptosis of up to 3 mm on the paretic side. Isolated involvement of the muscles innervated by either the superior or the inferior oculomotor branch points to an orbital process, often trauma or tumor.

Six months to a year after the occurrence of an oculomotor lesion, clinical findings of *aberrant regeneration* may be seen. They include elevation of the lid on down-gaze (pseudo-Graefe lid sign) or on adduction, but lid depression during abduction. This horizontal gaze-lid synkinesis is similar to but of opposite direction from the lid synkinesis observed in Duane retraction syndrome (reviewed below), in which the palpebral fissure narrows on adduction. The pupil may remain fixed to light but may respond to accommodation (pseudo-Argyll-Robertson pupil) or constrict on adduction or down-gaze. Longstanding lesions such as meningiomas or aneurysms may present as an aberrant regeneration of the third nerve without a history of a previous third nerve palsy. Ischemic neuropathy almost never causes this syndrome.

TROCHLEAR NERVE (CRANIAL NERVE IV)

ANATOMY. The trochlear *nucleus* lies caudal to the oculomotor nuclear group and at the level of the inferior colliculus. The nerve *fascicles* decussate in the dorsal midbrain and emerge from the brainstem near the dorsal midline, immediately below the inferior colliculi. The nerve then runs anteriorly over the lateral aspect of the midbrain in the *perimesencephalic cistern*. After traveling on the undersurface of the tentorial edge, it pierces the dura at a point slightly below the point of entry of the oculomotor nerve in the *cavernous sinus*. The trochlear nerve reaches the superior orbital fissure to innervate the superior oblique muscle (see Fig. 6-4).

LOCALIZATION OF LESIONS. Lesions of the trochlear nerve commonly follow trauma. Its long course around the mesencephalon, near the edge of the tentorium, makes this nerve particularly vulnerable. Ischemic neuropathy caused by diabetes or other vasculopathies can affect any segment of the trochlear nerve. With other lesions, precise localization depends on the damage done to neighboring structures. Expanding lesions in the dorsal midbrain may betray themselves by causing an upward gaze palsy. As the nerve courses anterolaterally around the midbrain, involvement of the superior cerebellar peduncle before the decussation may be manifest by ipsilateral cerebellar signs. A contralateral hemiparesis, predominantly involving the leg, would locate the lesion more anteriorly where the nerve swings around the cerebral peduncle. Tentorial meningiomas can cause the syndromes just described. Guillain-Barré syndrome usually affects other ocular motor nerves as well. Lesions in the cavernous sinus or superior orbital fissure may involve all the ocular motor nerves and the ophthalmic branch of the trigeminal nerve with subsequent retroorbital pain on the affected side. Motion of the superior oblique may be restricted by a tenosynovitis, usually painful, that prevents the tendon from passing freely through the trochlear pulley. Forced duction can be used to unmask this mechanical restriction of depression on adduction. Myokymia of the superior oblique muscle may cause transient diplopia.

Involvement of the trochlear nerve is commonly sought in the presence of a third nerve palsy. In this instance, adduction weakness prevents the superior oblique from depressing the eye. However, if the superior oblique is functional, it will intort the eye (upper pole will turn toward the nose) when the patient is asked to look down.

ABDUCENS NERVE (CRANIAL NERVE VI)

ANATOMY. The paired abducens nucleus is located in the lower pons, separated from the floor of the fourth ventricle by the genu of the facial nerve (see Fig. 14-2). Here abducens motoneurons are intermixed with internuclear neurons that send their axons across the midline to the opposite medial longitudinal fasciculus, where they ascend through the pons and midbrain to end in the third nerve nucleus. Thus, the abducens nuclear complex coordinates the action of both eyes to produce horizontal gaze. Axons of the abducens motoneurons course anteriorly in the pons, through the medial lemniscus and medial to the facial nerve fascicles, to emerge in the horizontal sulcus between the pons and medulla, lateral to the corticospinal bundles. The abducens nerve then ascends on the belly of the pons in the *prepontine cistern* and enters *Dorello's canal* beneath Grueber's ligament (see Fig. 6-4). In the lateral wall of the *cavernous sinus*, it lies between the carotid artery medially and the ophthalmic branch of the trigeminal nerve laterally (see Fig. 6-4). In their course from the pericarotid plexus to the ophthalmic branch of the trigeminal nerve, the pupil's sympathetic fibers join the abducens nerve for a few millimeters. After passing through the *superior orbital fissure*, the abducens nerve innervates the lateral rectus muscle.

LOCALIZATION OF LESIONS. Lesions affecting the *abducens nucleus* cause not only an ipsilateral lateral rectus paresis but also a horizontal gaze palsy to the same side because the abducens interneurons are involved.

Lesions of the abducens nucleus early in life can cause Möbius syndrome or Duane retraction syndrome. In addition to horizontal gaze disturbances, patients with Möbius syndrome have a facial diplegia and may have other cranial nerve abnormalities. Duane retraction syndrome is characterized by a narrowing of the palpebral fissure on adduction and appears in three forms. In the most common, abduction is limited but adduction is normal. Some patients have impaired adduction but normal abduction, and others have impairment of both. These patients seldom complain of diplopia, although this symptom may develop later in life. In this case, an old abducens palsy can then be diagnosed by noticing retraction of the globe as the patient attempts to look toward the paretic side.

Pontine tegmental lesions will be discussed in greater detail in the section on central disturbances of eye movements. Acute lesions of the low *dorsolateral pons* cause an ipsilateral gaze palsy, facial paresis, and terminal dysmetria. A more extensive unilateral lesion will also cause contralateral hemiparesis (Foville syndrome). More *anterior paramedial* lesions spare the abducens nucleus but affect the fascicles, resulting in ipsilateral abducens and facial weakness with contralateral hemiparesis (Millard-Gubler syndrome). Such lesions are often ischemic, but they may be tumors, particularly gliomas and metastases, granulomas, multiple sclerosis plaques, or lesions of Wernicke's encephalopathy. Lesions that affect the abducens nerve in the *prepontine cistern* may compress the ipsilateral corticospinal bundles and result in contralateral hemiparesis. However, extramedullary tumors can be quite large and yet fail to give any long tract signs. More often, stretching or compression of the trigeminal root will result in ipsilateral facial pain that may have all the characteristics of trigeminal neuralgia. A frequent cause of isolated abducens involvement at this level is increased intracranial pressure. Cerebellopontine angle tumors seldom involve the abducens nerve. Compressive lesions in the prepontine cistern include atherosclerotic elongation of the basilar artery, aneurysms, meningomas of the clivus, chordomas, and nasopharyngeal carcinomas. Here the nerve is also exposed to trauma, meningitis, meningeal carcinomatosis, and the peripheral demyelination of the Guillain-Barré syndrome.

Based on neurologic findings alone, it may be difficult at times to determine whether the nerve has been lesioned at the subarachnoid space or in its *petrous portion*, in Dorello's canal. Concomitant involvement of the trigeminal nerve is more likely if the lesion is in the petrous portion. There may be other clinical findings pointing to disease in the petrous bone, such as an otic discharge from chronic otitis media or mastoiditis, or deafness. An infection that spreads to the tip of the petrous bone may result in a classic Gradenigo syndrome, which includes abducens nerve paresis, ipsilateral facial (usually retroorbital) pain, and deafness. Trauma and tumors (cholesteatomas, schwannomas, carcinomas) may also injure the nerve at this level.

Retroorbital pain, involvement of other ocular motor nerves and, occasionally, an ipsilateral Horner syndrome point to the *cavernous sinus* as the site of the lesion. Similar findings may be encountered with more anterior lesions in the *superior orbital fissure*. However, tumors in this location may betray their presence by proptosis [9].

Pituitary adenomas, nasopharyngeal carcinomas, craniopharyngiomas, and metastases most commonly affect the abducens nerve at the cavernous sinus and superior orbital fissure [18]. Tolosa-Hunt syndrome, which is caused by inflammatory processes of various (often unclear) etiologies involving the cavernous sinus, responds promptly to steroids. It presents with ocular motor weakness and retroorbital pain. Facial sensation and visual acuity may be diminished. Sudden onset of headache and dysfunction of multiple ocular motor nerves on either one or both sides, with or without retroorbital pain or visual impairment, suggests the possibility of pituitary apoplexy, a sudden enlargement of the sella by bleeding into a pituitary adenoma. In the orbit, trauma, tumors, and inflammatory processes can cause abducens weakness. The abducens nerve may be involved anywhere along its course by an ischemic neuropathy related to diabetes or to other processes that cause small vessel disease, such as collagen-vascular disease and parainfectious or postinfectious arteritides.

A *pseudo-palsy of the sixth nerve* may result from excessive convergence. The most common variety is *spasm of the near triad* (see below, Convergence System), which is seen in some hysterical patients. When instructed to look sideways or to follow an object with both eyes, these patients generate convergence movements instead of gazing to the side, resulting in apparent weakness of the abducting eye. The miosis that occurs as the patient seems to attempt lateral gaze reveals the true nature of the problem. Occluding one eye or turning the head passively (doll's eye maneuver) often results in a full range of motion [31]. Less often, a pseudo-sixth palsy may result from midbrain lesions [4, 21].

The Pupil

SYMPATHETIC AND PARASYMPATHETIC INNERVATION. Pupillary size depends on the balance between sympathetic and parasympathetic tone. Sympathetic innervation, which dilates the pupil, proceeds ipsilaterally from the hypo-

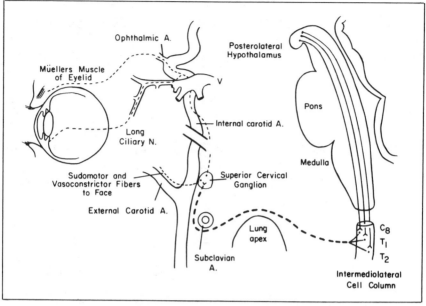

FIG. 7-4. *Sympathetic innervation of the pupil. The first-order neuron is located in the posterolateral hypothalamus. The second-order neuron is in the intermediolateral cell column of the low cervical and upper thoracic cord. The third-order neuron is in the superior cervical ganglion.*

thalamus through the lateral tegmentum of the brainstem, the intermediolateral nucleus of the cord at the C8–T2 segments, the sympathetic chain to the superior stellate ganglion, the carotid plexus, and the ophthalmic branch of the trigeminal nerve, reaching the pupil through the long ciliary nerves (see Figs. 6-4 and 7-4). From the Edinger-Westphal nucleus in the rostral portion of the third nerve nuclear complex, parasympathetic tone reaches the constrictor of the pupil through the third nerve, synapsing first in the ciliary ganglion, which is located behind the globe in the orbit (Figs. 6-4 and 7-5). The pupillomotor fibers probably course in the periphery of the oculomotor nerve, immediately internal to the epineurium, and are situated dorsally in the subarachnoid segment of the oculomotor nerve [21a].

Except for midbrain lesions and some unusual cases of bilateral miosis due to sympathetic damage, structural lesions impinging on the pupillomotor pathways are often unilateral and result in pupillary inequality. An abnormally small pupil (miosis) is a sign of a lesion in the sympathetic pathway. A large pupil (midriasis) suggests that the lesion affects the parasympathetic pathway. Because this pathway courses for the most

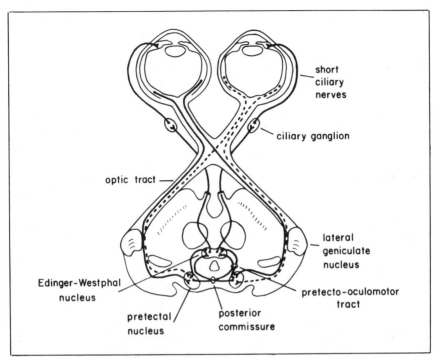

FIG. 7-5. *Parasympathetic innervation of the pupil and pathway for the light reflex.*

part with the third nerve, lesions affecting it are often accompanied by a lesser or greater degree of weakness of the extraocular muscles innervated by the oculomotor nerve and by an impaired light reflex (Fig. 7-5). Ptosis can accompany lesions on either pathway; it tends to be rather severe with third nerve lesions but is mild and certainly incomplete with lesions of the sympathetic pathway, which result in lack of tone of Mueller's muscle. Classically, oculosympathetic paralysis results in a *Horner syndrome*, which comprises the triad of miosis, ptosis, and anhidrosis of the forehead [28]. However, anhidrosis is inconstant after postganglionic lesions. Theoretically, because the sympathetic fibers that innervate the forehead follow the external carotid artery, lesions distal to the carotid bifurcation would be unaccompanied by anhidrosis of the forehead (Fig. 7-4). This is, however, an unreliable sign. Miosis may not be perceptible if the patient with a Horner syndrome is in a state of high sympathotonic activity, such as marked fear or anxiety. In these cases, high levels of circulating norepinephrine dilate the pupil. Enophthalmos may be part of a Horner syndrome. Pallor of the iris, resulting in different colors of the two irides (heterochromia irides), may accompany oculosympathetic paralysis that was sustained early in life.

PUPILLARY INEQUALITY (ANISOCORIA). Pupillary asymmetry is often the point of departure for diagnosis of lesions in the pupillomotor pathways [29]. However, between 15 and 30 percent of the normal population have a difference in pupillary size of 0.4 mm or greater (simple anisocoria) [28]. Several steps are taken to diagnose the cause of pupillary asymmetry [29].

If both pupils react well to light, the patient may have *simple anisocoria;* otherwise, it is likely that the smaller pupil is the abnormal one and that the anisocoria will become more pronounced when the lights in the examining room are turned off. While this is being done, one should look for a "dilatation lag" of the smaller pupil. If present, there may be more pupillary asymmetry 5 seconds after the lights are turned off than 15 seconds afterward. A dilatation lag implies poor sympathetic tone and is therefore indicative of a *Horner syndrome.* The diagnosis can be confirmed by instilling in both eyes one drop of a 10% cocaine solution. Another drop is instilled 1 minute later, and the result is read in 45 minutes. The normal pupil dilates after cocaine instillation, which blocks the reuptake of norepinephrine, but in Horner syndrome the pupil fails to dilate. Antihypertensive medications prevent pupillary dilatation by cocaine. A solution of 1% hydroxyamphetamine instilled at least 2 days after the cocaine test, will dilate a pupil in Horner syndrome only if the lesion is central to the superior cervical ganglion. A central Horner syndrome commonly occurs following acute (vascular) lesions of the lateral pons or medulla. It is part of the lateral medullary syndrome of Wallenberg. Pancoast tumors of the pulmonary apex often involve the sympathetic chain. A postganglionic Horner syndrome may accompany ipsilateral carotid artery disease, but carotid stenosis may instead give rise to a dilated, poorly reactive pupil, perhaps because of ischemia of the iris [9]. Inflammatory, neoplastic, or vascular disease of the cavernous sinus may result in ipsilateral retroorbital pain and a Horner syndrome (Reader's paratrigeminal neuralgia) [11].

If one of the pupils, generally the larger one, reacts poorly to light, the diagnosis can be narrowed to four possibilities:

1. Damage to the parasympathetic outflow, through the *third nerve,* of the Edinger-Westphal nucleus.
2. *Adie's tonic pupil,* which is due to neuronal loss in the ciliary ganglion and is often accompanied by loss of ankle jerks [16].
3. *Damage to the iris,* due to ischemia, trauma, or an inflammatory process.

4. Midriasis induced by the instillation of an *atropinic drug.* Unilateral midriasis may attend the use of transdermal scopolamine to prevent motion sickness [5].

Lesions in the Edinger-Westphal nucleus or anywhere along the course of the third nerve (see Oculomotor Nerve, above) may give rise to ipsilateral pupillary dilation. Nuclear lesions involve both eyes. Pupillary irregularity or eccentricity (sector palsy of the iris sphincter) may result from lesions anywhere along the third nerve or in the midbrain but not from pharmacologic blockade. Pupillary dilatation and unresponsiveness, with relatively preserved extraocular muscle function, is characteristic of compression of the third nerve in the subarachnoid space, usually by the temporal uncus or by a posterior communicating artery aneurysm [18a]. By contrast, lesions of the third nerve in the cavernous sinus often spare pupillary function, and pupillary sparing is the rule with ischemic diabetic oculomotor neuropathy [21a].

Cholinergic supersensitivity, which is characteristic of Adie's pupil, mediates pupillary constriction when 0.1% pilocarpine is instilled. A stronger solution of pilocarpine (1%) will cause constriction in the case of a third nerve lesion but will not modify pupillary size if the anisocoria is due to an atropinic drug or to iris damage. In the latter case, the iris may transilluminate, or its margin may appear torn on ophthalmoscopy or when it is examined with the slit-lamp.

SUPRANUCLEAR CONTROL OF EYE MOVEMENTS

The complex and precise array of eye movements that secure clear vision results from the interaction of a number of neural systems. Their combined output plays on the ocular motor nuclei in the brainstem; thus the term *supranuclear* is appropriate to designate these systems. Many eye movements are involuntary—for instance, the fine corrective movements that keep the eye in the appropriate orbital position, despite ongoing head motion. Input for these corrective movements comes from the vestibular nuclei (vestibular system) or from the retina (optokinetic and smooth pursuit systems). The systems that permit a moving target to remain sharply focused in the fovea (smooth pursuit and vergence systems) are also largely involuntary, although the person may choose to glance or not to glance at a particular object. The system that produces voluntary eye movements is called the saccadic system.

In the next section we will briefly review the function, anatomy, characteristics, and bedside testing of each of these systems. Gaze palsies, the most characteristic clinical manifestations of disturbances in the supranuclear control of eye movements, will be dealt with last. *Gaze* in this section refers to the position of the eyes in space.

Vestibular System. To be clearly perceived, images of the outside world have to slide over the retina at a speed of no more than a few degrees per second. Otherwise, things would appear blurry and fuzzy, like a photograph taken with a low shutter speed while the camera is moving. Without the appropriate corrective system something similar would happen to the eye, anchored in the orbit and constantly jerked by manifold head movements. The vestibular system drives the eye with the same velocity but in a direction opposite to the disruptive head motion. Thus, the eye globe, like a gyroscope, keeps its stable position despite orbital movements.

THE VESTIBULOOCULAR REFLEX. The reflex by which the vestibular system perceives head movement and, with a latency of about 10 msec, makes the eyeball move in the opposite direction is called the vestibuloocular reflex.

LABYRINTH AND VESTIBULAR NUCLEUS. The sensory arc of the reflex begins at the semicircular canals of the inner ear. Each of the three (horizontal, anterior, and posterior) semicircular canals is stimulated by movements in its plane and also induces eye movements in its plane (Flouren's law). The corresponding semicircular canals of both ears are yoked in such a way that when the head rotates, one canal increases its rate of firing while the corresponding canal in the opposite ear slows its rate. The impulses travel by way of the vestibular nerve to the ipsilateral vestibular nuclear complex in the pontomedullary junction (see Fig. 14-2). When a vestibular nucleus is excited it tends to deviate the eyes toward the contralateral side. However, each vestibular nuclear complex has neurons that increase their rate of firing with ipsilateral head rotations and others that increase their discharge rate with contralateral rotations. This feature, coupled with the existence of a vestibular commissure in the vicinity of the vestibular nuclei, may explain why vestibular function recovers when one side is damaged. From the vestibular nucleus the signal for horizontal eye movements is relayed to the abducens nucleus in the contralateral side of the lower pons.

OCULAR MOTOR NUCLEI AND THE MEDIAL LONGITUDINAL FASCICULUS. The abducens nucleus has two types of neurons: motor neurons for the sixth cranial nerve and internuclear neurons of the abducens nucleus [26]. The axons of the internuclear neurons cross to the contralateral side in the lower pons and, after ascending in the medial longitudinal fasciculus (MLF), synapse in the portion of the oculomotor nucleus that innervates the medial rectus (Fig. 7-6). Thus, a vestibular impulse originating in the labyrinth will be relayed from the ipsilateral vestibular nucleus to the contralateral abducens and ipsilateral oculo-

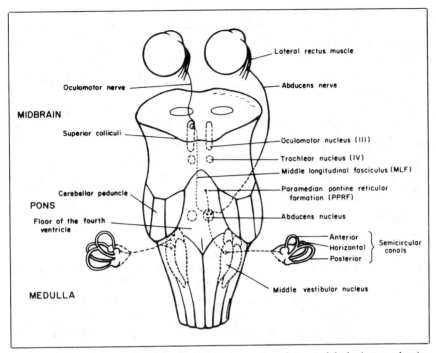

FIG. 7-6. *Horizontal gaze mechanisms. Right lateral gaze. Dorsal aspect of the brainstem, showing the pontine center for lateral gaze and the pathways mediating the vestibuloocular reflex.*

motor neurons, resulting in deviation of the eyes to the contralateral side. A similar pathway, but with a crossed and an uncrossed component, mediates the vertical vestibular eye movements. Ascending fibers course in the MLF and in the brachium conjunctivum, synapsing in the areas of the trochlear or oculomotor nuclei where the muscles involved in the appropriate movement are represented.

HEAD POSITION. In addition to information about angular acceleration registered by the semicircular canals, the labyrinth provides information about the static position of the head. This information is registered by the utricle and the saccule, situated on planes perpendicular to each other, and reaches the extraocular muscles through pathways akin to the ones used by signals from the semicircular canals.

CALORIC TESTING, NYSTAGMUS. The slow eye motions induced by the vestibular system cannot be appreciated in ordinary conditions. However, they become quite obvious when there is an imbalance between the vestibular nuclei in certain pathologic conditions. An imbalance can be easily produced by instilling a few milliliters of cold water in the external auditory canal while the head is kept at a 30-degree angle with the horizontal plane. This maneuver results in a slowing of the firing rate of the horizontal semicircular canal on the side of the infusion. Consequently, the eyes tend to deviate slowly to where the cold water has been infused. However, quick corrective jerks in a direction opposite the slow motion keep the eyes looking in the direction willed by the individual who is alert. The resultant repetitive eye movement with slow and quick components in opposite directions is termed *nystagmus*. Spontaneous nystagmus is a frequent sign of vestibular dysfunction. It will be discussed below. In a comatose patient, the quick jerks are absent and the eyes remain for 10 to 25 seconds deviated toward the side that has been cooled.

SYMPTOMS OF VESTIBULAR DYSFUNCTION

VERTIGO. Vestibular disease is often manifest by the presence of vertigo, the illusory sensation of movement of the patient himself or of the environment. The latter has been experienced by anyone subjected to a sustained angular movement (e.g., in a merry-go-round). When rotation ceases, the environment seems to move in the opposite direction for a few seconds. Vertigo is often accompanied by nausea and even vomiting. Nausea is much more common and severe when vertigo results from affection of the peripheral vestibular apparatus.

Lesions of the semicircular canals induce rotatory sensations, whereas disease of the otolith system (utricle and saccule) produces linear sensations of tilt or levitation. In acute vertigo due to labyrinthine disease, the diseased side may for some hours or even days be the more active of the two (irritative phase), but it soon becomes less active (paretic phase). When the eyes are closed, the patient feels a sensation of rotation toward the side opposite a paretic labyrinth. By contrast, in the paretic phase the eyes tend to deviate slowly toward the side of the lesion, and to this side the patient tends to past-point and to fall when standing with his eyes closed. A patient with severe vertigo feels most comfortable lying on one side, usually with the affected ear uppermost. Deafness accompanies recurrent vertigo in cases of Meniere's disease. In patients with labyrinthine disease, acoustic stimuli may induce vertigo and nystagmus (Tullio's phenomenon), perhaps through utricular stimulation.

Vertigo induced by a specific head position is often related to the entity known as benign paroxysmal positional vertigo. In this case, the Nylén-Bárány maneuver may elicit a characteristic pattern of nystagmus. From a sitting position the patient quickly lies down, with the head turned toward one shoulder and hanging down at 30 degrees to the horizontal plane. The maneuver is then repeated, turning the head to the opposite shoulder. If the maneuver is positive, after a latency period of about 10 seconds the patient experiences discomfort and begins to exhibit nystagmus, with a more pronounced vertical component in the upper eye and a rotatory component in the lower eye. The slow phase of nystagmus is directed downward. The nystagmus increases for about 10 seconds and then tends to fatigue. If at this point the patient is asked to sit up, a milder episode, with nystagmus beating in the opposite direction, may occur. This pattern of nystagmus suggests stimulation of the posterior semicircular canal of the lower ear. In some cases, detached otoliths may come to rest on the cupula of the dependent posterior semicircular canal, thereby generating the syndrome. With peripheral vestibular disease, this maneuver is positive only when the head is turned to one of the two sides and becomes less effective if repeated several times. A central lesion should be suspected when (1) the maneuver is positive with the head turned to either side; (2) the pattern of nystagmus is atypical, appearing immediately after the shift in position and remaining for as long as the head is down; (3) the nystagmus is unaccompanied by nausea or a sense of discomfort; and (4) repetition does not cause blunting of the effects. Mild transient nystagmus in one head position may be elicited by the Nylén-Bárány maneuver in normal subjects.

Vertigo may occur with ischemia of the vestibular structures in the brainstem, but when it progresses to infarction, other signs of brainstem damage (such as gaze palsies, hemiparesis, or a hemisensory loss) become apparent as well.

OSCILLOPSIA. Oscillopsia is the subjective feeling of unsteadiness of the visually perceived environment, which seems to move back and forth. Often it is increased by movement of the head, as when walking, and then it is related to impairment of the vestibular system that stabilizes images in the retina. Oscillopsia in the vertical plane may result from bilateral MLF involvement. Conditions that may cause oscillopsia even when the head remains still include acquired pendular nystagmus, paresis of an extraocular muscle, and epilepsy. Superior oblique myokymia can induce transient monocular oscillopsia.

Full-Field Optokinetic Reflex. The vestibuloocular reflex becomes fatigued after about 30 seconds. A different system is required to maintain the eyes on target during prolonged head motion in the same direction, such as when one is driving along a road next to a pine forest. The image of the trees, apparently moving in the direction opposite the car, act as signals that reach the vestibular nuclei from the retina. The intermediate pathway probably includes the pretectal area, the nucleus reticularis tegmenti pontis, and the medial pontine nuclei. The slow eye movement, contrary to the direction of the car, tends to stabilize the image of the trees in the retina, allowing the driver to see them sharply. This is the so-called optokinetic reflex. However, more meaningful for safety is that the eyes be on the road that lies ahead. Thus, they are repeatedly directed forward by quick ocular jerks, called saccades, which will be discussed later. This optokinetic reflex requires that the moving object fill most of the visual field (full-field stimulation) and differs from smooth pursuit of a target that is being followed while it is projected in the macular region of the retina. In humans, smooth pursuit probably plays a greater role than the full-field optokinetic reflex in stabilizing images in the retina. However, when the pathway that mediates pursuit (see Smooth Pursuit System) is damaged, the more primitive full-field pursuit mechanism can be elicited [2]. Unlike foveal pursuit, full-field pursuit builds up slowly (10 to 20 seconds) and decays gradually after the stimulus is terminated (optokinetic after-nystagmus).

Lesions of the anterior visual pathways decrease optokinetic responses. Unilateral vestibular lesions cause a directional preponderance of optokinetic nystagmus, with increased slow-phase velocity toward the side of the lesion. Reversed optokinetic nystagmus is characteristically found in patients with benign congenital nystagmus (see below, Pendular Nystagmus). In this case, the quick component beats in the direction of the slowly moving optokinetic target. This actually represents the patient's own gaze-modulated spontaneous nystagmus shifted to the primary position of gaze by optokinetic stimulation [15].

Smooth Pursuit System. An object is seen with most detail when its image falls in the fovea, located in the posterior pole of the retina. Two oculomotor systems allow visual images to remain in the fovea: smooth pursuit, as the object moves vertically or horizontally, and vergence eye movements (convergence and divergence) as the object moves along the depth axis of the visual field, particularly as it approaches the subject. As the eyes keep the interesting image in the fovea, the background may be blurred, just as it appears in a photograph of a skier when the photographer is able to follow him with the eye of the camera as the skier rushes past down the slope.

Images moving away from the fovea constitute the strongest stimuli for smooth pursuit. At the bedside, hand-held optokinetic drums or tapes provide an adequate stimulus for the foveal-pursuit system. The smooth pursuit system cannot follow objects that move faster than 30 to

40 degrees per second, the lower range being more characteristic of elderly persons [27]. Faster moving objects elicit quicker eye movements, termed saccades. Saccades are under the control of the will, but smooth eye movements cannot be voluntarily produced and need a visual object to be traced. When a person tries to move the eyes slowly, a number of short quick saccades results. However, some individuals can elicit slow smooth eye movements by tracking their own slowly moving finger in darkness.

As an object of interest moves in front of the subject, both the head and the eyes may turn to keep it in the macula. However, in order to do this, the vestibuloocular reflex, discussed above, must be inhibited. Otherwise, as the head moves in the direction of the object, the eyes would be pulled in the opposite direction. The neural command for the head and eyes to follow an object inhibits at the same time the vestibuloocular reflex. Thus, abnormalities of the pursuit system may be expressed by an inability to inhibit the vestibuloocular reflex.

The anatomic pathways involved in the smooth pursuit system remain partially unknown. After visual information has been received from the peristriate cortex, impulses arising in the superior parietal lobule (area 7) and perhaps in the frontal eye fields (area 8) reach the ipsilateral paramedian pontine reticular formation (PPRF) and the mesencephalic reticular formation, which originate commands for horizontal and vertical eye movements (Fig. 7-7). It is unclear whether this pathway is uncrossed or has a double decussation (rostrally in the mesencephalic decussation of Meynert and caudally with the fibers from the frontal eye fields to the pons at the pontomesencephalic junction). Superior collicular input may also be important.

Frontal lesions spare the pursuit system. Parietal lesions decrease the amplitude and velocity of smooth pursuit toward the side of the lesion [2]. This deficit is most evident after hemispherectomy [8, 25]. The cerebellar flocculus plays an important role in the production of smooth pursuit. Unilateral cerebellar damage results in impaired pursuit in the direction of the involved side [6]. This deficit is transient. Bilateral damage causes permanent impairment of smooth pursuit eye movements.

How well the smooth pursuit system works depends on the degree of attention elicited by the object being followed. Many drugs, including chloral hydrate, barbiturates, phenytoin, diazepam, alcohol, methadone, and marijuana impair smooth pursuit, rendering it jerky or slow or abolishing it altogether.

Patients with lesions that impair pursuit are often unable to inhibit the vestibuloocular reflex [6]. For instance, a patient with a left hemispherectomy, resulting in impaired pursuit to the left, when rotating to the

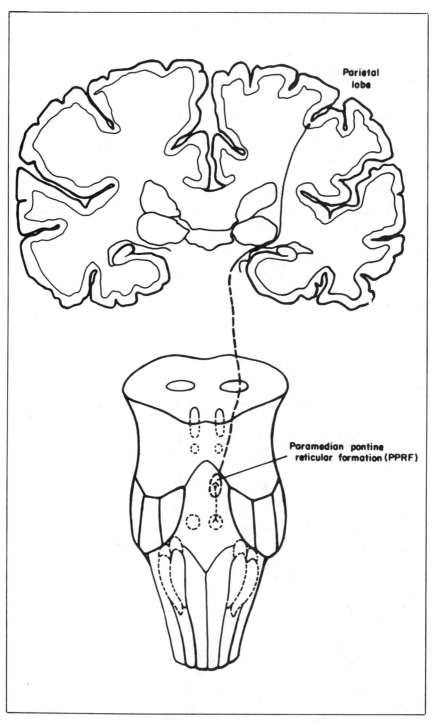

FIG. 7-7. *Smooth pursuit system. Horizontal eye movements. Diagrammatic and markedly simplified representation of the parietopontine pathway mediating ipsilateral slow tracking. Activation of the PPRF induces ipsilateral deviation of the eyes (see Fig. 7-6).*

right followed smoothly an object turning along with him [8]. However, when rotating to the left he had to make quick refixations to catch up with the target because the vestibuloocular reflex that in this situation tends to deviate the eyes to the right was not properly compensated for by foveal fixation and smooth pursuit. Inadequate suppression of the vestibuloocular reflex can be easily assessed by looking for quick refixations as the patient gazes at a finger in his outstretched arm while he is being rotated in a wheelchair [33].

Saccadic System. Most obvious among the eye movements are the quick refixations called saccades. Their purpose is to place in the fovea objects of interest, which often have first been registered by the peripheral retina. For instance, someone attending a lecture would tend to make a quick, saccadic eye movement to gaze on a person who just walked in through a side door. Any other sensory stimulus, particularly noise, can also elicit saccades. Saccadic eye movements are also used to inspect a complex scene such as a painting. A fairly complicated array of short refixations then takes place, as the diverse details of the painting are calibrated by placing them successively in the macular region. This task can be impaired by lesions of the frontal or parietal lobes. In addition to these types of saccades, a person may produce saccades at will or on command and can inhibit the tendency to glance at an object perceived by the peripheral retina. Other types of saccadic eye movements include the quick, corrective phase of vestibular and optokinetic nystagmus. On a command such as "look to your right," saccades are produced with greater ease if the head as well as the eyes are turned in the appropriate direction. Turning the eyes while keeping the head still is somewhat more difficult.

Alertness is required for the production of saccades. The slow phase of the vestibuloocular reflex can be elicited in a comatose patient by the doll's head maneuver or by caloric stimulation. The eyes are then slowly driven by the vestibular reflex, but there are no corrective jerks.

MECHANICAL PROPERTIES OF SACCADIC EYE MOVEMENTS. Saccades are produced by a combination of two mechanical elements: (1) a *pulse*, which, overcoming the resistance of the orbital tissues and the inertia of the globe, changes the position of the eye in the orbit, and (2) a *step* or change in tonic contraction of the orbital muscles, which, overcoming the elasticity of the orbital tissues, keeps the eye in the new position. A greater effort is required to keep the eye in a rather eccentric position.

A subject asked to switch his gaze from one object to another will produce saccades of larger amplitude when the objects are farther apart.

The amplitude of the saccade is expressed by the degrees of the angle it subtends. The velocity of a saccade is expressed in degrees per second. There is an invariate relation between the size and the peak velocity of saccades. Larger displacements in the orbit require faster saccades.

Saccades subtending a few degrees have velocities as low as 100 degrees per second, whereas large refixations may reach peak velocities of 600 degrees per second. Elderly subjects [27] and those who are drowsy, inattentive, or medicated produce slower saccadic eye movements. The predictability of the target, as in a test situation in which the subject looks alternately at either of two targets, increases velocity. Following the signal to switch gaze, there is a latency of about 200 msec before the saccade takes place.

Saccades are ballistic movements. They proceed according to their preprogrammed velocity. Once initiated, they cannot be stopped or modified in midflight. However, the brain can use information received as little as 70 msec before an upcoming saccade to modify it. In the production of saccades, the brain apparently makes use of a sensory map of the visual environment and of the coordinates of the orbit. The neural mechanisms involved in the production of saccades compare the ocular position desired with the actual position and calculate the pulse and step to be generated to reach the desired position. Disease of these neural mechanisms will result in saccades that have an abnormal velocity or erroneous amplitude (dysmetria) or fail to keep the eye steady in the desired position.

ANATOMY OF THE SACCADIC SYSTEM. Two parallel neural pathways control the production of saccades: a frontal system, concerned with voluntary gaze, and a collicular system, which redirects the gaze to novel stimuli appearing in the periphery of the visual fields.

FRONTAL SYSTEM. Neurons concerned with eye movements are located in the dorsal portion of the second frontal gyrus, in the so-called frontal eye field (FEF, area 8). The FEF receives projections from the peristriate, parietal, and superior temporal cortex, and from the pulvinar and dorsomedial thalamic nuclei. Stimulation of the frontal eye field causes a saccade to the contralateral side. From the second frontal gyrus the impulses proceed caudally in a pathway that runs in the anterior limb of the internal capsule and medial portion of the cerebral peduncle, decussates at the pontomesencephalic junction, and ends in the contralateral paramedian pontine reticular formation (PPRF) (Fig. 7-8).

The PPRF, located anterior and lateral to the MLF, extends from the pontomesencephalic junction to the abducens nucleus. Impulses from the frontal eye fields are relayed to the high pontine PPRF, which coordinates both vertical and horizontal saccades. Signals for horizontal saccades proceed to the ipsilateral PPRF in the lower pons, from which they finally reach the abducens nuclear complex. Abducens motor neurons and abducens interneurons that deliver the signal to the medial rectus area of the contralateral third nerve nucleus mediate a saccade to the same side of the pons but contralateral to the frontal eye field that originated the chain of command (Figs. 7-6 and 7-8).

Bilateral stimulation of homologous points of both frontal eye fields is required to produce vertical movements. The impulses reach the high pontine PPRF and through a para-MLF pathway are conveyed to the mesencephalic reticular formation. The rostral interstitial nucleus of the MLF, located in the prerubral field of the ventral diencephalomesencephalic junction, rostral to the tractus retroflexus and ventral to the nucleus of Darkschewitsch (Fig. 7-3), coordinates down-gaze [3]. Bilateral lesions here cause down-gaze palsy [13, 19, 30]. The right and left rostral interstitial nuclei are joined by a commissure. They project to the nucleus of Cajal (Fig. 7-3), at the diencephalomesencephalic junction, and to the ipsilateral oculomotor nucleus. Up-gaze is mediated by the rostral interstitial nucleus of the MLF and by the interstitial nucleus of Cajal, which projects to the contralateral third nerve nucleus through the posterior commissure in the pretectal area, just rostral to the superior colliculi. Bilateral lesions of the pretectal area, or unilateral lesions that affect the posterior commissure, cause paresis of upward gaze [1].

COLLICULAR SYSTEM. The superior colliculus has a sensory portion, located dorsally, and a motor portion, located ventrally or deep. Retinal fibers reach directly the sensory portion, where the contralateral hemifield is represented in detail. This part of the superior colliculus projects to the lateral geniculate body and to the pulvinar of the thalamus. By contrast, the motor portion receives its input from the pericalcarine primary visual cortex and projects to the subthalamic region and to the brainstem. This projection probably converges on the PPRF in a manner analogous to that described for the projection from the frontal eye fields. The superior colliculus tends to deviate the eyes to the contralateral side, particularly when a novel stimulus appears in the visual field. Partial lesions of the striate cortex, which impair vision severely, may nonetheless leave unaffected the ability to produce saccades to novel stimuli in a portion of the visual field that is blind ("blind sight"). This phenomenon is mediated by the superior colliculus, perhaps using extrastriatal pathways. Collicular lesions cause an increase in saccadic latency, mild hypometria (saccades that fall short of the target), and a paucity of saccades when scanning a scene, but not in darkness. There is also a paucity of saccades in response to stimuli appearing in the periphery of the visual field.

Combined lesions of the frontal eye field and the ipsilateral superior

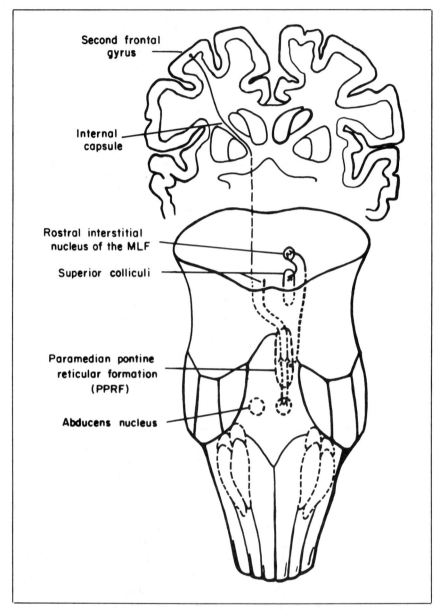

FIG. 7-8. *Saccadic system. Coronal section through the frontal lobe and dorsal view of the brainstem showing the frontopontine and colliculopontine pathways subserving horizontal saccadic eye movements. The rostral PPRF and the rostral interstitial nucleus of the MLF mediate vertical eye movements. Although only one side is represented, bilateral co-firing is needed for the production of vertical eye movements (see text).*

colliculus cause severe and permanent impairment of saccades to the contralateral side. Although purely frontal lesions spare smooth pursuit, combined lesions of this type severely impair smooth pursuit to the side of the lesion.

CEREBELLUM. The cerebellum also plays a role in the control of saccadic eye movements [6]. Lesions in the fastigial nucleus result in hypermetric saccades, whereas floccular lesions cause postsaccadic drift, or inability to maintain the globe in the newly acquired eccentric position after saccade. In addition, vermial cerebellar lesions impair an interesting adaptive capability of the saccadic system. Normally, if lateral rectus weakness develops in a subject, the involved eye makes abducting saccades that fall short (hypometric saccades). If the sound eye is then patched, the saccadic system is readjusted after as little as 3 days, so that the abducting saccades produced by the affected eye fall on target (are orthometric), whereas the adducting saccades of the other eye become hypermetric.

Other structures, such as the parietal lobe (mentioned above) also influence saccadic movements. Prolongation of latency and a paucity of saccades directed to the contralateral side have been attributed to a pulvinar lesion [34].

ABNORMAL SACCADES. Lesions in the structures that mediate the production of saccades may result in inappropriate saccades, poor initiation of saccades, inaccurate saccades (hypermetric or hypometric), and saccades that are too slow or too fast.

1. Inappropriate saccades, or *saccadic intrusions,* interfere with macular fixation of an object of interest. There are several types of inappropriate saccades: (1) *Square wave jerks* take the eyes off the target and are followed after about 200 msec by a corrective saccade. Small square wave jerks may appear normally in the young and the elderly, but when larger than 1 or 2 degrees they are pathologic, resulting from a variety of disorders including cerebral lesions, cerebellar system disease, progressive supranuclear palsy, Huntington's chorea, and schizophrenia. (2) *Macrosquare wave jerks* are similar to square wave jerks but are of larger amplitude (20–40 degrees). They have been noticed in multiple sclerosis and pontocerebellar atrophy. (3) *Ocular flutter* is a burst of to-and-fro horizontal saccades without an intersaccadic interval. (4) *Opsoclonus* is similar to ocular flutter, except that in opsoclonus the eyes move in all directions. The term *saccadomania* has been used to designate this chaotic succession of conjugate eye movements. Like ocular flutter, opsoclonus indicates brainstem or cerebellar disease.

These movements have been observed in patients with viral encephalitis, trauma, neuroblastoma, intracranial tumor, hydrocephalus, thalamic hemorrhage, or toxic encephalopathy induced by lithium, chlordecone, or thallium.

2. *Impaired initiation* of saccades, with abnormally increased latencies, can be the consequence of disease anywhere in the pathways mediating saccade production that were described above. Saccades toward the side contralateral to the lesion are delayed with frontal or collicular damage. Pontine lesions impair saccades to the side of the injury. In all these cases the saccades tend to be hypometric as well. A striking disorder of saccade initiation is *ocular apraxia*, characterized by an inability to look to either side on command, although random saccades and the quick phases of nystagmus are normal. This abnormality is part of the Balint syndrome (see Chapter 19). It can be congenital, but when acquired later in life it indicates bilateral hemispheric disease, often parietal. Impaired scanning of a complex picture, leading to bizarre interpretations of visual scenes, is also characteristic of these patients and of patients with bilateral frontal disease.

3. Inaccurate or *dysmetric saccades* usually point to brainstem or cerebellar disease [6]. Lesions of the superior vermis and fastigial nucleus cause hypermetria toward the side of the lesion. Also, patients with a hemispheric lesion resulting in a homonymous field defect may make hypermetric saccades toward the side of the field defect in order to visualize objects placed in that direction.

4. *Abnormal saccadic velocity* may have various causes. Saccades that appear to be too *fast* usually represent a normal-velocity saccade stopped in midflight. They are characteristically found in myasthenia gravis, when muscle fatigue prevents the saccade from evolving to completion. *Slow* saccades occur in the direction of a paretic extraocular muscle or in the adducting eye with an ipsilateral MLF lesion. In these cases the range of motion is limited (hypometric saccades). When the range of motion is full, slow saccades usually result from bilateral PPRF disease and have been described with olivopontocerebellar atrophy, Huntington's chorea, Wilson's disease, ataxia telangiectasia, progressive supranuclear palsy, and lipid storage disorders. Drowsy, inattentive, or sedated patients may also have slow saccades.

Convergence System. Convergence and divergence movements of the eyes bring about binocular vision. Like convergence, divergence is not a purely passive process but requires active contraction of eye muscles. Both eye movements aim at placing a point of the visual field in homologous points of both retinas, most often the maculas. Disparity between the location of an image in both retinas results in diplopia. Near objects elicit convergence, whereas distant ones elicit divergence of the axes of both eyes. Vergence movements are accompanied by accommodation of the lens to prevent the blur that results from a poorly focused image. An object approaching the subject in the sagittal plane induces the "near-triad," composed by convergence, rounding of the lens (accommodation), and constriction of the pupil (miosis). Vergence movements are much slower than saccades or pursuit, proceeding over a period as long as 1 second.

The neuronal groups or pathways involved in convergence remain poorly understood. Stimulation of areas 19 or 22 of the occipital cortex may induce some of the elements of the near-triad. Vergence movements involve fine coordination between the abducens and the oculomotor nuclei, but for vergence the link between these nuclei probably courses outside the MLF, because MLF lesions respect convergence. A group of oculomotor internuclear neurons located dorsal to the caudal portion of the oculomotor complex projects to both abducens nuclei and may play a role in convergence.

Vergence movements can be produced voluntarily in the absence of the appropriate visual stimulus (disparity of images in the retina). On the other hand, both hemispheres must perceive the retinal disparity for the visual stimulus to elicit convergence. A patient with a split corpus callosum was able to converge to near stimuli on both sides of the sagittal plane but not to those in the midsagittal plane. To explain this case, it can be postulated that stimuli in the midsagittal plane are projected on the temporal retina of both eyes, therefore reaching each hemisphere separately.

During convergence, the pupillary sphincter constricts the pupil, as parasympathetic impulses from the Edinger-Westphal nucleus reach the pupil by way of the third nerve and ciliary ganglion. Lesions affecting the midbrain, third nerve, or ciliary ganglion may cause paresis of the iris sphincter. In these cases the light reflex tends to be involved earlier and to a greater extent than convergence (light-near dissociation) because the contingent of pupillomotor fibers mediating convergence outnumbers the ones mediating the light reflex [16]. Adie's tonic pupil exemplifies this differential innervation. Damage to the ciliary ganglion and ulterior reinnervation of the iris results in a large pupil that is unresponsive or poorly responsive to light but tonically responsive to accommodation. Contraction and, particularly, relaxation are slow. Another example of pupillary abnormality showing light-near dissociation is the Argyll-Robertson pupil, which is characteristic of tertiary syphilis but now results more often from diabetes (diabetic pseudo-tabes). Argyll-

Robertson pupils are small and irregular and, unlike Adie's pupil, fail to constrict when 0.1% pilocarpine is instilled in the eye. Atropine causes dilation. The site of the lesion responsible for Argyll-Robertson pupils is unclear. It has often been localized to the periaqueductal gray and posterior commissure areas.

As mentioned below, vertical gaze abnormalities with midbrain lesions are often accompanied by abnormalities of vergence movements. Most often convergence is lost, but convergence-retraction nystagmus may be seen on attempted up-gaze.

Gaze Palsies. An understanding of the different systems that coordinate eye movements clarifies why lesions at different levels of the brain spare some systems while affecting others. The resulting pattern of eye movements is helpful for lesion localization. Alternative pathways account for different severity of the deficit related to a single lesion or to several lesions. For instance, a unilateral lesion in the frontal eye field (area 8) causes only a transient gaze palsy, but simultaneous involvement of the ipsilateral superior colliculus causes severe impairment of contralateral saccadic eye movements.

CONJUGATE GAZE PALSIES. A conjugate gaze palsy is one in which both eyes are symmetrically restricted in their excursion to one side, up, or down.

HORIZONTAL GAZE PALSY. Unilateral restriction of voluntary gaze to one side is usually due to contralateral frontal or ipsilateral pontine damage.

Frontal Lesions. Frontal lesions causing a gaze palsy tend to be rather acute, and the resulting palsy is transient. In the acute phase, the patient generally has a hemiparesis, which involves predominantly the arm, and "looks toward the lesion," away from the hemiparesis. If the process, most often due to brain infarction, evolves favorably, the gaze palsy resolves in a few days, although impaired initiation and hypometria of voluntary saccades may remain chronically. There may be a tendency for the eyes to become deviated toward the side of the hemiparesis (spastic gaze). This tendency can be elicited by asking the patient to close his eyes while the eyelids are kept forcibly open. Epileptogenic lesions in the frontal eye fields may cause transient deviation of the eyes and head to the contralateral side (the patient then "looks" away from the lesion). However, in most cases, as soon as the focal seizure ceases, the patient tends to look to the involved side. Hemorrhages deep in a cerebral hemisphere, particularly those involving the thalamus, can also cause eye deviation to the side of the hemiparesis, opposite the lesion ("wrong way eyes") [9, 17].

As regards optokinetic nystagmus elicited with a tape, the quick component toward the side contralateral to the lesion is impaired, but smooth pursuit is preserved if the lesion spares the parietal lobe.

Pontine Lesions. In a frontal gaze palsy, the eyes can be brought toward the paretic side by using the oculovestibular reflex (doll's eye maneuver). By contrast, in pontine lesions the eyes look toward the hemiparesis (although hemiparesis is an inconstant finding) and cannot be brought to the paretic side using the doll's eye maneuver or ipsilateral cold caloric stimulation. Smooth pursuit is also absent outside the limited range of motion.

VERTICAL GAZE PALSY. Bilateral lesions or involvement of commissural structures are required to impair vertical gaze. Large lesions in the upper pontine tegmentum cause paresis of both horizontal and vertical gaze, largely because of affection of the oculomotor and trochlear nuclei, thereby causing also weakness of the medial recti. As a rule, these patients are in coma (see Chap. 21).

Upgaze Palsy. This condition results from lesions in the pretectal region, usually with damage to the posterior commissure [1, 20]. Lesions of the dorsal midbrain not only cause impairment of all upward eye movements (although the vestibuloocular reflex and Bell's phenomenon may sometimes be spared) but other ocular findings as well. This constellation of findings has been variously designated as the Parinaud syndrome, Sylvian aqueduct syndrome, pretectal syndrome, dorsal midbrain syndrome, and Koerber-Salus-Elschnig syndrome. The upper eyelid may be retracted, baring the sclera above the cornea (Collier's "tucked lid" sign). Bilateral ptosis may result when the lesion extends ventrally. The pupils are large and react poorly to light, but accommodation is often spared (light-near dissociation). Down-gaze saccades, although present, tend to be restricted, more so than pursuit. Downward vestibuloocular movements are spared. A sign of dorsal midbrain compression in hydrocephalic infants is a tonic downward deviation of the eyes while the retracted eyelids expose the epicorneal sclera ("setting sun" sign). Convergence and divergence are often impaired. In some patients, convergence spasm may result in slow or restricted abduction ("midbrain pseudosixth") [4]. Attempted up-gaze may result in convergence-retraction nystagmus, with quick adducting-retraction jerks. This phenomenon can be elicited at the bedside by having the patient watch a downward-moving optokinetic drum. In this case, the normal upward corrective saccades are replaced by convergence-retractory nystagmus, which is made up not by convergence movements but by opposed adducting saccades, at least in some cases [22]. As mentioned above, true convergence is often absent. The retraction of the eye into the orbit results from irregular cofiring from several extraocular muscles. Tumors are most often responsible for damage of the dorsal midbrain. Hydrocephalus is another common etiologic agent. Less likely causes include cerebral hemorrhage or infarction, multiple sclerosis, trauma, lipid storage diseases, Wilson's disease, Whipple's disease, syphilis, and tuberculosis. Upward gaze is often limited in Parkinson's disease.

Down-gaze Palsy. Selective down-gaze palsy has been reported after bilateral lesions in the junction between the midbrain and the diencephalon, involving the area that lies ventral to the Sylvian aqueduct and dorsomedial to the red nucleus [30]. Damage to the rostral interstitial nucleus of the middle longitudinal fasciculus and its projections to the third nerve nuclear group is probably critical. Unlike the situation with dorsal midbrain lesions, infarcts in the territory of the paramedian thalamomesencephalic artery, a proximal branch of the posterior cerebral artery (see Table 17-2 and Fig. 17-21), represent the most common cause. Down-gaze is involved early in progressive supranuclear palsy.

DISCONJUGATE GAZE PALSIES

HORIZONTAL GAZE

The Medial Longitudinal Fasciculus Syndrome or Internuclear Ophthalmoplegia (INO). Clinically, this syndrome is characterized by adduction weakness on the side of the MLF lesion and nystagmus of the abducting eye. However, unless the lesion is quite high, reaching the midbrain, convergence is preserved. Adduction weakness results from disruption of the signals carried by the MLF — signals coming from the internuclear abducens nucleus and destined for the oculomotor nucleus. The pathogenesis of nystagmus in the abducting eye is unclear. It may represent the effects of adaptation to the contralateral medial rectus weakness. Bilateral INO is most often seen with multiple sclerosis. Unilateral INO may result from infarction. Other causes include Wernicke's encephalopathy, trauma, and encephalitis. The pattern of extraocular muscle weakness with myasthenia gravis and postinfectious neuritis can mimic INO.

The "One and a Half" Syndrome. In these cases (combined unilateral horizontal gaze palsy and internuclear ophthalmoplegia) [9, 23, 32] there is a conjugate gaze palsy to one side ("one") and impaired adduction on looking to the other side ("one and a half"). As a result, the only horizontal movement remaining is abduction of one eye, which exhibits nystagmus in abduction. Vertical movements and convergence are spared. The responsible lesion involves the PPRF and the adjacent MLF on the side of the complete gaze palsy. In some cases, deviation of the eyes toward this side can be accomplished with the vestibuloocular reflex, implying the presence of a lesion in the higher pons that spares the abducens nucleus.

A somewhat similar syndrome may result from two separate lesions involving both MLFs and the roots of the abducens nerve on the side of the unilateral horizontal "gaze" palsy. However, in this case, if the "gaze" palsy is incomplete, the eyes would move disconjugately in the direction of the gaze palsy [23]. A true gaze palsy due to unilateral PPRF damage causes concomitant paresis of both eyes. The one and a half syndrome is most often caused by multiple sclerosis [32], infarcts, hemorrhages, and tumors.

VERTICAL GAZE

Skew Deviation. Although vertical misalignment of the eyes may be caused by lesions of the ocular motor nerves or muscles (e.g., with myasthenia gravis), the term *skew deviation* is reserved for cases resulting from supranuclear derangements. Skew deviation can accompany lesions at different areas of the brainstem. Peripheral vestibular disease can cause contralateral hypertropia, in which the contralateral eye is higher than the ipsilateral eye [14]. Lateral pontomedullary lesions affecting the vestibular nuclei may result in skew deviation with the lower eye on the side of the lesion. By contrast, the eye on the side of a unilateral MLF lesion tends to be higher.

Lesions in the neighborhood of the posterior commissure occasionally are manifest with a skew deviation, in which the ipsilateral eye is higher or there is slowly alternating skew deviation in irregular periods lasting from 10 to 60 seconds [7]. In patients with downbeat nystagmus (see below), the skew deviation may change with the direction of horizontal gaze.

NYSTAGMUS

The to-and-fro ocular movement that takes place as an individual watches the tree line when driving alongside a forest was described above as optokinetic nystagmus. This type of *jerk nystagmus*, with a slow drift and a quick corrective component, is more common than *pendular nystagmus*, in which the eyes move with the same speed in both directions.

Fine nystagmus that may not be noticed by simple inspection of the eyes may be detected on fundoscopic examination. It is important to take into account that the direction in which the retinal vessels can be seen to oscillate is opposite the direction in which the globe oscillates. Changes in the amplitude of nystagmus when the patient fixates on an object serve to separate some varieties of nystagmus. Thus nystagmus should be observed during fixation and after removing fixation by having the patient wear Frenzel lenses or by recording eye movements in the dark. A simple maneuver is to observe the rate and amplitude of the nystagmus on fundoscopic examination with a hand-held ophthalmoscope while the patient fixates with the other eye. Then, as the lights of the examining room are turned off, thereby removing fixation, any changes in nystagmus are noticed.

Nystagmus induced by optokinetic or vestibular stimuli is physiologic. Nystagmus in extreme lateral or vertical gaze (end-point nystagmus) can also be found in normal persons. It tends to wane easily and belongs to the variety described below as "gaze-evoked" nystagmus. The next paragraphs will deal primarily with the localizing value of the pathologic varieties of nystagmus.

Jerk Nystagmus. Nystagmus is generally named according to the direction of the fast, corrective component. Thus, horizontal nystagmus to the left implies that there is a tendency for the eyes to slowly drift to the right, corrected by quick saccades to the left that bring the eyes back to where the patient wishes to look. Actually, it is analysis of the slow component that proves most helpful for the anatomic diagnosis of nystagmus. The slow component may have a uniform velocity or may reduce or gain speed as the eyes move in the direction of the slow component. Although the velocity characteristics of nystagmus cannot be appreciated with the naked eye, the easy availability of electrooculography makes it advisable to follow this classification.

CONSTANT VELOCITY NYSTAGMUS. This type of nystagmus may appear with disease of the peripheral or central vestibular system, with cerebellar disease involving the flocculus, and with cerebral hemisphere disease.

VESTIBULAR NYSTAGMUS. Both central and peripheral vestibular lesions induce a tendency for the eyes to drift in a direction parallel to the plane in which the diseased canal lies.

Horizontal nystagmus with the slow component toward the lesion results from unilateral horizontal canal or total labyrinthine destruction. In the latter case there is a torsional component causing the upper part of the globe to rotate toward the lesioned side. Although constant for a particular position of gaze, the slow-phase velocity is greater when the eyes are turned in the direction of the quick component (Alexander's law). Hence, depending on the intensity of a unidirectional nystagmus, it may be graded from 1 to 3. First-degree nystagmus is present only when gazing in the direction of the quick component. If it is present also in midposition, it is considered to be second-degree nystagmus, whereas third-degree nystagmus appears in all directions of gaze. Because both peripheral and central vestibular nystagmus may vary with head position and movement, it is useful to perform postural testing as outlined earlier. Two main differences identify peripheral and central vestibular nystagmus. Fixation suppresses peripheral but not central nystagmus. Also, peripheral nystagmus particularly when vertical has usually a torsional component. Pure vertical or torsional nystagmus is central.

Vertical nystagmus may be particularly helpful for the diagnosis. *Downbeat nystagmus* tends to be greatest when the patient looks down and to one side. It often accompanies posterior fossa lesions near the craniocervical junction, such as Arnold-Chiari malformation, tumors, and multiple sclerosis. Deficient drive by the posterior semicircular canals, whose central projections cross in the floor of the fourth ventricle, has been postulated as an explanation for this type of nystagmus. However, bilateral floccular and uvonodular lesions also cause downbeat nystagmus. By contrast, damage to the central projections of the anterior semicircular canals, which tend to deviate the eyes superiorly, has been suggested to explain *upbeat nystagmus*. The central projections of the anterior semicircular canals run in the brachium conjunctivum. Anterior vermial cerebellar lesions often cause upbeat nystagmus, but it has been reported also with involvement of the perihypoglossal and inferior olivary nuclei of the medulla and with processes that affect the brainstem diffusely. Wernicke's encephalopathy, drug intoxication, and meningitis may also cause upbeat nystagmus.

PURSUIT-IMBALANCE NYSTAGMUS. Parietal lobe lesions may cause the eyes to drift slowly toward the intact side when the person is watching a moving target. Correcting saccades need then be made toward the side of the lesion. Floccular cerebellar lesions may cause a similar deficit.

EXPONENTIALLY CHANGING VELOCITY NYSTAGMUS

GAZE-EVOKED NYSTAGMUS. In this disorder, the eyes fail to remain in an eccentric position of gaze but drift to midposition. The velocity of the slow component decreases as the eyes approach midposition. Cerebellar lesions may result in this type of nystagmus, which is more pronounced when the patient looks toward the lesion. Cerebellopontine angle tumors may cause Bruns's nystagmus, a combination of ipsilateral large-amplitude, low-frequency nystagmus that is due to impaired gaze holding, and contralateral small-amplitude, high-frequency nystagmus that is due to vestibular impairment. Horizontal gaze-evoked nystagmus has greater amplitude in the abducting eye when there is an MLF lesion. Asymmetrical gaze-evoked nystagmus may also be due to muscle disease (myasthenia gravis). *Rebound nystagmus* is seen in some patients with cerebellar disease. After keeping the eyes eccentric for some time, the original gaze-evoked nystagmus may wane and actually reverse direction, so that the slow component is directed centrifugally and it becomes obvious if the eyes are returned to midposition.

CONGENITAL NYSTAGMUS. Congenital nystagmus is a benign finding, which results from an arrested process occurring early in life. It is seldom familial and most often idiopathic. Metabolic derangements and structural anomalies of the brain, including abnormalities of the eye or the anterior visual pathways, have been occasionally responsible. More important, when it is found later in life it must be distinguished from other forms of nystagmus that have a potentially treatable cause. Unlike gaze-evoked nystagmus, congenital nystagmus has a slow phase with a velocity that increases exponentially as the eyes move in the direction of the slow phase. Often, congenital nystagmus is wholly pendular or has both pendular and jerk components. Although irregular, it is generally conjugate and horizontal even on up-gaze or down-gaze; visual fixation accentuates it and active eyelid closure or convergence attenuates it. The nystagmus decreases in an eye position ("null region") that is specific for each patient. Despite the constant eye motion, these patients do not experience oscillopsia. When they are tested with a hand-held optokinetic tape or drum, the quick phase of the elicited nystagmus generally follows the direction of the tape (reversed optokinetic nystagmus) [15].

LATENT NYSTAGMUS. Latent nystagmus is common and generally congenital. It appears when one eye is covered. The eyes then develop conjugate nystagmus, the viewing eye having a slow phase directed toward the nose.

Pendular Nystagmus. Pendular nystagmus is often congenital (see preceding section). Acquired pendular nystagmus may be either wholly horizontal or wholly vertical, or have both components. It may be disconjugate, have a circular or elliptical trajectory, and be accompanied by oscillopsia and palatal myoclonus. Damage to the dentatorubroolivary pathways (Guillain-Mollaret triangle) may be responsible for some cases of acquired pendular nystagmus, which is most often encountered in patients with multiple sclerosis or brainstem infarction. It may also appear with blindness or monocular loss of vision, in which case it may be monocular. Blind patients may have *windmill nystagmus*, in which there are repeated oscillations in the vertical plane alternating with repeated oscillations in the horizontal plane.

See-Saw Nystagmus. See-saw nystagmus refers to a cyclic movement of the eyes: while one rises and intorts, the other falls and extorts; the vertical and torsional movements are then reversed, completing the cycle. Responsible lesions are generally in the inferior portion of the third ventricle (parasellar tumors) or midbrain (infarction). The interstitial nucleus of Cajal may play a role in the production of this type of nystagmus.

Periodic Alternating Nystagmus. Periodic alternating nystagmus can be congenital, but it is often acquired and has a localizing value similar to that of downbeat nystagmus, pointing to possible disease at the craniocervical junction. The eyes exhibit primary position nystagmus, which, after 60 to 90 seconds, stops for a few seconds and then starts beating in the opposite direction. A few beats of downbeat nystagmus may appear in the interval between alternating sidebeat nystagmus. This type of nystagmus has been described with tumors, trauma, encephalitis, multiple sclerosis, and vascular disease.

Convergence-Retraction Nystagmus. Convergence-retraction nystagmus was included with the discussion of vertical gaze palsy because these two entities are often associated. In this disorder of ocular motility, repetitive adducting saccades, which are often accompanied by retraction of the eyes into the orbit, occur spontaneously or on attempted up-gaze. Sliding an optokinetic tape downward in front of the patient's eyes may also elicit convergence-retraction nystagmus. Mesencephalic lesions affecting the pretectal region are most likely to cause this type of nystagmus.

Lid Nystagmus. Lid nystagmus refers to eyelid twitches that are synchronous with the fast phase of horizontal nystagmus. It has been ascribed to lateral medullary disease.

In this chapter we have discussed the clinical findings resulting from disease in the ocular motor systems and the likely anatomic localization of the responsible lesions. For an account of the eye findings that result from localized damage of the different areas of the brainstem, see Chapters 14 and 21.

REFERENCES

1. Auerbach, S. H., De Piero, T. J., and Romanul, F. Sylvian aqueduct syndrome caused by unilateral midbrain lesion. *Ann. Neurol.* 11:91, 1982.
2. Baloh, R. W., Yee, R. D., and Honrubia, V. Optokinetic nystagmus and parietal lobe lesions. *Ann. Neurol.* 7:269, 1980.
3. Bender, M. B. Brain control of conjugate horizontal and vertical eye movements. *Brain* 103:23, 1980.
4. Caplan, L. R. "Top of the basilar" syndrome. *Neurology* 30:72, 1980.

5. Chiaramonte, J. S. Cycloplegia from transdermal scopolamine. *N. Engl. J. Med.* 306:174, 1982.

6. Cogan, D. G., Chu, F. C., and Reingold, D. B. Ocular signs of cerebellar disease. *Arch. Ophthalmol.* 100:755, 1982.

7. Corbett, J. J., et al. Slowly alternating skew deviation: Description of a pretectal syndrome in three patients. *Ann. Neurol.* 10:540, 1981.

8. Estanol, B., et al. Oculomotor and oculovestibular functions in a hemispherectomy patient. *Arch. Neurol.* 37:365, 1980.

9. Fisher, C. M. Some neuro-ophthalmological observations. *J. Neurol. Neurosurg. Psychiat.* 30:383, 1967.

9a. Glaser, J. S. *Neuro-ophthalmology.* Hagerstown, Md.: Harper & Row, 1978.

10. Greenberg, H. S., et al. Metastasis to the base of the skull: Clinical findings in 43 patients. *Neurology* 31:530, 1981.

11. Grimson, B. S., and Thompson, H. S. Reader's syndrome. A clinical review. *Surv. Ophthalmol.* 24:199, 1980.

12. Growdon, J. H., Winkler, G. F., and Wray, S. H. Midbrain ptosis. A case with clinicopathologic correlation. *Arch. Neurol.* 30:179, 1974.

13. Halmagyi, G. M., Evans, W. A., and Hallinan, J. M. Failure of downward gaze. The site and nature of the lesion. *Arch. Neurol.* 35:22, 1978.

14. Halmagyi, G. M., Gresty, M. A., and Gibson, W. P. R. Ocular tilt reaction with peripheral vestibular lesion. *Ann. Neurol.* 6:80, 1979.

15. Halmagyi, G. M., Gresty, M. A., and Leech, J. Reversed optokinetic nystagmus (OKN): Mechanism and clinical significance. *Ann. Neurol.* 7:429, 1980.

16. Harriman, D. G. F., and Garland, H. The pathology of Adie's syndrome. *Brain* 91:401, 1968.

17. Keane, J. R. Contralateral gaze deviation with supratentorial hemorrhage. *Arch. Neurol.* 32:119, 1975.

18. Keane, J. R. Bilateral sixth nerve palsy. Analysis of 125 cases. *Arch. Neurol.* 33:681, 1976.

18a. Kissel, J. T., et al. Pupil-sparing oculomotor palsies with internal carotid-posterior communicating artery aneurysms. *Ann. Neurol.* 13:149, 1983.

19. Jacobs, L., Anderson, P. J., and Bender, M. B. The lesions producing paralysis of downward but not upward gaze. *Arch. Neurol.* 28:319, 1973.

20. Leigh, R. J., and Zee, D. S. *The Neurology of Eye Movements.* Philadelphia: F. A. Davis, 1983.

21. Masdeu, J., et al. Pseudo-abducens palsy with midbrain lesions. *Trans. Am. Neurol. Assoc.* 105:184, 1981.

21a. Nadeau, S. E., and Trobe, J. D. Pupil-sparing in oculomotor palsy: A brief review. *Ann. Neurol.* 13:143, 1983.

22. Ochs, A. L., et al. Opposed adducting saccades in convergence-retraction nystagmus. *Brain* 102:497, 1979.

23. Pierrot-Deseilligny, C., et al. The "one-and-a-half" syndrome. Electro-oculographic analyses of five cases with deductions about the physiological mechanisms of lateral gaze. *Brain* 104:665, 1981.

24. Selhorst, J. B., et al. Midbrain corectopia. *Arch. Neurol.* 33:193, 1976.

25. Sharpe, J. A., Lo, A. W., and Rabinovitch, H. E. Control of the saccadic and smooth pursuit systems after cerebral hemidecortication. *Brain* 102:387, 1979.

26. Spector, R. H., and Troost, B. T. The ocular motor system. *Ann. Neurol.* 9:517, 1981.

27. Spooner, J. W., Sakala, S. M., and Baloh, R. W. Effect of aging on eye track-
    ing. *Arch. Neurol.* 37:575, 1980.
28. Thompson, B. M., et al. Pseudo-Horner's syndrome. *Arch. Neurol.* 39:108,
    1982.
29. Thompson, H. S., and Pilley, S. F. J. Unequal pupils: A flow chart for sort-
    ing out the anisocorias. *Surv. Ophthalmol.* 21:45, 1976.
30. Trojanowski, J. Q., and Lafontaine, M. H. Neuroanatomical correlates of
    selective downgaze paralysis. *J. Neurol. Sci.* 52:91, 1981.
31. Troost, B. T., and Troost, E. G. Functional paralysis of horizontal gaze. *Neu-
    rology* 29:82, 1979.
32. Wall, M., and Wray, S. H. The one-and-a-half syndrome. A unilateral dis-
    order of the pontine tegmentum: A study of 20 cases and review of the
    literature. *Neurology* (Cleveland) 33:971, 1983.
33. Zee, D. S. Suppression of vestibular nystagmus. *Ann. Neurol.* 1:207, 1977.
34. Zihl, J., and Cramon, D. V. The contribution of the second visual system to
    directed visual attention in man. *Brain* 102:835, 1979.

Chapter 8

THE LOCALIZATION OF LESIONS AFFECTING CRANIAL NERVE V (THE TRIGEMINAL NERVE)

Paul W. Brazis

ANATOMY OF CRANIAL NERVE V
(TRIGEMINAL NERVE)

The trigeminal nerve is a mixed nerve that provides sensory innervation to the face and mucous membranes of the oral and nasal cavities and motor innervation to the muscles of mastication [2, 6].

Motor Portion. The motor nucleus of the trigeminal nerve is situated in the middle of the pons, medial to the main sensory nucleus of the trigeminal nerve, near the floor of the fourth ventricle. It receives its supranuclear control by corticobulbar fibers originating in the lower third of the precentral gyrus. These bilateral connections travel through the corona radiata, internal capsule, and cerebral peduncle and decussate in the pons before supplying the motor nuclei.

The *motor root*, or *portio minor*, exits from the motor nucleus, passes through the substance of the pons, and emerges from the anterolateral aspect of the pons anterior and medial to the larger *sensory root* (the *portio major*). The motor root then passes forward in the posterior fossa and pierces the dura mater beneath the attachment of the tentorium to the tip of the petrous portion of the temporal bone. It then enters a cavity in the dura mater overlying the apex of the petrous bone *(Meckel's cave)*, travels beneath the *trigeminal (gasserian) ganglia,* and leaves the skull via the *foramen ovale.* After leaving the skull, the motor root joins the *mandibular (third) division* of the trigeminal nerve to form the *mandibular nerve,* which supplies the masticatory muscles: the masseter, temporalis, and medial and lateral pterygoid muscles. In addition, motor fibers are given off to the tensor tympani, tensor veli palatini, and mylohyoid muscles, and to the anterior belly of the digastric muscle.

Sensory Portion. The pseudounipolar perikarya of the sensory portions of the trigeminal nerve is in the *semilunar or gasserian ganglion,* which is situated near the apex of the petrous bone in the middle cranial fossa. From this ganglion, the fibers of the sensory root (portio major) enter the substance of the pons, course dorsomedially, and terminate in three major nuclear complexes within the brainstem: *the nucleus of the spinal tract of the trigeminal nerve, the main (or principal) sensory nucleus, and the mesencephalic nucleus.*

On entering the pons, many of the sensory fibers descend as a bundle, *the spinal tract of the trigeminal nucleus,* to the caudal end of the medulla and into the spinal cord (as far as the third or fourth cervical level), where the bundle fuses with Lissauer's tract. As the spinal tract descends, it gives off fibers to the medially located *nucleus of the spinal tract of the trigeminal nerve,* which also descends into the upper cervical cord. This nucleus may be divided into three sections: the nucleus oralis, interpolaris, and caudalis. The fibers of the ophthalmic division of the trigeminal nerve travel in the most ventral part of the spinal tract and extend most caudally (i.e., terminate in the trigeminal nucleus in series with the second cervical sensory level). The fibers of the mandibular division of the trigeminal nerve travel in the most dorsal part of the spinal tract and terminate in the most rostral level of the spinal nucleus of the trigeminal nerve. In another possible sensory somatotopic spinal nucleus representation, the midline facial areas (nose and mouth) are represented rostrally in the spinal nucleus while the more lateral facial sensation fibers terminate in more caudal spinal nucleus regions. This pattern of termination may account for the "onion-skin" pattern of facial sensory loss and the perioral numbness that occurs with more rostral spinal nucleus and tract lesions.

The spinal nucleus of the trigeminal nerve receives fibers that convey the sensations of pain, temperature, and soft touch from the face and mucous membranes. From the spinal nucleus, ascending fibers travel mainly ipsilaterally in the trigeminothalamic tract to terminate in the ventral posteromedial (VPM) and intralaminar nuclei of the thalamus.

Other fibers from the portio major enter the pons and ascend and enter the *main sensory nucleus of the trigeminal nerve*. This nucleus is located in the lateral pons, posterolateral to the motor nucleus of the trigeminal nerve. Fibers entering this nucleus are concerned with tactile and proprioceptive sensation. The main sensory nucleus gives off ascending fibers that terminate in the thalamus. These fibers travel in the *ventral crossed trigeminothalamic (quintothalamic) tract* or *trigeminal lemniscus*, which ascends with the medial lemiscus, and in the *uncrossed dorsal trigeminothalamic tract*. Both of these fiber tracts terminate predominantly in the VPM nucleus of the thalamus.

The third sensory trigeminal nucleus, the *mesencephalic nucleus*, extends cephalad from the main sensory nucleus to the superior colliculus of the mesencephalon. This nucleus receives proprioceptive impulses from the masticatory muscles and from muscles supplied by other motor cranial nerves.

The sensory root (portio major) of the trigeminal nerve leaves the pons in association with the motor root (portio minor) and expands in Meckel's cave to form the trigeminal (gasserian) ganglion. This ganglion lies near the cavernous sinus and internal carotid artery and gives rise to three nerve trunks: the *ophthalmic, maxillary, and mandibular divisions of the trigeminal nerve.*

OPHTHALMIC DIVISION. This division lies in the lateral wall of the *cavernous sinus* in close association with the third (oculomotor), fourth (trochlear), and sixth (abducens) cranial nerves. With these three nerves, the ophthalmic division enters the orbit through the *superior orbital fissure*. Before leaving the cavernous sinus, this division divides into tentorial, lacrimal, frontal, and nasociliary branches.

The ophthalmic division supplies the skin of the nose, the upper eyelid, the forehead and scalp (as far back as the lambdoidal suture in the midline and for 8 cm lateral to the midline), the upper half of the cornea, conjunctiva, and iris, the mucous membranes of the frontal, sphenoidal, and ethmoidal sinuses and the upper nasal cavity and septum, the lacrimal canals, and the dura mater of the anterior cranial fossa, falx cerebri, and tentorium cerebelli.

MAXILLARY DIVISION. This division passes through the inferolateral portion of the *cavernous sinus* and then leaves the skull through the foramen rotundum to enter the *sphenopalatine fossa*. Next, it enters the orbit through the inferior orbital fissure (as the *infraorbital nerve*) and, after traveling through the infraorbital canal, reaches the face by way of the *infraorbital foramen*.

The maxillary division supplies the skin of the lateral nose, upper lip, and cheek, the lower half of the cornea, conjunctiva, and iris, the mucous membranes of the maxillary sinus, lower nasal cavity, hard and soft palates, and upper gum, the teeth of the upper jaw, and the dura mater of the middle cranial fossa (through the middle or recurrent meningeal nerve).

MANDIBULAR DIVISION. The mandibular division joins the motor root of the trigeminal nerve to form the *mandibular nerve*. This nerve leaves the skull through the *foramen ovale* and travels in the infratemporal fossa, dividing finally into several terminal branches.

In addition to the muscles listed previously (see above, Motor Portion), the mandibular nerve supplies the skin of the lower lip, lower jaw, chin, tympanic membrane, auditory meatus, and upper ear, the mucous membranes of the floor of the mouth, the lower gums, and the anterior two-thirds of the tongue (*not* taste sensation, which is carried by the facial nerve), the teeth of the lower jaw, and the dura mater of the posterior cranial fossa.

CLINICAL EVALUATION OF
CRANIAL NERVE V FUNCTION

Sensory Evaluation. Exteroceptive sensation (pain, light touch, heat, and cold) is tested on the face and mucous membranes. Each of the three trigeminal divisions is tested individually and compared with the opposite side. Lesions of individual divisions (distal to the gasserian ganglion) result in sensory loss confined to the cutaneous supply of that division with relatively little overlap into the cutaneous area of another division. Lesions at or proximal to the gasserian ganglion result in sensory loss that affects the whole ipsilateral face. Lesions within the brainstem or upper cervical cord may result in an onionskin distribution of sensory loss (see later discussion), whereas dissociation of sensation on the face (pain and temperature vs. touch sensation) differentiates lesions affecting the spinal tract and nucleus of the trigeminal nerve from lesions affecting the main sensory nucleus.

The cutaneous area over the angle of the mandible is supplied by the second and third cervical roots (by way of the great auricular nerve) and not by the trigeminal nerve. Therefore, a hemifacial sensory loss that spares the angle of the jaw is probably organic, whereas one that includes this area may be of hysterical origin or related to an intramedullary lesion.

Motor Evaluation. The trigeminal nerve supplies the muscles of mastication. These are tested by having the patient clench his jaw (masseters and temporalis) move his jaw from side to side against resistance (lateral pterygoids), and protrude the jaw. With nuclear or infranuclear lesions of the motor division of the trigeminal nerve, the temporalis and masseter muscles on the side of the lesion do not contract when the jaw is clenched, the jaw deviates to the paralyzed side when the mouth is opened (due to contraction of the contralateral intact lateral pterygoid muscle), and the jaw cannot be deviated toward the nonparalyzed side (due to ipsilateral lateral pterygoid paresis). Atrophy and fasciculation of the masticatory muscles may also be evident.

Other muscles supplied by the trigeminal nerve (mylohyoid, anterior belly of the digastric, tensor tympani, tensor veli palatini) are difficult to evaluate clinically. However, flaccidity of the floor of the mouth may be evident on palpation due to mylohyoid and digastric paralysis, and paralysis of the tensor tympani may result in difficulty in hearing high notes.

Reflex Evaluation. The important reflexes conveyed by the trigeminal nerve include the corneal reflex and the jaw jerk (masseter reflex). The afferent arc of the *corneal reflex* travels through the ophthalmic (upper cornea) and maxillary (lower cornea) divisions of the trigeminal nerve. The efferent arc moves through the ipsilateral (direct reflex) and contralateral (consensual reflex) facial nerve to the orbicularis oculi muscles. Lesions of the trigeminal nerve result in loss of the ipsilateral and contralateral responses. These lesions may involve the peripheral or ponto-medullary trigeminal pathways; however, a suprasegmental modulation of this reflex also exists, because a parietal lobe lesion may result in a contralateral loss of the corneal reflex. The *jaw jerk* or *masseter reflex* involves contraction of the masseter and temporalis muscles when the patient's lower jaw is tapped. The afferent arc is through the 1a motor fibers in the mandibular division of the trigeminal nerve that run to the mesencephalic nucleus of the trigeminal nerve. The efferent arc also moves through mandibular fibers that originate in the motor nucleus of the trigeminal nerve. Lesions anywhere along this reflex arc result in depression of the ipsilateral jaw reflex, whereas bilateral supranuclear lesions result in an accentuated response. The masseter reflex may be investigated electrophysiologically (latency, approximately 8.4 msec) by using a reflex hammer to trigger a recording device and recording the response in the masseter muscles.

Another reflex mediated partly by trigeminal pathways is the *blink reflex* (glabellar reflex, orbicularis oculi reflex) [9, 13, 20, 21]. Percussion over the supraorbital ridge results in bilateral contraction of the orbicularis oculi muscles. Electrophysiologically, this reflex may be elicited by electrical stimulation of the supraorbital nerve. The response consists of an initial ipsilateral component (R_1 response) of relatively short latency, perhaps mediated by the ipsilateral main sensory nucleus of the trigeminal nerve (afferent arc) and by the ipsilateral facial nerve (efferent arc). This R_1 response has no apparent clinical correlate. It is followed by a bilateral orbicularis oculi contraction (R_2 response) with a longer latency that correlates clinically with the bilateral blinking of the eyes. This response is perhaps mediated by the spinal nucleus of the trigeminal nerve (bilateral) with motor connections through the corresponding facial nerve to the orbicularis oculi muscle. By studying the blink reflex electrically, subtle peripheral and central lesions of the trigeminal and facial nerves may be uncovered.

LOCALIZATION OF LESIONS
AFFECTING CRANIAL NERVE V

Supranuclear Lesions. Supranuclear control of trigeminal motor function is bilateral. Corticobulbar fibers originate in the lower frontal motor cortex, descend through the corona radiata, internal capsule, and cerebral peduncle, and then decussate in the pons to supply the motor nucleus of the trigeminal nerve. Lesions interrupting this pathway may result in contralateral trigeminal motor paresis (e.g., deviation of the jaw "away from" the lesion), but because of the bilateral innervation, paresis is mild. Bilateral upper motor neuron lesions (pseudobulbar palsy) result in profound trigeminal motor paresis, often with an exaggerated jaw reflex. Mastication is then markedly impaired. Thalamic lesions may result in anesthesia of the contralateral face. Parietal lesions may be associated with depression of the contralateral corneal reflex, even when facial sensation is otherwise intact.

Nuclear Lesions. The motor and sensory nuclei of the trigeminal nerve may be involved by lesions (e.g., tumor, arteriovenous malformation, demyelinating disease, vascular disease, syringobulbia) that affect the pons, medulla, and upper cervical cord. These nuclear lesions involve other brainstem structures, and therefore brainstem lesions of the trigeminal nuclei are diagnosed by "the company they keep" (e.g., long tract signs, other cranial nerve involvement, and so on).

Lesions affecting the dorsal midpons may affect the *motor nucleus of the trigeminal nerve.* Ipsilateral paresis, atrophy, and fasciculations of the muscles of mastication thus occur. A pontine localization of this masticatory paresis is suggested by associated findings that may include contralateral hemiplegia (due to affection of the basis pontis), ipsilateral hemianesthesia of the face (due to affection of the main sensory nucleus of the trigeminal nerve), contralateral hemisensory loss of the limbs and trunk (due to spinothalamic tract affection), and ipsilateral tremor (due to affection of the brachium conjunctivum). Internuclear ophthalmoplegia (secondary to medial longitudinal fasciculus damage) and an ipsilateral Horner syndrome (due to involvement of descending sympathetic fibers) may also occur. Pontine syndromes are more thoroughly discussed in Chapter 14.

The nucleus of the spinal tract of the trigeminal nerve extends from the caudal end of the medulla to the third or fourth cervical spinal cord level. Therefore, lesions affecting the lateral medulla or upper cervical cord result in ipsilateral facial analgesia, hypesthesia, and thermoanesthesia. Because the lateral spinothalamic tract lies in close proximity to the trigeminal spinal nucleus, the hemifacial sensory disturbance is often associated with contralateral trunk and extremity hypalgesia and thermoanesthesia. With upper (rostral) spinal nuclear lesions, the entire trigeminal cutaneous distribution is affected. However, lower medullary or upper cervical spinal nuclear lesions result in a sensory disturbance that affects the peripheral (lateral) forehead, cheek, and jaw (onion-skin pattern of sensory loss). This onion-skin segmental distribution reflects the rostral-caudal somatotopic arrangement of the cutaneous distribution of the spinal nucleus (e.g., perioral area—rostral; lateral face—caudal).

The spinal nucleus of the trigeminal nerve is characteristically affected in the *lateral medullary (Wallenberg) syndrome,* which is most often secondary to brainstem infarction due to vertebral artery or posterior inferior cerebellar artery occlusion. This syndrome consists of the following signs:

1. Ipsilateral facial hypalgesia and thermoanesthesia (due to trigeminal spinal nuclear involvement).
2. Contralateral trunk and extremity hypalgesia and thermoanesthesia (due to damage to the spinothalamic tract).
3. Ipsilateral palatal, pharyngeal, and vocal cord paralysis with dysphagia and dysarthria (due to involvement of the nucleus ambiguus).
4. Ipsilateral Horner syndrome (due to affection of the descending sympathetic fibers).
5. Vertigo, nausea, and vomiting (due to involvement of the medullary vomiting centers and vestibular nuclei).
6. Ipsilateral cerebellar signs and symptoms (due to involvement of the inferior cerebellar peduncle).

Lesions affecting the *mesencephalic nucleus of the trigeminal nerve* cause no apparent neurologic signs and symptoms except perhaps depression of the ipsilateral jaw jerk (masseter reflex).

Lesions Affecting the Preganglionic Trigeminal Nerve Roots. In its cisternal course, the preganglionic trigeminal nerve root may be damaged by tumor (meningioma, schwannoma, metastasis, nasopharyngeal carcinoma), infection (granulomatous, infectious, or carcinomatous meningitis), trauma, or aneurysm. Sensory root atrophy may selectively occur with systemic lupus erythematosus, scleroderma, and Sjögren's syndrome [1, 12]. Trigeminal involvement is manifested by ipsilateral facial pain, paresthesias, numbness, and sensory loss. The corneal reflex is depressed, and a trigeminal motor paresis may occur. Preganglionic trigeminal nerve involvement is suggested by involvement of the neighboring cranial nerves (especially cranial nerves VI, VII, and VIII).

The trigeminal roots may be involved by extension of pathologic processes (usually acoustic neuroma or meningioma) located in the cerebellopontine angle [8]. Ipsilateral facial pain, paresthesias, and sensory loss, masticatory paresis, and a depressed corneal reflex are then associated with ipsilateral tinnitus, deafness, and vertigo (due to involvement of cranial nerve VIII). Facial nerve paralysis, ipsilateral ataxia and nystagmus (due to involvement of the cerebellar peduncles and cerebellum), ipsilateral lateral rectus paralysis (due to abducens nerve involvement), and, rarely, affection of cranial nerves IX through XII may also occur.

Trigeminal Neuralgia (Tic Douloureux, Fothergill's disease) refers to a syndrome of sudden, excruciating pains in the distribution of one or more of the divisions (usually the maxillary or mandibular) of the trigeminal nerve [6, 7]. Although often called idiopathic, this pain syndrome may be seen with pathology affecting the brainstem, preganglionic root, gasserian ganglion, and peripheral trigeminal nerve. Many cases are probably due to compression or irritation of the entry zone of the trigeminal nerve root (e.g., by a multiple sclerosis plaque or an aberrant blood vessel) [4, 11, 16, 19].

Lesions Affecting the Gasserian Ganglion. Lesions of the middle cranial fossa (e.g., tumor, herpes zoster, trauma, abscess) [5, 17] may directly damage the gasserian ganglion in Meckel's cave. Pain, often severe and paroxysmal, is the most characteristic finding and may be hemifacial or involve only select divisions of the trigeminal nerve (especially the maxillary and mandibular divisions). Paresthesias and numbness may also occur, often starting close to the midline on the upper lip and chin and progressing laterally to involve the anterior ear. Sensory loss occurs in the division or divisions affected, and unilateral pterygoid and masseter paresis may occur. Other cranial nerves (especially the abducens nerve) may also be affected.

Raeder's Paratrigeminal Syndrome. This syndrome is composed of two essential components—unilateral oculosympathetic paresis and evidence of trigeminal involvement on the same side [15, 18, 22]. The former consists of meiosis and ptosis but differs from the typical Horner syndrome in that facial anhidrosis is absent because the sudomotor fibers to the face that travel extracranially with the external carotid artery are spared. The unilateral head, facial, or retroorbital pain related to trigeminal dysfunction may be associated with evidence of involvement of other cranial nerves (e.g., cranial nerves IV and VI). This syndrome is usually due to lesions in the middle cranial fossa, especially in the region between the trigeminal ganglion and the internal carotid artery, near the petrous apex. It may also be caused by lesions of the gasserian ganglion. The usual etiologies include tumor, aneurysm, trauma, and infection.

Gradenigo Syndrome. Lesions located at the apex of the temporal bone, especially osteitis or leptomeningitis associated with otitis media, may cause damage to the ophthalmic division of the trigeminal nerve and the nearby abducens nerve (Gradenigo syndrome). Pain and sensory disturbance in the upper part of the face (ophthalmic distribution) are then associated with ipsilateral lateral rectus palsy. Oculosympathetic paresis (without anhidrosis) may also occur ipsilaterally if the lesions extend to involve sympathetic fibers. Other etiologies for this syndrome include trauma and tumor.

The Cavernous Sinus Syndrome. Lesions within the cavernous sinus (e.g., tumor, carotid aneurysm, trauma, carotid-cavernous fistula, infection) may damage the ophthalmic and maxillary divisions of the trigeminal nerve and the abducens, trochlear, and oculomotor nerves. Total unilateral ophthalmoplegia, usually starting with abducens nerve involvement (lateral rectus palsy) is then associated with pain, paresthesias, and sensory loss in the distribution of the ophthalmic and, less often, the maxillary divisions of the trigeminal nerve. Occasionally, oculosympathetic paresis (without anhidrosis) may also occur. Because the mandibular nerve is spared, no masticatory paresis is evident.

The Superior Orbital Fissure Syndrome. Through the superior orbital fissure pass the abducens, trochlear, and oculomotor nerves as well as the ophthalmic division of the trigeminal nerve. Thus, lesions at the superior orbital fissure (e.g., tumor, trauma, aneurysm, infection) may cause complete (external and internal) ophthalmoplegia associated with pain, paresthesias, and sensory loss in the ophthalmic cutaneous distribution. Occasionally, oculosympathetic paresis (without anhidrosis) may occur due to involvement of the sympathetic fibers. Exophthalmos due to blockade of the ophthalmic veins, and blindness, due to extension of the pathologic process to involve the optic canal, may also occur.

Except for the occasional involvement of the maxillary division of the trigeminal nerve in the cavernous sinus syndrome, the superior orbital fissure syndrome and the cavernous sinus syndrome usually cannot be differentiated clinically without the use of neuroradiologic procedures.

LESIONS AFFECTING THE PERIPHERAL BRANCHES OF THE TRIGEMINAL NERVE

The *ophthalmic division* of the trigeminal nerve may be damaged in the middle cranial fossa, at the temporal bone apex, at the lateral wall of the cavernous sinus, in the superior orbital fissure, or distally in the face. Localization of ophthalmic branch lesions in the former regions is made by associated cranial nerve findings, whereas very distal (e.g., facial) lesions result in sensory disturbances that are confined to the cutaneous supply of the ophthalmic division or its branches (e.g., the nasociliary, frontal, and lacrimal nerves).

The *maxillary division* of the trigeminal nerve may be damaged at the lower lateral wall of the cavernous sinus, at the foramen rotundum, in the pterygopalatine fossa, in the floor of the orbit, at the infraorbital foramen, or in the face. Lesions affecting this nerve in the cavernous sinus usually affect other cranial nerves as well. More distal lesions (e.g., infraorbital nerve damage secondary to maxillary fracture) result in sensory disturbances that are confined to the cutaneous supply of the maxillary nerve.

The *mandibular division* of the trigeminal nerve may be damaged in the foramen ovale, in the zygomatic fossa, or in the face. Lesions affecting these regions result in sensory disturbances confined to the cutaneous supply of the maxillary division associated with ipsilateral masticatory paralysis. A syndrome of isolated mental neuropathy *(the syndrome of the numb chin)* [3, 10, 14] consists of pain, swelling, and numbness in the jaw (lower lip, chin, and mucous membrane on the inside of the lip). This syndrome is usually seen in patients with systemic cancer (especially lymphoreticular neoplasms and carcinoma of the breast). This syndrome is usually due to metastatic lesions of the mental canal of the jaw.

The peripheral branches of the trigeminal nerve are most often damaged in isolation by tumors or by fractures of the facial bones or skull.

REFERENCES

1. Ashworth, B., and Tait, G. B. W. Trigeminal neuropathy in connective tissue disease. *Neurology (Minneap.)* 21:609, 1971.
2. Brodal, A. *Neurological Anatomy In Relation to Clinical Medicine* (3rd ed.). New York: Oxford University Press, 1981. Pp. 508–532.
3. Calverley, J. R., and Mohnac, A. Syndrome of the numb chin. *Arch. Intern. Med.* 112:819, 1963.
4. Chakravorty, B. G. Association of trigeminal neuralgia with multiple sclerosis. *Arch. Neurol.* 14:95, 1966.
5. Cuneo, H. M., and Rand, C. W. Tumors of the Gasserian ganglion. Tumor of the left Gasserian ganglion associated with enlargement of the mandibular nerve. A review of the literature and case report. *J. Neurosurg.* 9:423, 1952.
6. DeJong, R. N. *The Neurologic Examination Incorporating the Fundamentals of Neuroanatomy and Neurophysiology* (4th ed.). Hagerstown, Md.: Harper & Row, 1979. Pp. 163–177.
7. Gardner, W. J. Trigeminal neuralgia. *Clin. Neurosurg.* 15:1, 1968.
8. Gonzalez Revilla, A. Differential diagnosis of tumors at the cerebellopontine recess. *Bull. Johns Hopkins Hosp.* 83:187, 1948.
9. Goor, C., and Ongerboer de Visser, B. W. Jaw and blink reflexes in trigeminal nerve lesions. *Neurology* 26:95, 1976.
10. Horton, J., et al. The numb chin in breast cancer. *J. Neurol. Neurosurg. Psychiat.* 36:211, 1973.
11. Jannetta, P. J., and Rand, R. W. Arterial compression of the trigeminal nerve at the pons in patients with trigeminal neuralgia. *J. Neurosurg.* 26 (Suppl.): 159, 1967.

12. Kaltreider, H. B., and Talal, N. The neuropathy of Sjögren's syndrome: Trigeminal nerve involvement. *Ann. Intern. Med.* 70:751, 1969.
13. Kimura, J. Electrically elicited blink reflex in diagnosis of multiple sclerosis. *Brain* 98:413, 1975.
14. Massey, E. W., Moore, J., and Schold, S. C. Mental neuropathy from systemic cancer. *Neurology* 31:1277, 1981.
15. Mokri, B. Raeder's paratrigeminal syndrome—Original concept and subsequent deviations. *Arch. Neurol.* 39:395, 1982.
16. Olafson, R. A., Rushton, J. G., and Sayre, G. P. Trigeminal neuralgia in a patient with multiple sclerosis. An autopsy report. *J. Neurosurg.* 24:755, 1966.
17. Olive, I., and Svien, H. J. Neurofibromas of the fifth cranial nerve. *J. Neurosurg.* 14:484, 1957.
18. Raeder, S. G. "Paratrigeminal" paralysis of oculo-pupillary sympathetic. *Brain* 47:149, 1924.
19. Rushton, J. G., and Olafson, R. A. Trigeminal neuralgia associated with multiple sclerosis. Report of 35 cases. *Arch. Neurol.* 13:383, 1965.
20. Rushworth, G. Observations on blink reflexes. *J. Neurol. Neurosurg. Psychiat.* 25:93, 1962.
21. Shahani, B. T., and Young, R. R. Human obicularis oculi reflexes. *Neurology* 22:149, 1972.
22. Smith, J. L. Raeder's paratrigeminal syndrome. *Am. J. Ophthalmol.* 46:149, 1958.

Chapter 9

THE LOCALIZATION OF LESIONS AFFECTING CRANIAL NERVE VII (THE FACIAL NERVE)

Paul W. Brazis

ANATOMY OF CRANIAL
NERVE VII (FACIAL NERVE)

Cranial nerve VII (the facial nerve) (Fig. 9-1) is a predominantly motor nerve that supplies the facial mimetic musculature *(the motor division)* [4, 31]. In addition, sensation and parasympathetic fibers are carried in a minor root called *the nervus intermedius (of Wrisberg)*.

Motor Division. Fibers of this division arise from the *motor facial nucleus,* which lies in the caudal pons, dorsal to the superior olive, medial to the nucleus of the spinal tract of cranial nerve V (trigeminal nerve), and anterolateral to the nucleus of cranial nerve VI (abducens nerve). The *intrapontine roots* arise from the motor nucleus dorsally and run rostrally and dorsally (the ascending intrapontine root) to the level of the nucleus of cranial nerve VI. The root then sweeps over the dorsal surface of the abducens nucleus (as the *genu of the facial nerve*) and then passes ventrolaterally and caudally through the pons to emerge on the lateral aspect of the brainstem.

The supranuclear control of facial movements occurs through corticobulbar fibers originating in the lower third of the precentral gyrus. These fibers course through the corona radiata, the genu of the internal capsule, and the medial cerebral peduncle to reach the pons. In the pons the majority of fibers decussate, ending in the facial motor nucleus of the contralateral side. The ventral part of the facial nucleus, which innervates the lower two-thirds of the face, has a predominantly crossed supranuclear control. The dorsal portion, which supplies the upper third of the face, has bilateral supranuclear control.

This schema of supranuclear facial muscle control holds true for voluntary facial movements. Emotional involuntary movements and voluntary facial movements may be clinically dissociated, and therefore a separate supranuclear pathway for the control of involuntary movements probably exists. These fibers probably originate in the globus pallidus, hypothalamus, and thalamus and do not descend in the internal capsule in their course to the facial motor nuclei.

Nervus Intermedius (of Wrisberg). The nervus intermedius is the sensory and parasympathetic division of the facial nerve. It carries preganglionic parasympathetic fibers to the submaxillary ganglion (postganglionic fibers go to the submandibular and sublingual glands) and to the pterygopalatine or sphenopalatine ganglion (postganglionic fibers go to the lacrimal, palatal, and nasal glands) and also receives sensory fibers from the *geniculate ganglion*. This latter ganglion receives fibers that carry taste sensation from the anterior two-thirds of the tongue and also receives afferents from the mucosa of the pharynx, nose and palate and

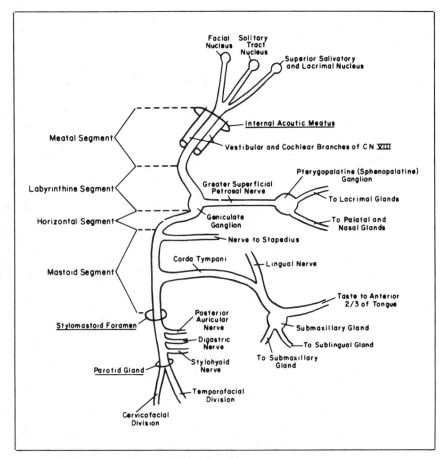

FIG. 9-1. *Anatomy of cranial nerve VII (facial nerve).*

from the skin of the external auditory meatus, lateral pinna, and mastoid.

The parasympathetic fibers arise in the *superior salivatory nucleus* of the dorsal pons, those controlling lacrimation arising from an associated nuclear mass, the *lacrimal nucleus.* The gustatory afferents end primarily in the *nucleus of the tractus solitarius* of the medulla, and the exteroceptive afferents end in the *nucleus of the spinal tract of cranial nerve V* in the medulla. Some proprioceptive afferents from the facial musculature also travel in the facial nerve and have their perikarya in the mesencephalic trigeminal nucleus.

The sensory fibers of the nervus intermedius travel through the substance of the pons lateral to the motor fibers. Together with the motor divisions of cranial nerve VII medially and cranial nerve VIII (auditory nerve) laterally, the nervus intermedius leaves the pons in the cerebello-pontine angle and enters the internal auditory meatus.

Anatomy of the Peripheral Course of the Facial Nerve. After emerging from the ventrolateral pons, the motor division and the nervus interme-dius proceed laterally in the cerebellopontine angle in company with cranial nerve VIII. Cranial nerve VII then enters the *internal auditory meatus* of the temporal bone together with the auditory nerve and the in-ternal auditory artery and vein. Within the temporal bone, four portions of the facial nerve can be distinguished.

THE MEATAL (CANAL) SEGMENT (7–8 mm). On entering the meatus, the motor di-vision lies on the superoanterior surface of cranial nerve VIII with the nervus intermedius between them. Within this segment, the facial nerve runs in close association with the vestibular and cochlear divisions of cranial nerve VIII. There are no major branches from this segment of the facial nerve.

THE LABYRINTHINE SEGMENT (3–4 mm). At the lateral end of the internal audi-tory meatus, the motor division and the nervus intermedius enter the *facial or fallopian* canal in the petrous bone. The labyrinthine segment runs at nearly a right angle to the petrous pyramid and courses antero-laterally above the labyrinth to reach the *geniculate ganglion,* which con-tains the pseudounipolar perikarya of the sensory fibers of the nervus intermedius. The first major branch of the facial nerve, the *greater superfi-cial petrosal nerve,* arises from the geniculate ganglion. This nerve is com-posed of preganglionic parasympathetic efferents that innervate the lacrimal, palatal, and nasal glands by way of the pterygopalatine (sphe-nopalatine) ganglion. The greater superficial petrosal nerve also con-tains sensory cutaneous afferent fibers from the skin of the external auditory meatus, lateral pinna, and mastoid.

THE HORIZONTAL (TYMPANIC) SEGMENT (12–13 mm). From the geniculate gan-glion, the facial nerve runs horizontally backward below and medial to the horizontal semicircular canal. No major branches of the facial nerve originate from this segment.

THE MASTOID (VERTICAL) SEGMENT (15–20 mm). At the posterior aspect of the middle ear (sinus tympani) the facial nerve again changes course and bends inferiorly as the mastoid segment. The *nerve to the stapedius muscle* originates near the upper end of this segment. The other major branch of this segment is the *chorda tympani,* which has a variable location of origin. The chorda tympani joins the lingual nerve and contains preganglionic parasympathetic fibers (originating in the superior salivatory nucleus), which innervate the submandibular and sublingual glands by way of the submaxillary ganglion. The chorda tympani also contains afferent taste fibers from the anterior two-thirds of the tongue destined for the nucleus of the solitary tract.

After giving off the chorda tympani, cranial nerve VII exits the facial canal through the *stylomastoid foramen*. Near its exit, it gives rise to the *posterior auricular nerve* (to the occipitalis, posterior auricular, and transverse and oblique auricular muscles), the *digastric branch* (to the posterior belly of the digastric muscle), and the *stylohyoid branch* (to the stylohyoid muscles). The facial nerve then pierces the parotid gland and divides into the *temporofacial and cervicofacial divisions*. The former divides into temporal, zygomatic, and upper buccal branches, and the latter divides into lower buccal, mandibular, and cervical branches. These branches supply all facial mimetic muscles and the platysma muscle.

CLINICAL EVALUATION OF CRANIAL NERVE VII FUNCTION

Motor Function. The motor functions of the facial innervated muscles [9] are assessed by facial inspection and tests of facial mobility. The patient is asked to raise the eyebrows, wrinkle the brow, close the eyes (orbicularis oculi), show his teeth while repeating a sentence with several labial consonants (orbicularis oris), blow out the cheeks (buccinator), and retract the chin (platysma). Any asymmetries of contraction are noted. The stylohyoid, posterior belly of the digastric, occipitalis, and auricular muscles cannot be adequately tested. Weakness of the stapedius muscle may be detected by the subjective complaint of hyperacusis, especially for low tones that sound louder on the affected side (because the stapedius muscle no longer contracts adequately to tighten the ossicular chain and protect the inner ear from loud noises).

Sensory Function. The sensory examination of cranial nerve VII essentially consists of evaluation of taste on the anterior two-thirds of the tongue. Each half of the protruded tongue is tested with the four fundamental tastes (sweet, sour, salty, and bitter), and any asymmetries are documented.

Reflex Function. The most important of the facial reflexes are the corneal and palpebral reflexes, which are depressed on the side of a lower motor neuron-type facial nerve lesion [9, 21]. Consensual reflexes are spared. Orbicularis oculi (glabellar), orbicularis oris, and palpebral reflexes may also be depressed with infranuclear lesions.

Parasympathetic Function. Infranuclear facial nerve lesions may result in increased or impaired lacrimation that may be noted subjectively by the patient and can be tested by hanging litmus or filter paper on each lower lid *(Schirmer's test)*. Excessive salivation may also be noted with infranuclear lesions. Otherwise, facial parasympathetic function is difficult to test objectively at the bedside.

LOCALIZATION OF LESIONS AFFECTING CRANIAL NERVE VII

Supranuclear Lesions (Central Facial Palsy). In supranuclear corticobulbar lesions, there is contralateral paresis of the lower portion of the face with relative sparing of upper facial function. The upper part of the face is spared because its supranuclear control has both ipsilateral and contralateral components, whereas the lower face has mainly or solely contralateral supranuclear connections. The muscles around the mouth are especially affected, but there is occasional paresis of the lower or even the upper orbicularis oculi.

On occasion, there may be a dissociation between voluntary lower facial movements *(volitional facial palsy)* and emotional lower facial movements *(emotional* or *mimetic facial palsy)* [5, 26]. Volitional lower facial paresis without emotional paresis (e.g., one side of the orbicularis oris may be paretic when the patient speaks, or he may be unable to retract the angle of his mouth on command but does so when spontaneously laughing or crying) may occur with corticobulbar interruption from lesions of the lower precentral gyrus, internal capsule, cerebral peduncle, or upper pons (above the facial nucleus). The occurrence of the reverse dissociation (emotional or mimetic facial paresis without volitional facial paresis) supports the assumption that "voluntary" and "mimetic" supranuclear fibers travel separately before they exert their influence on the facial nucleus. The mimetic fibers probably do not travel in the internal capsule; most likely, they arise in the globus pallidus, thalamus, and hypothalamus and descend in the central tegmental tract to the facial nucleus. A lesion affecting these structures may thus cause a mimetic facial paresis. A cortical component of this pathway must also exist because frontal lobe lesions that occur anterior to the precentral gyrus may also cause mimetic paresis.

Bilateral upper motor neuron lesions result in facial diplegia associated with other manifestations of pseudobulbar palsy (e.g., spastic tongue, uninhibited laughter and crying).

Nuclear and Fascicular Lesions (Pontine Lesions). Lesions within the pons may affect either the nucleus of the facial nerve or its emerging roots (fascicles). These lesions usually affect neighboring structures such as the abducens nerve or nucleus (lateral rectus paralysis), the para-median pontine reticular formation (paralysis of conjugate gaze to the ipsilateral side), the corticospinal tract (contralateral hemiplegias), and occasionally the spinal tract and nucleus of the trigeminal nerve and the spinothalamic tract (ipsilateral facial and contralateral body sensory disturbances). The association of involvement of these intraparenchymal structures with a facial palsy indicates a pontine lesion.

Nuclear and fascicular lesions of the facial nerve result in a *peripheral type* of facial nerve palsy [10, 11, 14, 22, 32]. This consists of unilateral paralysis of all mimetic facial muscles with facial asymmetry at rest and with motion. The patient cannot frown or raise his eyebrow on the affected side, close his eye (orbicularis oculi palsy), retract the angle of the mouth (orbicularis oris palsy), puff out the cheek (buccinator palsy), or tighten the chin (platysma palsy). With mild peripheral affection, only blink asymmetry (incomplete blink on the side of the paresis) may be evident. On attempting to close the eye on the affected side, the eyeball will deviate up and slightly outward *(Bell's phenomenon)* owing to relaxation of the inferior rectus and contraction of the superior rectus (a normal phenomenon that becomes visible because of the paralysis of eye closure). The cheek puffs out during respiration and food tends to accumulate between the teeth and the cheek on the affected side owing to buccinator paralysis. This peripheral type of facial paralysis will also result in depressed facial reflexes (e.g., corneal and palpebral reflexes) on the affected side with intact consensual reflexes and ipsilateral hyperacusis.

MILLARD-GUBLER SYNDROME. This syndrome is caused by a lesion located in the ventral pons that destroys the fascicles of the facial and abducens nerves and the corticospinal tract. It is thus characterized by:

1. Ipsilateral peripheral-type facial paralysis.
2. Ipsilateral lateral rectus paralysis (diplopia with failure to abduct the ipsilateral eye).
3. Contralateral hemiplegia.

FOVILLE SYNDROME. This syndrome is caused by a lesion located in the pontine tegmentum that destroys the fascicle of the facial nerve, the paramedian pontine reticular formation, and the corticospinal tract. It is characterized by:

1. Ipsilateral peripheral-type facial paralysis.
2. Paralysis of conjugate gaze to the side of the lesion.
3. Contralateral hemiplegia.

Posterior Fossa Lesions (Cerebellopontine Angle Lesions). In this location, the motor division of the facial nerve is in close proximity to the nervus intermedius and the eighth cranial nerve. Lesions in this location (e.g., acoustic neuroma, meningioma) result in:

1. Ipsilateral peripheral-type facial nerve paralysis (including loss of taste over the ipsilateral anterior two-thirds of the tongue) without hyperacusis (due to associated eighth cranial nerve affection).
2. Ipsilateral tinnitus, deafness, and vertigo.

Cerebellopontine angle lesions frequently extend to involve other neighboring structures including the trigeminal nerve (ipsilateral facial pain and sensory changes), the cerebellar peduncles and cerebellum (ipsilateral ataxia and nystagmus), and the abducens nerve (ipsilateral rectus paralysis). Affection of cranial nerves IX through XII may rarely occur.

Lesions Affecting the Meatal (Canal) Segment of the Facial Nerve in the Temporal Bone. In this location, the facial nerve is closely associated with the auditory nerve, and thus lesions will cause clinical findings similar to those seen with the cerebellopontine angle syndrome: unilateral facial motor paralysis, impairment of taste over the ipsilateral anterior two-thirds of the tongue, impaired lacrimation, and deafness (rather than hyperacusis). This syndrome is most often caused by temporal bone fracture and primary or secondary tumors.

Lesions Affecting the Facial Nerve Within the Facial Canal Distal to the Meatal Segment but Proximal to the Departure of the Nerve to the Stapedius Muscle. Lesions at this location involve the motor division of the facial nerve and the nervus intermedius. There is no deafness or other cranial nerve involvement. Ipsilateral facial motor paralysis, loss of taste over the anterior two-thirds of the tongue, and hyperacusis result. If the lesion is proximal to the greater superficial petrosal nerve, lacrimation is impaired; if it is distal to this branch, lacrimation is normal. When the geniculate ganglion is injured, pain in the region of the eardrum may occur. Infection of the geniculate ganglion by herpes zoster results in facial paralysis, hyperacusis, and loss of taste associated with geniculate neuralgia and herpetic vesicles on the eardrum and in the external auditory meatus *(Ramsay-Hunt syndrome)* [17, 18].

Lesions Affecting the Facial Nerve Within the Facial Canal Between the Departure of the Nerve to the Stapedius and the Departure of the Chorda Tympani. Lesions at this location cause facial motor paralysis with loss of taste on the anterior two-thirds of the tongue. Because the lesion is distal to the nerve to the stapedius, hearing is spared (no hyperacusis).

Lesions Affecting the Facial Nerve in the Facial Canal Distal to the Departure of the Chorda Tympani. Lesions at this location (e.g., lesions at the stylomastoid foramen) cause facial motor paralysis without associated hyperacusis or loss of taste.

Lesions Distal to the Stylomastoid Foramen. Lesions in this location produce isolated facial motor paralysis. Individual motor branches of the facial nerve may be affected, thus causing paralysis of individual facial muscles (e.g., an isolated lesion affecting the temporofacial division of the facial nerve). In this location, the fibers of the facial nerve may be involved by inflammation of the retromandibular lymph nodes or by tumors or infections (e.g., sarcoidosis, infectious mononucleosis) of the parotid gland. The facial nerve or its branches are also susceptible to facial trauma (e.g., by obstetric forceps).

ABNORMAL FACIAL MOVEMENTS AND THEIR LOCALIZATION

Abnormal facial movements may be classified* as follows:

1. Dyskinetic movements
2. Dystonic movements
3. Hemifacial spasm
4. Postparalytic spasm and synkinetic movements
5. Miscellaneous movements
   a. Facial myokymia
   b. Focal seizures
   c. Tics and habit spasms
   d. Fasciculations
   e. Myoclonus

Dyskinetic Movements. Oral-facial dyskinesia may express itself as a constellation of involuntary movements of the face, jaw, lip, and tongue [28] including:

1. Facial grimaces, distortions, expressions, and twitches
2. Wide opening, tight closing, up and down movements, and lateral deviation of the jaw

*Gupta, S. Personal communication, 1982.

3. Puckering, pursing, and opening and closing movements of the lips
4. Protrusion, writhing, and distorted posturing of the tongue

Oral-facial dyskinesias may occur spontaneously (especially in the elderly) but are usually side effects of neuroleptic drug use or are associated with various extrapyramidal diseases (e.g., Huntington's chorea, Wilson's disease).

Dystonic Movements (Blepharospasm and Blepharospasm with Oromandibular Dystonia). Blepharospasm is an involuntary, spasmodic closing of the eyes that is always bilateral and symmetrical and that may be episodic or sustained. The spasm may spread to involve other facial and cranial musculature. This condition usually indicates the presence of extrapyramidal disease (e.g., Parkinson's disease, progressive supranuclear palsy) and is distinguished from other facial movement disorders by its symmetry.

Idiopathic blepharospasms may be associated with oromandibular dystonia as in *Meige's syndrome (Brueghel syndrome)* [6, 19, 23, 25, 33, 34]. This syndrome consists of a combination of blepharospasm plus oromandibular dystonia, manifested by sustained grimacing around the mouth, platysma contraction, and sustained neck flexion. This disorder may spread beyond the facial and nuchal musculature to involve one or both arms and the trunk. It is of unknown etiology, but basal ganglia dysfunction, perhaps with a dopaminergic predominance, may be involved [34].

Hemifacial Spasm. Hemifacial spasm [3, 20, 36] may be cryptogenic or postparalytic (occurring after Bell's palsy or traumatic facial nerve injury). It consists of clonic intermittent spasms of the orbicularis oculi muscle and may involve all other muscles innervated by the facial nerve on that side [12]. The stapedius muscle may be affected (intermittent clicking is heard ipsilaterally). These contractions are irregular, intermittent, and usually unilateral. When bilateral, they are asynchronous and asymmetrical on the two sides of the face.

Lesions causing hemifacial spasm reportedly occur anywhere from the facial nucleus to the stylomastoid foramen [13]. Lesions located in the cerebellopontine angle (e.g., tumors and aneurysms) that compress or angulate the facial nerve are the most common cause, but intrapontine (multiple sclerosis) and intratemporal lesions have also been described. Cross-talk (ephaptic conduction) among facial nerve fibers may mediate this disorder [13, 15, 16].

23. Marsdeu, C. D. Blepharospasm—oromandibular dystonia syndrome (Brueghel's syndrome)—A variant of adult-onset torsion dystonia? *J. Neurol. Neurosurg. Psychiat.* 39:1204, 1976.
24. Mateer, J. E., Gutmann, L., and McComas, C. F. Myokymia in Guillain-Barré syndrome. *Neurology (Clev.)* 33:374, 1983.
25. Meige, H. Les convulsions de la face, uneforme clinique de convulsion faciale, bilaterale et mediane. *Rev. Neurol. (Paris)* 20:237, 1910.
26. Monrad-Krohn, G. H., and Refsum, S. *The Clinical Examination of the Nervous System* (12th ed.). London: H. K. Lewis, 1964.
27. Negri, S., Carceni, T., and Lorenzi, L. D. Facial myokymia in brainstem tumour. *Eur. Neurol.* 14:108, 1976.
28. Paul, H. A. Oral-facial dyskinesia. *Arch. Neurol.* 26:506, 1972.
29. Radu, E. W., Skorpil, V., and Kaeser, H. E. Facial myokymia. *Eur. Neurol.* 13:499, 1975.
30. Spiller, W. G. Contracture occurring in partial recovery from paralysis of the facial nerve and other nerves. *Arch. Neurol. Psychiat.* (Chic.) 1:564, 1919.
31. Sunderland, S., and Cossar, D. F. The structure of the facial nerve. *Anat. Rec.* 116:147, 1953.
32. Taverner, D. Bell's palsy. A clinical and electromyographic study. *Brain* 78:209, 1955.
33. Tolosa, E. S., and Klawans, H. L. Meige's disease—A clinical form of facial convulsion, bilateral and medial. *Arch. Neurol.* 36:635, 1979.
34. Tolosa, E. S., and Lai, C. Meige disease: Striatal dopaminergic preponderance. *Neurology* 29:1126, 1979.
35. Tenser, L. B. Myokymia facial contractures in multiple sclerosis. *Arch. Intern. Med.* 136:81, 1976.
36. Wartenberg, R. *Hemifacial Spasm: A Clinical and Pathophysiological Study.* New York: Oxford University Press, 1952.
37. Wassertom, W. R., and Starr, A. Facial myokymia in the Guillain-Barré syndrome. *Arch. Neurol.* 34:576, 1977.

Chapter 10

THE LOCALIZATION OF LESIONS AFFECTING CRANIAL NERVE VIII (THE VESTIBULOCOCHLEAR NERVE)

José Biller and Paul W. Brazis

ANATOMY OF CRANIAL NERVE VIII

The eighth cranial nerve consists of two separate functional components: the *auditory nerve* and the *vestibular nerve*. The auditory nerve receives information from the cochlea, the organ of hearing. The vestibular nerve derives its input from the *saccular and utricular macules* (which
sense *linear* acceleration) and the cristae of the semicircular canals
(which sense *angular* acceleration of the head). Because of this functional
dualism, the two vestibulocochlear nerve components will be discussed
separately.

The Auditory Pathways. The auditory pathway may be simplistically divided into a four-tiered neuronal network, as follows [7, 38, 43]:

FIRST-ORDER NEURONS. The auditory receptors are the *hair cells* of the organ
of Corti. The structure of the cochlea is such that those hair cells that are
located at the cochlear apex are stimulated by low tones, whereas those
located at the base are stimulated by high tones. The first-order neurons
of the auditory pathway have their cell bodies in the *spiral ganglion of the
cochlear nerve,* which lies in *Rosenthal's canal* at the base of the bony spiral
lamina. The afferent components of these cells make contact with the
hair cells of the cochlea, the majority converging on the inner hair cells
and a smaller number diverging to make contact with the outer hair
cells. When the hair cells are activated, impulse transmission is triggered
in fibers with their perikarya in the spiral ganglion; these fibers then enter the brainstem, at the level of the ventral cochlear nuclei, as the cochlear nerve.

SECOND-ORDER NEURONS. On entry into the brainstem, the afferent cochlear nerve fibers bifurcate, innervating the *dorsal nucleus* and the *anteroventral* and *posteroventral* nuclei of the cochlear nuclear complex. This
innervation follows a tonotopic pattern in which the more dorsal aspects
of these nuclei receive fibers that have innervated "high-frequency"
(basal) hair cells, whereas the ventral aspects receive fibers from "low-
frequency" (apical) hair cells. The dorsal and ventral cochlear nuclei contain the second-order neurons and give rise to several projections to the
contralateral brainstem that ascend as the *lateral lemniscus.* These projections include the *dorsal acoustic striae* (from the dorsal cochlear nucleus),
the *intermediate acoustic striae* (from the dorsal part of the ventral cochlear
nucleus), and the *ventral acoustic striae* (from the ventral cochlear nucleus), which is part of the trapezoid body. The lateral lemniscal fibers
ascend, with some fibers terminating in the lateral lemniscal nuclei
along the way, and terminate in the *inferior colliculus.* (The ventral acous-

tic striae also terminate in the ipsilateral and contralateral reticular formation, the superior olivary nuclei, and the nuclei of the trapezoid body.)

THIRD-ORDER NEURONS. The *inferior colliculus* (part of the midbrain tectum) contains the third-order neurons and serves as the central relay in the auditory pathway receiving ascending and descending input. Fibers from the lateral lemniscus end in the central nucleus of the inferior colliculus, which has a tonotopic organization. The projections from the inferior colliculus terminate in the *medial geniculate body,* with low-frequency fibers ending in the apical-lateral areas and high-frequency fibers ending in the medial portions.

FOURTH-ORDER NEURONS. The medial geniculate body gives rise to geniculotemporal fibers. The majority of these fibers terminate in lamina IV of the primary auditory cortex (area 41), located in the transverse temporal gyri of Heschl, while others end in the association auditory cortex (area 42). The primary auditory cortex terminations conform to a tonotopic pattern with the high tones terminating medially and low tones laterally.

There is a high degree of commissural connections all along the auditory pathway, with the exception of the medial geniculate body. The bilaterality of representation has obvious significance when unilateral brainstem lesions are considered. Another important consideration is that from the inferior colliculus upward, there are two different projection systems. The first (including the central nucleus of the inferior colliculus, portions of the medial geniculate, and the primary auditory cortex) is referred to as a core system, which is a direct auditory pathway with a tonotopic organization. The other (including the pericentral region of the inferior colliculus, the nonlaminated portions of the medial geniculate body, and the secondary auditory cortex) is referred to as a belt projection, which has less tonotopic organization and serves as a polymodal system that receives both auditory and nonauditory information.

There are also several descending auditory pathways that run parallel to the ascending fibers and are integrated in the feedback control of auditory input. These include corticogeniculate fibers, corticocollicular fibers, geniculocollicular fibers, collicular efferents, and an efferent cochlear bundle from the superior olivary complex to the hair cells of the spiral organ of Corti.

The Vestibular System. The vestibular system monitors angular and linear accelerations of the head. These accelerations are transduced into neuronal signals within a specialized structure, the *membranous laby-*

rinth. The labyrinth consists of the three semicircular canals, the utricle, and the saccule [1, 8]. Linear acceleration is monitored by specialized receptors, the *macules,* of the utricle and saccule, whereas angular acceleration is monitored by the *cristae* in the ampullae of the semicircular canals. These receptors are themselves composed of numerous hair cells that serve as transducers that convert mechanical movements of their sensory hairs into changes of receptor potentials in the hair cells themselves and in their afferent neurons.

The *semicircular canals* are three in number and are arranged at right angles in order to detect angular accelerating movements of the head. These canals include the *horizontal canal* (with an outward convexity), the *anterior or superior canal* (with an upward convexity), and the *posterior or inferior canal* (with a backward convexity). When the head is in the erect position, the horizontal canal is almost horizontal (there is a slight inclination down and back, forming a 30-degree angle with the horizontal), and the superior and posterior canals are arranged in two different vertical planes that form a 45-degree angle with the frontal and sagittal planes. Thus, the horizontal canals of both labyrinths are in the same plane, while the superior canal on one side is in the same plane as the posterior canal of the opposite side.

The utricle and saccule are arranged at right angles also, with the utricle horizontal to the base of the skull and the saccule parallel to the sagittal plane. Therefore, horizontal head movements stimulate the utricle linearly, whereas tilting the head activates the saccule.

When the cristae or macules are stimulated, potentials are developed in their afferent nerve endings, the cell bodies of which lie in the *vestibular ganglion (of Scarpa).* These impulses are then transmitted through the nerve fibers that make up the *vestibular nerve.*

The information from the membranous labyrinth is transmitted in a different manner in two different components of the vestibular nerve. The superior portion of the nerve carries input from the anterior and horizontal semicircular canals and from the utricle, whereas the inferior portion of the nerve transmits information from the posterior semicircular canal and the saccule. The vestibular nerve enters the brainstem at the pontomedullary level, bifurcates into ascending and descending fascicles, and terminates in the *vestibular nuclei* (the superior nucleus of Bechterew, the lateral nucleus of Deiters, the medial nucleus of Schwalbe, and the inferior or descending nucleus of Roller). The semicircular canals relate preferentially to the superior and medial vestibular nuclei, whereas the macular fibers project mainly to the medial and inferior vestibular nuclei. Other afferents in the vestibular nerve enter the cerebellum by way of the inferior cerebellar peduncle and terminate in the vestibulocerebellum.

Most of the vestibular nuclei output is concerned with feedback integration with the cerebellum, spinal cord, and brainstem. The main vestibular connections include the following structures:

THE MEDIAL LONGITUDINAL FASCICULUS (MLF). Through the MLF the vestibular nuclei exert an influence on conjugate eye movements and on head and neck movements. Although all of the vestibular nuclei make contributions to the MLF, only the superior nucleus projects to the ipsilateral MLF; other nuclei send fibers to the contralateral MLF.

THE MEDIAL VESTIBULOSPINAL TRACT. Through this tract the medial vestibular nucleus exerts an excitatory and inhibitory effect on the cervical and upper thoracic levels of the contralateral spinal cord.

THE LATERAL VESTIBULOSPINAL TRACT. This pathway originates in the lateral vestibular nucleus and projects to the ipsilateral spinal cord. The fibers destined for the cervical cord arise from the rostroventral portion of the lateral vestibular nucleus, whereas the lumbosacral fibers originate from the dorsocaudal portion. The lateral vestibulospinal pathway facilitates extensor trunk tone and the action of antigravity axial muscles, reflecting the input the vestibular nucleus receives from the utricular "gravity detector."

THE CEREBELLUM. The vestibular nuclei (primarily the inferior and medial nuclei) project to the ipsilateral flocculonodular lobe and uvula and to the fastigial nucleus.

THE RETICULAR FORMATION. Through its cerebellar projections, the vestibular nuclei influences the reticular formation (especially the lateral reticular nucleus and the nucleus reticularis pontis caudalis).

The vestibular nuclei also project fibers back to the hair cells of the membranous labyrinth, these fibers probably serving a modulating function.

The cortical representation of vestibular function is located in the postcentral gyrus near areas 2 and 5 of the cerebral cortex. Other receptive areas include the frontal lobe (area 6) and the superior temporal gyrus.

CLINICAL EVALUATION OF
CRANIAL NERVE VIII FUNCTION

Sensorineural Deafness. The term *sensorineural deafness* refers to a deficit in perceiving either tones or speech that is due to a lesion central to the oval window. This deficit may therefore involve the cochlea (sensory), the cochlear nerve and nuclei (neural), or the central auditory pathways. Sensorineural deafness may be bilateral and progressive (e.g., presbyacusis, ototoxic drugs), unilateral and progressive (e.g., Meniere's disease, acoustic neuroma), or unilateral (rarely bilateral) and acute (e.g., impaired blood flow to the cochlea, viral infection, perilymphatic fistula, or, rarely, acoustic neuroma) [29, 30, 31, 39].

Individuals suffering from sensorineural hearing loss frequently have difficulty hearing high-pitched sounds and vowels (e and i to a greater extent than a, o, or u). Formal audiometric testing usually reveals a loss of speech discrimination that is out of proportion to associated pure tone deafness [11, 20].

Besides the hearing difficulty, patients with sensorineural pathology often complain of *tinnitus*, which varies in both pitch and intensity. The evaluation of the individual with complaints of hearing loss commences with a thorough examination of the external auditory canal and inspection of the tympanic membranes. Next, it must be determined whether the observed hearing loss is due to a sensorineural process or a *conductive* disturbance (i.e., the lesion is located between the environment and the organ of Corti). In bedside qualitative assessment of hearing loss a tuning fork (256 or 512 Hz because lower frequencies introduce a component of vibration into the testing) is used to distinguish between these two types of hearing loss. Later, more formal quantitative audiologic tests are performed.

There are three major tuning fork tests for evaluation of hearing loss.

THE WEBER TEST. A vibrating tuning fork is placed over the midline of the skull or forehead, over the nasal bone, or over the anterior upper incisors. Normally, the vibrations are perceived equally in both ears (no lateralization) because bone conduction is equal bilaterally. In conductive deafness, the vibrations are louder in the deaf ear (lateralized to the diseased ear). In sensorineural hearing loss, the sound is louder in the normal ear (lateralized to the normal ear).

THE RINNE TEST. The stem of the vibrating tuning fork is applied to the mastoid bone. When the patient no longer hears the vibration, the instrument is placed next to the ear with the tines parallel to the sagittal plane of the skull, 1 inch from the external auditory meatus. In normal individuals, because air conduction is better than bone conduction, the vibrations are perceived in the ear after they are no longer perceived at the mastoid. With conduction deafness, bone conduction is better than air conduction, and therefore the tuning fork cannot be heard when it is placed next to the ear. With sensorineural hearing loss, air and bone conduction are diminished to a similar extent, and air conduction remains greater than bone conduction. When performing the Rinne test it is advisable to mask the hearing in the opposite ear (by a Bárány noisemaker or finger rubbing).

THE SCHWABACH TEST. As in the Rinne test, the tuning fork is held against the mastoid process until the patient is unable to perceive any sound. The examiner then places the tuning fork over his own mastoid bone and thus compares his bone conduction to that of the patient. If the examiner hears the tuning fork after the patient no longer hears it, a sensorineural hearing loss is suspected.

In summary, in sensorineural hearing loss:

1. The Weber test lateralizes to the normal ear.
2. The Rinne test is positive (air conduction is better than bone conduction).
3. The Schwabach test demonstrates that the patient's bone conduction is worse than the examiner's.

In conductive hearing loss:

1. The Weber test lateralizes to the diseased ear.
2. The Rinne test is negative (bone conduction is better than air conduction).
3. The Schwabach test is normal or prolonged (the patient may hear the tuning fork longer than the examiner).

Vertigo and Vestibular Function. The clinical evaluation of the patient affected with dizziness or vertigo focuses on four areas [6, 12, 18, 19, 48, 49]:

DEFINITION OF CHARACTERISTICS OF SYMPTOMS. *Dizziness* is an imprecise term meaning different things to different people (e.g., lightheadedness, faintness, disequilibrium, disturbance of consciousness, true vertigo). *Vertigo* is a hallucination of motion that may be subjective (the patient feels that he is spinning) or objective (the environment seems to be spinning). Vegetative symptoms such as nausea, vomiting, pallor, and sweating are frequently present in patients affected with vertigo.

ASSOCIATED AUDITORY SYMPTOMS. If unilateral hearing loss occurs with vertigo, primary ear disease is suggested. A feeling of "fullness" in the ear may occur with external middle or inner ear pathology. *Autophony,* or the perception of the reverberation of the patient's own voice in the affected ear, occurs only with external or middle ear disease.

Tinnitus (ringing in the ears), which is associated with vertigo, may be paroxysmal or continuous but has little localizing significance; however, tinnitus is more frequently noted with peripheral than central lesions. Low roaring tinnitus suggests cochlear hydrops, whereas high-pitched tinnitus suggests presbyacusis or an acoustic tumor. Pulsatile tinnitus is usually a subjective appreciation of the patient's normal heartbeat but may occur with glomus jugulare tumors and intracranial or cervical aneurysms.

ASSOCIATED SYMPTOMS SUGGESTING CENTRAL NEUROLOGIC DYSFUNCTION. Symptoms and signs suggesting brainstem, cerebellar, or cranial nerve dysfunction localize the responsible lesion to the central pathways. Associated auditory hallucinations suggest temporal lobe disease.

ETIOLOGIC SEARCH. An accurate history should investigate for associated viral infection, head or cervical trauma, toxin or drug exposure, alcohol abuse, endocrine and metabolic diseases, cardiovascular disease, or previous syphilitic infection (congenital or acquired).

The *physical examination* in the vertiginous patient should include a complete otologic and audiologic evaluation and a complete neurologic evaluation. This examination should stress the following:

1. Blood pressure evaluation in both arms (including tests for postural changes), with a search for bruits and cardiac arrhythmias.
2. A detailed cranial nerve examination, including tuning fork evaluation of hearing.
3. Cerebellar testing, especially evaluation for nystagmus, gait and station abnormalities, and ataxia.
4. Provocative tests designed to induce symptoms: postural changes, head turning, sudden turn while walking, hyperventilation, Nylén-Bárány test, Valsalva maneuver, and caloric testing.

LOCALIZATION OF LESIONS
CAUSING DEAFNESS AND VERTIGO

Localization of Lesions
Causing Sensorineural Deafness

CEREBRAL LESIONS. The human auditory cortex is located in the superior temporal gyrus near the Sylvian fissure (areas 41, 42, and 22 of Brodmann). This area is subdivided into an auditosensory region (area 41) and an auditopsychic region (areas 42 and 22).

Lesions of the auditory cortex do not lead to complete deafness even when they are bilateral. A slight hearing impairment may be seen with unilateral lesions, but this impairment is more a difficulty in localizing sounds. Unilateral dominant posterior temporal lesions or bilateral temporal lesions affecting Heschl's gyri may cause *pure word deafness,* an inability to understand spoken language despite normal auditory acuity; reading, writing, and naming are preserved [2, 24, 34].

Irritative lesions of the temporal cortex may result in subjective auditory hallucinations that may be simple (e.g., tinnitus) or complex (e.g., voices). The auditory sensations are most often referred to the contralateral ear and are more frequent with irritation of areas 42 and 22 than with irritation of area 41. Temporal lobe seizures may start with acoustic auras, which are often associated with vertiginous auras, suggesting an acoustic cortex locus of origin for the epileptiform phenomenon [10, 27, 32, 33].

BRAINSTEM LESIONS. In general, because of the binaural representation of the ascending auditory tracts above the level of the cochlear nuclei, lesions of the brainstem that affect the auditory pathways usually do not cause hearing impairment. Bilateral hearing loss may occur with severe bilateral brainstem lesions and has been described with lesions of the trapezoid bodies, pons, midbrain tegmentum, and medial geniculate bodies. Associated brainstem findings dominate the clinical picture. Neurologic localization may be assisted by brainstem auditory evoked potentials [13, 28, 40, 46].

PERIPHERAL NERVE LESIONS AND THE CEREBELLOPONTINE ANGLE SYNDROME. Peripheral cochlear nerve lesions produce partial or complete deafness, often associated with ipsilateral tinnitus. This deafness is most prominent for high-frequency tones and may be due to trauma (e.g., basal skull fracture), infections (e.g., syphilis, bacterial infections), drugs (e.g., streptomycin, neomycin), aneurysms of the anterior inferior cerebellar artery, or tumors (e.g., schwannoma or meningioma). Nearby cranial nerves (e.g., cranial nerves V, VI, VII, IX, X, and XI) may be affected by these processes, and their affection assists in localizing the lesion clinically.

The *cerebellopontine angle syndrome* is commonly caused by an acoustic neurinoma (schwannoma) [25], which typically originates in the vestibular portion of the eighth cranial nerve. These tumors usually show evidence of insidious cochlear nerve dysfunction characterized by unilateral high-pitched tinnitus and progressive sensorineural hearing loss with early loss of speech discrimination. In a small percentage of cases (less than 10%) deafness may occur suddenly, most likely due to intratumoral hemorrhage or internal auditory artery occlusion. With vestibular nerve involvement, vertigo and progressive unsteadiness develop. As the tumor grows, the internal auditory meatus progressively widens (on radiographs), and complete ipsilateral nerve deafness ensues (the tinnitus subsiding as the deafness progresses). With medial tumor growth, the neighboring cranial nerves are affected, and eventual brainstem and ipsilateral cerebellar compromise occurs with very large tumors. Eventually, hydrocephalus or signs of increased intracranial pressure (headache, nausea, vomiting, papilledema) develop.

The dysfunction of the neighboring cranial nerves that occurs varies according to the direction of growth of the acoustic tumor. With anterior extension, the trigeminal nerve (facial numbness, paroxysmal facial pain, depressed ipsilateral corneal reflex) and abducens nerve (horizontal diplopia) are compromised. With posteroinferior tumoral extension, cranial nerves IX and X (dysphagia, absent pharyngeal reflexes, vocal cord paralysis) and cranial nerve XI (ipsilateral sternocleidomastoid and trapezius paresis) are affected. In either case, the facial nerve is usually involved, resulting in facial paresis, loss of taste on the ipsilateral anterior two-thirds of the tongue, and, rarely, hemifacial spasm [3, 14, 16, 24, 26, 35, 36, 37, 44].

The Localization of Lesions Causing Vertigo. The localization of lesions causing vertigo may be approached by dividing these etiologies into three general categories: *peripheral* causes (vestibular labyrinth disease), *central* causes (dysfunction of the vestibular connections), and *systemic* causes (e.g., endocrine and metabolic diseases) [17, 19, 22, 48].

PERIPHERAL CAUSES OF VERTIGO. Peripheral vestibular syndromes are usually of short duration and are characterized by severe, often paroxysmal, vertigo that may be accompanied by auditory dysfunction (tinnitus and hearing loss). Nystagmus is often present and is characteristically unidirectional (fast-phase "away from" the side of the lesion) and horizontorotatory (never vertical or exclusively rotatory). This nystagmus is inhibited by visual fixation. The subjective environmental twirl, pastpointing, deviation of the outstretched hands, and Romberg fall are toward the slow phase of the nystagmus (toward the side of the lesion). The peripheral vestibular syndrome is thus *complete* (has all of the clinical elements of vestibular dysfunction—i.e., vertigo, nystagmus, deviation of the outstretched hands, Romberg sign, and so on) and *congruent* (all the "slow deviations" are toward the same side—i.e., ipsilateral to the responsible lesion).

POSITIONAL VERTIGO. Positional vertigo was first described by Bárány and is usually of a peripheral type (rarely secondary to central lesions). Most cases (50%) are "idiopathic" and are possibly due to degeneration of the macula of the otolith organ, but other causes of this syndrome include trauma, infection, fistula, vertebral artery occlusion, and rarely, cerebellar tumor. Paroxysmal vertigo in certain head positions is the most common complaint; the patient is asymptomatic between bouts. The Nylén-Bárány maneuver (briskly tilting the patient's head backward and turning it 45 degrees to one side) allows a differentiation between a peripheral and a central origin for positional vertigo, as follows:

With *peripheral lesions,* severe vertigo and nystagmus appear several seconds after the head position is changed (latency of response). This nystagmus is usually rotatory, with the fast component beating toward the diseased ear. The vertigo and nystagmus then fatigue and abate within 10 seconds after appearance (fatigability), and when the patient is rapidly brought back to a sitting position, vertigo recurs and nystagmus may occur in the opposite direction (rebound). With repetition of the maneuver, the symptoms and nystagmus become progressively less severe (habituation), and the reproducibility of the abnormalities is inconstant.

If a *central lesion* causes positional vertigo, vertigo and nystagmus begin immediately on changing the head position (no latency of response), and the response does not fatigue or demonstrate habituation with repetitive trials. The duration of the vertigo is usually no longer than 60 seconds, and the vertigo induced is relatively mild (vs. that seen with a peripheral lesion). The nystagmus is more often direction-changing than fixed and may be produced by more than one head position.

PERIPHERAL VESTIBULOPATHY. This term (recommended by Drachman [19]) describes acute or recurrent episodes of vertigo caused by extramedullary disorders of the vestibular system when precise knowledge of the site or nature of the responsible lesion is unknown. This term encompasses such entities as vestibular neuronitis, acute labyrinthitis, epidemic vertigo, and viral labyrinthitis.

Vestibular neuronitis is characterized by acute and severe vertigo, almost always associated with nausea and vomiting and lasting 7 to 10 days; it is not associated with cochlear symptoms or other neurologic dysfunction. This vertigo is generally unrelated to head position and may rarely be recurrent.

Acute labyrinthitis is similar to vestibular neuronitis except that there is associated tinnitus and hearing loss. This syndrome may follow systemic or ear infections (i.e., bacterial or viral labyrinthitis) or may occur in association with the use of ototoxic drugs such as aminoglycosides and diuretics (i.e., toxic labyrinthitis).

MENIERE'S DISEASE. This syndrome consists of episodic vertigo, fluctuating sensorineural hearing loss, tinnitus, and a sense of pressure or fullness in the ear. Meniere's disease is unilateral in 90 percent of cases and is "idiopathic" in 80 percent of patients (possibly due to an increased volume of endolymphatic fluid leading to distention of the semicircular canals—"endolymphatic hydrops"). Other etiologies for this syndrome include congenital syphilis, hypothyroidism, hyperlipidemia, diabetes, labyrinthine otosclerosis, dysproteinemia, labyrinthine concussion, and acoustic neurinoma [41, 42].

Patients with Meniere's disease (usual age of onset is 30–40 years) usually complain initially of severe fluctuating and episodic vertigo that is often associated with nausea and vomiting. However, tinnitus and hearing loss may precede the vertigo by months or years. Individual attacks last 30 minutes to 2 hours, and in the interim the patient is initially symptom-free. Eventually there is progressive deterioration of hearing, initially primarily for low tones, which culminates in complete deafness.

Two subtypes of Meniere's disease are recognized—*cochlear Meniere's disease* (in which vertigo is absent) and *vestibular Meniere's disease* (in which vertigo is prominent, but hearing loss and tinnitus are absent in the early stages). A variant of Meniere's disease, called *crisis of Tumarkin*, is characterized by acute episodes of vertigo during which muscle tone and power are lost and the patient falls to the ground without compromise of consciousness.

VERTIGO SECONDARY TO MIDDLE EAR DISEASE. Vertigo of the peripheral type may occur with acute or chronic ear infection, cholesteatoma, and congenital or acquired syphilis. Congenital syphilis should be suspected in patients presenting with the symptoms of bilateral Meniere's syndrome.

VERTIGO SECONDARY TO TRAUMA. Head or cervical trauma may result in vertigo owing to inner ear concussion, fracture of the temporal bone (damaging the eighth nerve or labyrinth), or "whiplash" injury.

CENTRAL CAUSES OF VERTIGO. In contrast to the peripheral vestibular syndrome, the central vestibular syndrome is usually prolonged (permanent or chronic) rather than of short duration. Signs and symptoms of neighboring structures secondary to dysfunction of the central brainstem and cerebellar structures are usually present, whereas auditory symptoms are less frequent. Vertigo in central syndromes is usually less severe, ill-defined, and continuous in nature; the associated nystagmus is bidirectional or unidirectional, may be exclusively horizontal, rotatory, or vertical, and is not altered by visual fixation. The directions of subjective environmental rotation, past-pointing, deviation of the outstretched hands, and Romberg fall are variable and are not significantly altered by changes in head position. The central vestibular syndrome is thus incomplete or partial (does not always consist of all elements of vestibular dysfunction—i.e., it may lack nystagmus, vertigo, or even deviation of the outstretched hands or body) and *incongruent* (the nystagmus and tonic deviations are variable in direction).

VASCULAR CAUSES OF THE CENTRAL VESTIBULAR SYNDROME. These include [4, 5, 15, 21, 23, 47]:

Transient Ischemic Attacks (TIAs). Vertigo may be a prominent symptom during a vertebrobasilar TIA. However, TIA is an unlikely cause for vertigo and dizziness unless other symptoms (diplopia, dysarthria, perioral paresthesias, drop attacks, visual field defects, and so on) are associated.

Labyrinthine Stroke. Labyrinthine stroke may occur secondary to thrombosis of the internal auditory artery or one of its branches. Vertigo, tinnitus, nausea, and vomiting result (mimicking other labyrinthine disorders), and, if the cochlear branch is also involved, deafness may occur.

Wallenberg Syndrome (Lateral Medullary Lesion). With lateral medullary infarction (usually due to vertebral artery or posterior inferior cerebellar artery occlusion), vertigo, nausea, vomiting, and nystagmus occur owing to vestibular nuclei damage. This vestibular involvement is superimposed on the other manifestations of this syndrome (see Chap. 14).

Other vascular causes of vertigo include basilar migraine, the subclavian steal syndrome, and cerebellar infarction or hemorrhage.

MULTIPLE SCLEROSIS. Vertigo is the presenting symptom in 7 to 10 percent of multiple sclerosis patients. This etiology for vertigo should be considered only after documentation of disseminated central nervous system lesions and a history of remissions and exacerbations of neurologic signs and symptoms.

CEREBELLOPONTINE ANGLE TUMOR. Vertigo is not a prominent symptom with cerebellopontine angle tumors but may be superimposed on the more common findings of slowly progressive hearing loss, tinnitus, imbalance, and other cranial nerve or cerebellar abnormalities.

VESTIBULAR EPILEPSY. Rarely episodic vertigo may be the sole manifestation of a seizure disorder, especially "temporal lobe" seizures. Other temporal lobe irritative phenomena (e.g., staring spells, automatisms, auditory hallucinations, episodes of deja-vu or jamais-vu) should be sought to confirm this as an etiology for vertiginous symptoms.

SYSTEMIC CAUSES OF DIZZINESS AND VERTIGO. Various systemic conditions may affect peripheral or central vestibular structures to produce dizziness or vertigo. These include:

CARDIOVASCULAR DISEASE. Arrhythmias, aortic stenosis, conges-

198

tive heart failure, cardiomyopathies, carotid sinus hypersensitivity, and other valvular lesions may be associated with dizziness and syncope.

HEMATOLOGIC DISORDERS. Polycythemia, anemia, and hyperviscosity syndromes may be associated with dizziness.

HYPOGLYCEMIA. Dizziness or faintness 30 to 40 minutes after a meal may be secondary to hypoglycemia.

HYPOTHYROIDISM. Hypothyroidism may be associated with episodic vertigo, sensorineural hearing loss, tinnitus, and cerebellar ataxia.

HYPERVENTILATION SYNDROME. Hyperventilation may account for episodes of lightheadedness that are frequently associated with circumoral and digital paresthesias.

MULTIPLE SENSORY DEFICITS. Dizziness in older patients (especially elderly diabetics) may result from a combination of sensory deficits including visual impairment, neuropathy, vestibular dysfunction, and cervical spondylosis. This dizziness is especially prominent during ambulation, especially when turning corners.

DRUGS. Dizziness is a common side effect of many drugs including analgesics, antiarrhythmics, anticonvulsants, antiinflammatory drugs, antibiotics (especially aminoglycosides), diuretics, and sedatives.

OCULAR DISORDERS. Vertigo and dizziness may occur in association with glaucoma, extraocular muscle paresis, the use of strong corrective lenses, and refractive abnormalities.

PSYCHIATRIC DISORDERS (PSYCHOGENIC DIZZINESS). Subjective dizziness (unassociated with hyperventilation) may occur with anxiety, depression, conversion reactions, and other psychiatric disturbances [45].

REFERENCES

1. Anson, B. J., Harper, D. G., and Winch, T. R. The vestibular system. Anatomic considerations. *Arch. Otolaryngol.* 85:497, 1967.
2. Antonelli, A., and Calearo, A. Further investigations on cortical deafness. *Acta Otolaryngol.* 66:97, 1968.
3. Bebin, J. Pathophysiology of Acoustic Tumors. *In* House, W. F., and Luetje, C. M. (Eds.). *Acoustic Tumors: Diagnosis.* Baltimore: University Park Press, 1979. Pp. 45–83.
4. Bergan, J. J., et al. Vascular implications of vertigo. *Arch. Otolaryngol.* 85:78, 1967.
5. Blau, J. N., and Spillane, J. A. Vertebro-basilar insufficiency and the ENT surgeon with an approach to the giddy patient. *Clin. Otolaryngol.* 6:73, 1981.
6. Brandt, T., and Daroff, R. B. The multisensory physiological and pathological vertigo syndromes. *Ann. Neurol.* 7:195, 1980.
7. Brodal, A. *Neurological Anatomy in Relation to Clinical Medicine* (2nd ed.). New York: Oxford University Press, 1975. Pp. 488–508.
8. Brodal, A. *Neurological Anatomy in Relation to Clinical Medicine* (2nd ed.). New York: Oxford University Press, 1975. Pp. 374–397.

9. Bocca, E., Calearo, A., and Cassinari, V. A new method for testing hearing in temporal lobe tumors. *Acta Otolaryngol.* 44:219, 1951.
10. Bocca, E., et al. Testing "cortical" hearing in temporal lobe tumors. *Acta Otolaryngol.* 45:298, 1955.
11. Calearo, C., and Antonelli, A. R. Audiometric findings in brainstem lesions. *Acta Otolaryngol.* 66:305, 1968.
12. Cawthorne, T., et al. Vestibular Syndromes and Vertigo. *In* Vinkin, P. S., and Bruyn, G. W. (Eds.). *Handbook of Clinical Neurology,* Vol. 2. Amsterdam: North-Holland Pub. Co., 1969. Pp. 358–391.
13. Chladek, V. Audiometric diagnosis of brainstem lesions. *Excerpta Med.* 11:22, 1969.
14. Crabtree, J. A., and Gardner, G. Radiographic Findings in Cerebellopontine Angle Tumors. *In* House, W. F., and Luetje, E. M. (Eds.). *Acoustic Tumors: Diagnosis.* Baltimore: University Park Press, 1972. Pp. 241–252.
15. Currier, R. D., Giles, C. L., and DeJong, R. N. Some comments on Wallenberg's lateral medullary syndrome. *Neurology* 11:778, 1961.
16. Cushing, H. *Intracranial Tumors.* Springfield, Ill.: Charles C Thomas, 1937.
17. Daroff, R. B. Evaluation of Dizziness and Vertigo. *In* Glaser, J. S. (Ed.). *Neuroophthalmology Symposium,* Vol. 9. St. Louis: C.V. Mosby, 1977. Pp. 39–54.
18. Dix, M. R. Modern tests of vestibular function, with special reference to their value in clinical practice. *Br. Med. J.* 270:317, 1969.
19. Drachman, D. A., and Hart, C. W. An approach to the dizzy patient. *Neurology* 22:323, 1972.
20. Eichel, B. S., Hedgecock, L. D., and Williams, H. L. A review of the literature on the audiologic aspect of neuro-otologic diagnosis. *Laryngoscope* 76:1, 1966.
21. Fields, W. S. Arteriography in the differential diagnosis of vertigo. *Arch. Otolaryngol.* 85:555, 1967.
22. Finestone, A. J. (Ed.). *Evaluation and Clinical Management of Dizziness and Vertigo.* Boston: John Wright Pub., 1982.
23. Fisher, C. M. Vertigo in cerebrovascular disease. *Arch. Otolaryngol.* 85:529, 1967.
24. Gilroy, J., and Lynn, G. E. Neuro-audiological abnormalities in patients with temporal lobe tumors. *J. Neurol. Sci.* 17:167, 1972.
25. Harner, S. G., and Laws, E. R. Diagnosis of acoustic neuroma. *Neurosurgery* 9:373, 1981.
26. Hart, R. G., and Davenport, J. Diagnosis of acoustic neuroma. *Neurosurgery* 9:450, 1981.
27. Heilman, K. M., Hammer, L. C., and Wilder, B. J. An audiometric defect in temporal lobe dysfunction. *Neurology* 23:384, 1973.
28. Jergen, J., and Jerger, S. Auditory findings in brainstem disorders. *Arch. Otolaryngol.* 99:342, 1974.
29. Ludman, H. Assessing deafness (ABC of ENT). *Br. Med. J.* 282:207, 1981.
30. Ludman, H. Deafness in adults (ABC of ENT). *Br. Med. J.* 282:128, 1981.
31. Ludman, H. Deafness in childhood (ABC of ENT). *Br. Med. J.* 282:381, 1981.
32. Lynn, G. E., et al. Neuro-audiological correlates in cerebral hemisphere lesions: Temporal and parietal lobe tumors. *Audiology* 11:115, 1972.
33. Lynn, G. E., and Gilroy, J. Neuro-audiological abnormalities in patients with temporal lobe tumors. *J. Neurol. Sci.* 17:167, 1972.
34. Lynn, G. E., and Gilroy, J. Central Aspects of Audition. *In* Northern, J. L. (Ed.). *Hearing Disorders.* Boston: Little, Brown, 1976. Pp. 102–116.

35. Marks, H. W. Acoustic neuroma: Experience with clinical diagnosis. *South. Med. J.* 75:985, 1982.
36. Mazurowski, W., Kus, J., and Wislawski, J. Clinical manifestations of cerebellopontine angle tumors. *Pol. Med. J.* 9:449, 1970.
37. Nedzelski, J., and Tator, C. Other cerebellopontine angle (nonacoustic neuroma) tumors. *J. Otolaryngol.* 11:248, 1982.
38. Noback, C. R., and Demarest, R. J. *The Human Nervous System. Basic Principles of Neurobiology* (3rd ed.). New York: McGraw Hill, 1981. Pp. 341–368.
39. Northern, J. L. (Ed.). *Hearing Disorders.* Boston: Little, Brown, 1976. Pp. 3–19.
40. Parker, W., Decker, R. L., and Richards, N. G. Auditory functions and lesions of the pons. *Arch. Otolaryngol.* 87:228, 1968.
41. Pulec, J. L. Meniere's disease: Results of a 2½ year study of the etiology, natural history and results of treatment. *Laryngoscope* 82:1703, 1972.
42. Pulec, J. L. Meniere's disease: Etiology, natural history, and results of treatment. *Otolaryngol. Clin. North Am.* 6:25, 1973.
43. Report on Workshop. Neuroanatomy of the auditory system. *Arch. Otolaryngol.* 98:397, 1973.
44. Revilla, A. G. Differential diagnosis of tumors of the cerebellopontine recess. *Bull. Johns Hopkins Hosp.* 83:183, 1948.
45. Schmidt, R. T. Personality and fainting. *J. Psychosom. Res.* 19:21, 1975.
46. Shapiro, I. Progression of auditory signs in pontine glioma. *Laryngoscope* 79:201, 1969.
47. Troost, B. T. Dizziness and vertigo in vertebrobasilar disease. Part II. Central causes and vertebrobasilar disease. *Current Concepts of Cerebrovascular Disease—Stroke* 14(6):25, 1979.
48. Troost, B. T. Vertigo. *Neurol. Neurosurg. Wkly. Update* 2(5):38, 1979.
49. Wolfson, R. J. Vertigo. *Otolaryngol. Clin. North Am.* 6(1):1, 1973.

Chapter 11

THE LOCALIZATION OF LESIONS AFFECTING CRANIAL NERVES IX AND X (THE GLOSSOPHARYNGEAL AND VAGUS NERVES)

Paul W. Brazis

ANATOMY OF CRANIAL NERVE IX
(GLOSSOPHARYNGEAL NERVE)

The *glossopharyngeal nerve* contains motor, sensory, and parasympathetic fibers. The nerve emerges from the medulla dorsal to the inferior olive in close relation with cranial nerve X (the vagus nerve) and the bulbar fibers of cranial nerve XI (the spinal accessory nerve) [4, 17, 18]. These three nerves then travel together through the jugular foramen. Within or distal to this foramen, the glossopharyngeal nerve widens at the *superior* and the *petrous ganglia* and then descends on the lateral side of the pharynx, passing between the internal carotid artery and the internal jugular vein. The nerve winds around the lower border of the *stylopharyngeus muscle* (which it supplies) and then penetrates the pharyngeal constrictor muscles to reach the base of the tongue.

The motor fibers originate from the rostral nucleus ambiguus and innervate the *stylopharyngeus muscle* (a pharyngeal elevator) and (with the vagus nerve) the *constrictor muscles of the pharynx.*

The *sensory fibers* carried in the glossopharyngeal nerve include taste afferents supplying the posterior third of the tongue and pharynx and general visceral afferents from the posterior third of the tongue, tonsillar region, posterior palatal arch, soft palate, nasopharynx, and tragus of the ear. By way of the tympanic branch of the glossopharyngeal nerve *(Jacobson's nerve)*, sensation is supplied to the tympanic membrane, eustachian tube, and mastoid region. Taste afferents [14] and general visceral afferent fibers have their cell bodies in the petrous ganglion and terminate mainly in the nucleus of the solitary tract (the rostral terminating fibers convey taste, and the caudal terminating fibers convey general visceral sensation); exteroceptive afferents have their cell bodies in the superior and petrous ganglia and terminate in the spinal nucleus of the trigeminal nerve. The glossopharyngeal nerve also carries chemoreceptive and baroreceptive afferents from the carotid body and carotid sinus, respectively, by way of the *carotid sinus nerve.*

The *parasympathetic fibers* carried in the glossopharyngeal nerve originate in the inferior salivatory nucleus, located in the periventricular gray matter of the rostral medulla, at the superior pole of the rostral nucleus of cranial nerve X. These parasympathetic preganglionic fibers leave the glossopharyngeal nerve at the petrous ganglion and travel by way of the *tympanic nerve* (coursing in the petrous bone) and the *lesser superficial petrosal nerve* to reach the *otic ganglion* (just below the foramen ovale), where they synapse. The postganglionic fibers then travel by way of the *auriculotemporal branch* of the trigeminal nerve carrying secretory and vasodilatory fibers to the *parotid gland.*

CLINICAL EVALUATION OF CRANIAL NERVE IX

Motor Function. Stylopharyngeal function [8] is difficult to assess. Motor paresis may be negligible with glossopharyngeal nerve lesions, although mild dysphagia may occur and the palatal arch may be somewhat lower at rest on the side of glossopharyngeal injury. (However, the palate elevates symmetrically with vocalization).

Sensory Function. The integrity of taste sensation may be tested over the posterior third of the tongue [14] and is lost ipsilaterally with nerve lesions. Sensation (pain, soft touch) is tested on the soft palate, posterior third of the tongue, tonsillar regions, and pharyngeal wall. These areas may be ipsilaterally anesthetic with glossopharyngeal lesions.

Reflex Function. The *pharyngeal* or *gag reflex* is tested [8] by stimulating the posterior pharyngeal wall, tonsillar area, or base of the tongue. The response is tongue retraction associated with elevation and constriction of the pharyngeal musculature. The *palatal reflex* consists of elevation of the soft palate and ipsilateral deviation of the uvula with stimulation of the soft palate. The afferent arcs of these reflexes probably involve the glossopharyngeal nerve, whereas the efferent arcs involve both the glossopharyngeal and vagus nerves. Unilateral absence of these reflexes is seen with glossopharyngeal nerve lesions.

Autonomic Function. Salivary secretion (from the parotid gland) may be decreased, absent, and occasionally increased with glossopharyngeal lesions, but these changes are difficult to demonstrate without specialized quantitative studies.

LOCALIZATION OF LESIONS AFFECTING
THE GLOSSOPHARYNGEAL NERVE

Lesions affecting the glossopharyngeal nerve usually also involve the vagus, and therefore syndromes affecting both nerves are much more common than nerve lesions occurring in relative isolation.

Supranuclear Lesions. Supranuclear lesions, if unilateral, result in no neurologic deficit because of bilateral corticobulbar input to the nucleus ambiguus. However, bilateral corticobulbar lesions (pseudo-bulbar palsy) result in severe dysphagia along with other pseudo-bulbar signs (e.g., pathologic laughter and crying, spastic tongue, explosive dysarthria). With stimulation, the gag reflex may be depressed or markedly exaggerated, resulting in severe retching and even vomiting.

Nuclear and Intramedullary Lesions. These lesions include syringobulbia, demyelinating disease, vascular disease, motor neuron disease, and malignancy. Such lesions commonly involve other cranial nerves, especially the vagus, and other brainstem structures (e.g., Wallenberg syndrome) and are thus localized by "the company they keep."

Extramedullary Lesions

CEREBELLOPONTINE ANGLE SYNDROME. The glossopharyngeal nerve may be injured [10] by lesions, especially acoustic tumors, occurring in the cerebellopontine angle. Here there may be glossopharyngeal involvement associated with tinnitus, deafness, and vertigo (cranial nerve VIII), facial sensory abnormalities (cranial nerve V), and occasionally other cranial nerve or cerebellar involvement.

JUGULAR FORAMEN SYNDROME (VERNET'S SYNDROME). Lesions at the jugular foramen, especially glomus tumors and basal skull fractures, injure cranial nerves IX, X, and XI, which travel through this foramen. This syndrome (Vernet's syndrome) consists of:

1. Ipsilateral trapezius and sternocleidomastoid paresis and atrophy (cranial nerve XI).
2. Dysphasia, dysphagia, depressed gag reflex, and palatal droop on the affected side associated with homolateral vocal cord paralysis, loss of taste on the posterior third of the tongue on the involved side, and anesthesia of the ipsilateral posterior third of the tongue, soft palate, uvula, pharynx, and larynx (cranial nerves IX and X).

LESIONS WITHIN THE RETROPHARYNGEAL AND RETROPAROTID SPACE. The glossopharyngeal nerve may be injured in the retropharyngeal or retroparotid space by neoplasms (e.g., nasopharyngeal carcinoma), abscesses, adenopathy, aneurysms, trauma, or surgical procedures (e.g., carotid endarterectomy). Resulting syndromes include the Collet-Sicard syndrome (affecting cranial nerves IX, X, XI, and XII) and Villaret's syndrome (affecting cranial nerves IX, X, XI, and XII, the sympathetic chain, and occasionally cranial nerve VII). The glossopharyngeal nerve may rarely be damaged in isolation by retropharyngeal or retroparotid space lesions resulting in a "pure" glossopharyngeal syndrome (mild dysphagia, depressed gag reflex, mild palatal droop, loss of taste on the posterior third of the tongue, glossopharyngeal distribution anesthesia).

Glossopharyngeal (Vagoglossopharyngeal) Neuralgia. Glossopharyngeal neuralgia [3, 6, 16, 20, 21] refers to pain (usually stabbing, sharp, and paroxysmal) located in the field of sensory distribution of the glosso-pharyngeal or vagus nerves. Patients usually describe an abrupt, severe pain in the throat or ear that lasts seconds to minutes and is often trig-gered by chewing, coughing, talking, swallowing, and eating certain foods (e.g., highly spiced foods). The pain may occasionally be more persistent and have a dull aching or burning quality. Other areas (e.g., larynx, tongue, tonsils, face, jaws) may also be affected by the pain, which is rarely bilateral (occurs in 2% of patients affected).

The attacks of glossopharyngeal pain may occasionally be associated with coughing paroxysms, excessive salivation, hoarseness, and, rarely, syncope [11, 19, 20]. The syncopal episodes may possibly result from re-flex bradycardia and asystole due to stimulation of the tractus solitarius and dorsal motor nucleus of the vagus by impulses originating in glosso-pharyngeal afferents.

Vagoglossopharyngeal neuralgia is often "idiopathic" and is thought to be possibly related to ephaptic excitation of the glossopharyngeal-vagus nerves; however, lesions in the posterior fossa or anywhere along the peripheral distribution of the glossopharyngeal nerve (e.g., tumor, infection, trauma) may also cause the syndrome. Multiple sclerosis is an extremely rare etiology for this syndrome (unlike its relatively common association with trigeminal neuralgia).

ANATOMY OF
CRANIAL NERVE X (VAGUS NERVE)

The *vagus nerve*, like the glossopharyngeal, contains motor, sensory, and parasympathetic nerve fibers [4, 7, 18]. The rootlets of the vagus nerve emerge from the lateral medulla dorsal to the inferior olive in close asso-ciation with the glossopharyngeal nerve. These vagal rootlets form a sin-gle trunk that leaves the skull by way of the *jugular foramen* in a dural sheath that also contains the spinal accessory nerve. Within, or just infe-rior to, the jugular foramen are the two vagal ganglia—the *jugular* (general somatic afferent) and the *nodose* (special and general visceral af-ferent). Between the two ganglia, the *auricular ramus (nerve of Arnold)* of the vagus nerve is given off; this branch then traverses the mastoid pro-cess and innervates the skin of the concha of the external ear. At this point the vagus also gives off the *meningeal ramus*, which runs to the dura mater of the posterior fossa, and the *pharyngeal ramus*, which forms the pharyngeal plexus with the glossopharyngeal nerve and which sends motor fibers to the muscles of the pharynx and soft palate (except the stylopharyngeus and tensor veli palatini muscles). The *superior laryn-geal nerve* arises from the vagus near the nodose ganglion and divides in-to a predominantly motor *external ramus* (to the cricothyroid muscle) and an *internal ramus* (which pierces the thyrohyoid membrane and sends sensory fibers to the larynx).

In the neck, the vagus nerve proper descends within a sheath common to the internal carotid artery and internal jugular vein. Within the neck, the vagus gives off the *cardiac rami,* which follow the carotids downward to the aorta and contribute fibers to the cardiac plexus. At the root of the neck, the *recurrent laryngeal nerves* are given off and pursue different courses on the two sides. The right recurrent laryngeal nerve bends upward behind the subclavian artery to ascend in the tracheoesophageal sulcus, whereas the left recurrent laryngeal nerve passes beneath the aortic arch to attain this sulcus. The recurrent laryngeal nerves then divide into anterior and posterior rami, which supply all of the muscles of the larynx except the cricothyroid muscle (supplied by the external ramus of the superior laryngeal nerve).

The vagus nerve enters the thorax, on the right side crossing over the subclavian artery and on the left side traveling between the left common carotid and subclavian arteries. The right nerve then passes downward near the brachiocephalic trunk and trachea and behind the right brachiocephalic vein and superior vena cava to the posterior lung root. The left nerve travels between the left common carotid and subclavian artery, passes over the aortic arch, and reaches the left lung root. In the posterior mediastinum both nerves send fibers to the pulmonary and esophageal plexuses and then enter the abdomen by way of the esophageal opening of the diaphragm (the left nerve in front of the esophagus, the right nerve behind it). The vagi terminate by innervating the abdominal viscera.

The *motor fibers* carried in the vagus nerve arise from the dorsal motor nucleus of the vagus and the nucleus ambiguus. The *dorsal motor nucleus of the vagus* is situated on the floor of the fourth ventricle lateral to the hypoglossal nucleus. This nucleus gives rise to preganglionic parasympathetic fibers that innervate the pharynx, esophagus, trachea, bronchi, lungs, heart, stomach, small intestine, ascending and transverse colon, liver, and pancreas. The *nucleus ambiguus* is located in the reticular formation of the medulla medial to the spinal tract and nucleus of the trigeminal nerve. Fibers from this nucleus supply all of the striated musculature of the soft palate, pharynx, and larynx except the tensor veli palatini (cranial nerve V) and stylopharyngeus (cranial nerve IX) muscles. The cortical centers for control of vagal motor function are located in the lower precentral gyri, with supranuclear innervation predominantly crossed but bilateral.

The *sensory fibers* carried in the vagus nerve have their perikarya in the jugular and nodose ganglia. Within the nodose ganglion are cells whose fibers carry *taste sensation* from the epiglottis, hard and soft palates, and pharynx. The axons of these ganglion cells terminate in the *nucleus solitarius* of the medulla. *General visceral sensations* from the oropharynx, larynx, and linings of the thoracic and abdominal viscera have their cells of origin in the nodose ganglion, which also projects to the *nucleus solitarius* (nucleus parasolitarius). *Exteroceptive* sensation from the concha of the ear is carried by the vagus (jugular ganglion) to terminate in the *descending (spinal) nucleus of the trigeminal nerve.*

CLINICAL EVALUATION OF CRANIAL NERVE X

Motor Function. The striated muscle of the soft palate, pharynx, and larynx is innervated by the vagus nerve [8]. The soft palate and uvula are examined at rest and with phonation; with phonation the palate should elevate symmetrically with no uvular deviation. Pharyngeal function [17] is evaluated by observing pharyngeal contraction during phonation and swallowing and by noting the character of the voice, by noting the ease of respirations and cough, and by direct observation of laryngeal movements during laryngoscopy.

With *unilateral* vagal lesions, there is ipsilateral flattening of the palatal arch; with phonation, the ipsilateral palate fails to elevate, and the uvula is retracted toward the nonparalyzed side. Dysphagia and articulation disturbances (a "nasal twang" to the voice) may occur, and during phonation only the normal upper pharynx will be elevated. The ipsilateral vocal cord will assume the cadaveric position (midway between adduction and abduction), and although voluntary coughing may be impaired, there is little dyspnea.

With *bilateral* vagal lesions, the palate droops bilaterally with no palatal movement on phonation. On speaking, air will thus escape from the oral to the nasal cavity, giving the voice a "nasal" quality. Bilateral pharyngeal involvement results in profound dysphagia, more pronounced for liquids, which tend to be diverted into the nasal cavity. The voice is hoarse and weak, coughing is poor or not possible, and respiration is severely embarrassed.

Sensory Function. Sensory function of the vagus nerve cannot be tested adequately because the area of supply overlaps that of other cranial nerves (e.g., the pinna), some structures are inaccessible (e.g., the meninges), and there is difficulty in testing the epiglottis for taste function.

Reflex Function. The afferent limb of the pharyngeal reflex (gag reflex) runs in the glossopharyngeal nerve, and the efferent limb runs in the glossopharyngeal and vagus nerves. Therefore, unilateral vagal lesions will depress the ipsilateral gag reflex by interrupting the efferent arc.

LOCALIZATION OF LESIONS
AFFECTING THE VAGUS NERVE

Supranuclear Lesions. Unilateral cerebral hemispheral lesions (lower precentral gyrus) rarely cause any vagal dysfunction because supranuclear control is bilateral. Rarely, dysphagia may occur with a unilateral precentral lesion [15].

Bilateral upper motor neuron lesions result in *pseudo-bulbar palsy*, in which dysphagia and dysarthria are prominent. The gag reflex may be depressed or exaggerated.

Nuclear Lesions and Lesions Within the Brainstem. Lesions of the nucleus ambiguus may occur with vascular insults (lateral medullary or Wallenberg syndrome), tumors, syringobulbia, motor neuron disease, and inflammatory disease. Nuclear lesions result in ipsilateral palatal, pharyngeal, and laryngeal paralysis that is usually associated with affection of other cranial nerve nuclei, roots, and long tracts. When only the more cephalad portion of the nucleus ambiguus is injured while the more caudal portion is spared, laryngeal function is spared *(palatopharyngeal paralysis of Avellis)* due to the somatotopic organization of this motor nucleus.

Lesions Within the Posterior Fossa. The vagus nerve may be damaged [10] on the portion that extends from its emergence from the medulla to its exit from the jugular foramen. Lesions at this location usually also involve the glossopharyngeal, spinal accessory, and hypoglossal nerves and include primary (e.g., glomus jugulare) and metastatic tumors, infections (e.g., meningitis, otitis), and trauma. The syndromes that occur most commonly include:

Syndrome	Cranial Nerves Involved
Jugular foramen syndrome of Vernet	IX, X, XI
Schmidt syndrome	X, XI
Hughlings Jackson syndrome	X, XI, XII
Collet-Sicard syndrome	IX, X, XI, XII

Lesions Affecting the Vagus Nerve Proper. The trunk of the vagus nerve may be injured in the neck and thorax by tumors, aneurysms of the internal carotid artery, trauma, and enlarged lymph nodes. These injuries result in complete ipsilateral vocal cord paralysis associated with unilateral laryngeal anesthesia.

Lesions of the Superior Laryngeal Nerve. The superior laryngeal nerve [9] may be damaged by trauma, surgery, or tumor. Lesions of this nerve result in few clinical findings because this branch is primarily sensory. However, the cricothyroid muscle is innervated by this branch, and its involvement may result in mild hoarseness with some decrease in voice strength.

Lesions of the Recurrent Laryngeal Nerve. The recurrent laryngeal nerve is susceptible to injury throughout its intrathoracic course by aneurysms of the aortic arch or subclavian artery, enlarged tracheobronchial lymph nodes, mediastinal tumors, and operative damage (e.g., thyroidectomy) [1, 13]. The left recurrent laryngeal nerve is longer than the right and is thus damaged more often.

Unilateral recurrent laryngeal nerve injury results in hoarseness that is often transient. Unilateral paralysis of all laryngeal muscles (except the cricothyroid, which is innervated by the superior laryngeal nerve) results, and on laryngoscopy the paralyzed vocal cord lies near the midline whereas the normal cord comes across to meet it when phonation is attempted. The adductor muscles of the larynx tend to be affected first with peripheral recurrent laryngeal nerve injury (Semon's law).

Bilateral recurrent laryngeal nerve palsies are usually noted after thyroidectomy and are always symptomatic. Bilateral adduction paralysis may produce severe approximation of the vocal cords associated with airway limitation, which often necessitates tracheostomy. Inspiratory stridor and dyspnea on exertion are common. The voice is weak but remains clear; when the cords cannot be brought into contact, aphonia results.

REFERENCES
1. Blackburn, G., and Salmon, L. F. Cord movements after thyroidectomy. *Br. J. Surg.* 48:371, 1960.
2. Blau, J. N., and Kapadia, R. Idiopathic palsy of the recurrent laryngeal nerve: A transient cranial mononeuropathy. *Br. Med. J.* 4:259, 1972.
3. Bohm, E., and Strange, R. R. Glossopharyngeal neuralgia. *Brain* 85:371, 1962.
4. Brodal, A. *Neurological Anatomy in Relation to Clinical Medicine* (3rd ed.). New York: Oxford University Press, 1981. Pp. 46–470.
5. Bulteau, E. The aetiology of bilateral recurrent laryngeal nerve paralysis. *Med. J. Aust.* 2:776, 1973.
6. Chawla, S. C., and Falconer, M. A. Glossopharyngeal and vagal neuralgia. *Br. Med. J.* 3:529, 1967.

7. Davis, J. N., et al. Diseases of the Ninth, Tenth, Eleventh, and Twelfth Cranial Nerves. *In* Dyck, P. J., Thomas, P. K., and Lambert, E. H. (Eds.). *Peripheral Neuropathy.* Philadelphia: W.B. Saunders, 1975. Pp. 614–622.
8. DeJong, R. N. *The Neurologic Examination Incorporating the Fundamentals of Neuroanatomy and Neurophysiology* (4th ed.). Hagerstown, Md.: Harper & Row, 1979. Pp. 225–240.
9. Droulias, C., et al. The superior laryngeal nerve. *Am. Surg.* 42:635, 1976.
10. Fay, T. Observation and results from intracranial section of the glossopharyngeus and vagus nerves in man. *J. Neurol. Psychopathol.* 8:110, 1927.
11. Garretson, H. D., and Elvidge, A. R. Glossopharyngeal neuralgia with asystole and seizures. *Arch. Neurol.* 8:26, 1963.
12. Gorman, J. B., and Woodward, F. D. Bilateral paralysis of the vocal cords: Management of twenty-five cases. *South. Med. J.* 58:34, 1965.
13. Hawe, P., and Lothian, K. R. Recurrent laryngeal nerve injury during thyroidectomy. *Surg. Gynecol. Obstet.* 110:488, 1960.
14. Lewis, D., and Dandy, W. E. The course of the nerve fibers transmitting sensation of taste. *Arch. Surg.* 21:249, 1930.
15. Meadows, J. C. Dysphagia in unilateral cerebral lesions. *J. Neurol. Neurosurg. Psychiat.* 36:853, 1973.
16. Orton, C. I. Glossopharyngeal neuralgia: Its diagnosis and treatment. *Br. J. Oral Surg.* 9:228, 1972.
17. Palmer, E. D. Disorders of the cricopharyngeus muscle: A review. *Gastroenterology* 71:510, 1976.
18. Peele, T. L. *The Neuroanatomic Basis for Clinical Neurology* (3rd ed.). New York: McGraw-Hill, 1977. Pp. 216–224.
19. Riley, H. A., et al. Glossopharyngeal neuralgia initiating or associated with cardiac arrest. *Trans. Am. Neurol. Assoc.* 68:28, 1942.
20. Rushton, J. G., Stevens, J. C., and Miller, R. H. Glossopharyngeal (vagoglossopharyngeal) neuralgia—A study of 217 cases. *Arch. Neurol.* 38:201, 1981.
21. Spurling, R. G., and Grantham, E. G. Glossopharyngeal neuralgia. *South. Med. J.* 35:509, 1942.

Chapter 12

THE LOCALIZATION OF LESIONS
AFFECTING CRANIAL NERVE XI
(THE SPINAL ACCESSORY NERVE)

Paul W. Brazis

ANATOMY OF CRANIAL NERVE XI
(SPINAL ACCESSORY NERVE)

This purely motor nerve [3, 6, 7] arises partly from the medulla *(cranial part or internal ramus)* and partly from the spinal cord *(spinal part or external ramus)*. The *cranial part* arises from cells situated in the caudal part of the nucleus ambiguus of the medulla. Its fibers emerge from the lateral medulla below the roots of the vagus. The *spinal part* arises from a column of cells (the *accessory nucleus*) that extends from the first to the fifth or sixth cervical cord segments in the dorsolateral part of the ventral horn of the spinal cord. These spinal fibers pass through the lateral funiculus of the cord, leaving the cord between the dentate ligament and the dorsal spinal roots. They then unite to form the spinal part and ascend in the subarachnoid space to enter the skull through the *foramen magnum.*

The cranial and spinal parts unite and exit from the skull through the *jugular foramen.* The cranial portion then separates as the *internal ramus* and joins the vagus nerve to supply the pharynx and larynx. The *external ramus* enters the neck between the internal carotid artery and the internal jugular vein. It then penetrates and supplies the *sternocleidomastoid muscle* and emerges near the middle of the posterior border of the muscle. The ramus then crosses the posterior cervical triangle to supply the *trapezius* muscle. In its course the nerve receives branches from the second, third, and fourth cervical nerves. The supranuclear innervation of the trapezius and sternocleidomastoid muscles probably originates in the lower precentral gyrus. The corticobulbar fibers to the trapezius are mainly crossed, and thus one cerebral hemisphere supplies the contralateral trapezius muscle. The course of the fibers controlling the sternocleidomastoid muscle is unknown, but the fibers are thought to terminate mainly in the *ipsilateral* nuclei. Geschwind [5] postulated three alternative pathways for this ipsilateral innervation:

1. The innervation may be truly ipsilateral with fibers descending ipsilaterally from hemisphere to nuclei.
2. The pathway may start in one hemisphere and cross the corpus callosum to the opposite hemisphere, which in turn controls movement on the contralateral side.
3. A double decussation may exist. That is, the pathway originates in one hemisphere, crosses to the opposite side of the brainstem or cord, and then undergoes a decussation back to the side ipsilateral to the hemisphere of origin. This last possibility is supported by the work of Bender et al. [2], which suggests that the pathway to the sternocleidomastoid muscle crosses from the hemisphere to the opposite pons and

then returns to the side of the cord ipsilateral to the hemisphere of origin.

Clinical Evaluation of Cranial Nerve XI Function. The spinal accessory nerve [4, 7] supplies two muscles, the sternocleidomastoid and the trapezius.

STERNOCLEIDOMASTOID MUSCLE. This muscle flexes the head and turns it from side to side. When one muscle contracts, the head is drawn toward the ipsilateral shoulder and rotated so that the occiput is pulled toward the side of the contracting muscle. The right sternocleidomastoid is thus tested by having the patient rotate his head to the left against resistance while the examiner notes the muscle's contraction by inspection and palpation. Both sternocleidomastoid muscles contracting simultaneously will flex the head (tested by exerting pressure on the patient's forehead while the patient attempts anteroflexion of the neck).

TRAPEZIUS MUSCLE. This muscle retracts the head and also elevates, rotates, and retracts the scapula. It also assists in raising the abducted arm above the horizontal. This muscle is tested by having the patient shrug his shoulders against resistance, comparing the two sides by observation and palpation.

LOCALIZATION OF LESIONS
AFFECTING CRANIAL NERVE XI

Lesions of the spinal accessory nerve result in paresis and atrophy of the sternocleidomastoid and the trapezius muscles. Unilateral paresis of the *sternocleidomastoid* does not affect the position of the head at rest. There is weakness in turning the head to the opposite side, and when the patient flexes the head, there is a slight rotation of the head toward the unaffected side because the action of the opposite sternocleidomastoid muscle is unopposed. Bilateral sternocleidomastoid paresis causes weakness of neck flexion with the head tending to fall backward when the patient attempts to stand erect.

Unilateral *trapezius* paresis due to spinal accessory nerve lesions affects predominantly the upper trapezius fibers (the part not supplied by the cervical plexus). The shoulder is lowered on the affected side at rest and the scapula is displaced downward and laterally with its vertebral border slightly winged. There is paresis of shoulder elevation and retraction, and the patient cannot raise the arm above the horizontal after it has been abducted by the supraspinatus and deltoid muscles. Bilateral trapezius paresis results in weakness of neck extension with the head tending to fall forward when the patient attempts to stand erect.

Because the spinal accessory nerve is a purely motor nerve (except for some proprioceptive afferent fibers), nerve lesions result in no sensory disturbance.

Supranuclear Lesions. In hemispheral lesions resulting in contralateral hemiplegia, the trapezius muscle on the side of the hemiplegia is paretic. However, the head is turned *away from* the hemiplegic side, thus indicating paresis of the sternocleidomastoid muscle on the side opposite the hemiplegia (i.e., ipsilateral to the cerebral lesion). Focal seizures, particularly those arising in areas 8 and 19 of the cerebral cortex, cause contraction of the ipsilateral sternocleidomastoid muscle as the head turns to the side contralateral to the epileptogenic lesion (adversive seizures). This further confirms the notion, discussed above, that the sternocleidomastoid muscle receives a strong input from the ipsilateral cerebral hemisphere.

Bender et al. [2] suggest that the pathway for sternocleidomastoid control crosses from the hemisphere to the opposite pons and then returns to the side of the cord ipsilateral to the hemisphere of origin. Geschwind [5] points out that this second decussation may well be located in the decussation of the pyramids and that the side of sternocleidomastoid paresis in relation to the side of the hemiplegia may be of localizing significance. That is, when the hemiplegic side is contralateral to the paretic sternocleidomastoid muscle, a hemispheric lesion is likely, the descending pathway being affected above its double decussation. On the other hand, hemiplegia associated with ipsilateral (to the hemiplegia) sternocleidomastoid paresis implies a lesion at or below the pontine level (i.e., after the first decussation on the descending pathway).

Nuclear Lesions. These relatively rare lesions result in paresis with prominent atrophy and fasciculations that affect the trapezius and sternocleidomastoid muscles. The motor neurons may be preferentially attacked (e.g., motor neuron disease) or may be involved by intraparenchymal high cervical cord–low medulla lesions (e.g., intraparenchymal tumor, syringomyelia). A nuclear localization is suggested by associated medullary or upper cervical cord dysfunction (see Chaps. 4 and 14).

Infranuclear Lesions

LESIONS WITHIN THE SKULL AND FORAMEN MAGNUM. Lesions of the spinal accessory nerve at the foramen magnum and within the skull also involve neighboring cranial nerves IX (glossopharyngeal), X (vagus), and XII (hypoglossal). Thus, the trapezius and sternocleidomastoid paresis is associated with dysphonia and dysphagia, loss of taste on the ipsilateral posterior third of the tongue, ipsilateral palatal paresis, an ipsilateral depressed gag reflex, ipsilateral vocal cord paralysis, and ipsilateral tongue paresis and atrophy (the protruded tongue deviates to the side of the lesion). A mass lesion in this location may also directly compress the upper cervical cord or lower medulla, resulting in "intramedullary" dysfunction. The most common etiologies for spinal accessory nerve involvement within the skull and foramen magnum include extramedullary neoplasms, meningitis, and trauma.

JUGULAR FORAMEN SYNDROME (VERNET'S SYNDROME) AND ASSOCIATED SYNDROMES. The spinal accessory nerve enters the jugular foramen accompanied by cranial nerve IX (glossopharyngeal nerve) and cranial nerve X (vagus nerve). Therefore, lesions at the jugular foramen (e.g., basal skull fracture, tumors, infections) result in a syndrome *(Vernet syndrome)* characterized by:

1. Ipsilateral trapezius and sternocleidomastoid paresis and atrophy.
2. Dysphonia and dysphagia with an absent or depressed gag reflex and a palatal droop on the affected side. The homolateral vocal cord is paralyzed.
3. Loss of taste over the posterior third of the tongue on the involved side.
4. Depressed sensation (e.g., anesthesia) on the posterior third of the tongue, soft palate, uvula, pharynx, and larynx.

Lesions affecting the spinal accessory nerve just after it leaves the skull (in the retroparotid or retropharyngeal space) may also involve cranial nerves IX, X, and XII and the nearby sympathetic chain in variable combinations. The resulting syndromes vary and may also be seen with lesions of multiple cranial nerves within the skull and even with intramedullary lesions. Involvement of all four of the lower cranial nerves (IX through XII) results in the *Collet-Sicard syndrome* (all findings are ipsilateral to the site of injury).

1. Paralysis of the trapezius and sternocleidomastoid (cranial nerve XI)
2. Paralysis of the vocal cord (cranial nerve X) and pharynx (cranial nerve IX)
3. Hemiparalysis of the tongue (cranial nerve XII)
4. Loss of taste on the posterior third of the tongue (cranial nerve IX)

TABLE 12-1. *Syndromes Involving Cranial Nerves IX Through XII*

Syndrome (Eponym)	Nerves Affected	Location of Lesion
Collet-Sicard	Cranial nerves IX, X, XI, XII	Retroparotid space usually; lesion may be intracranial or extracranial
Villaret	Cranial nerves IX, X, XI, XII plus sympathetic chain; cranial nerve VII occasionally involved	Retroparotid or retropharyngeal space
Schmidt	Cranial nerves X and XI	Usually intracranial before nerve fibers leave skull; occasionally inferior margin of jugular foramen
Jackson	Cranial nerves X, XI, and XII	May be intraparenchymal (medulla); usually intracranial before nerve fibers leave skull
Tapia	Cranial nerves X and XII (cranial nerve XI and the sympathetic chain occasionally involved)	Usually high in neck
Garcin (Hembase syndrome)	All cranial nerves on one side (often incomplete)	Often infiltrative; arising from base of skull (especially nasopharyngeal carcinoma)

5. Hemianesthesia of the palate, pharynx, and larynx (cranial nerves IX and X)

The descriptions of other syndromes involving cranial nerves IX through XII and the sympathetic chain vary widely in the literature; Table 12-1 describes some of these syndromes.

Clinical presentations vary depending on the nerves involved. When the sympathetic chain is affected, an ipsilateral Horner syndrome (meiosis, ptosis, and anhidrosis) will also occur.

LESIONS OF THE SPINAL ACCESSORY NERVE WITHIN THE NECK. The spinal accessory nerve may be injured in the neck by trauma, adenopathy, or neoplasm [1]. Nerve injury results in ipsilateral weakness of the sternocleidomastoid and trapezius muscles without affecting other cranial nerves. With injuries in the posterior cervical triangle distal to the sternocleidomastoid muscle, trapezius weakness occurs in isolation.

REFERENCES

1. Bell, D. S. Pressure palsy of the accessory nerve. *Br. Med. J.* 1:1483, 1964.
2. Bender, M. B., Shanzer, S., and Wagman, I. H. On the physiologic decussation concerned with head turning. *Confin. Neurol.* 24:169, 1964.
3. Brodal, A. *Neurological Anatomy In Relation to Clinical Medicine* (3rd ed.). New York: Oxford University Press, 1981. Pp. 457–459.
4. DeJong, R. N. *The Neurologic Examination Incorporating the Fundamentals of Neuroanatomy and Neurophysiology* (4th ed.). Hagerstown, Md.: Harper & Row, 1979. Pp. 241–248.
5. Geschwind, N. Nature of the decussated innervation of the sternocleidomastoid muscle. *Ann. Neurol.* 10:495, 1981.
6. Pearson, A. A., Sauter, R. W., and Herrin, G. R. The accessory nerve and its relation to the upper spinal nerves. *Am. J. Anat.* 114:371, 1964.
7. Strauss, W. L., and Howell, A. B. The spinal accessory nerve and its musculature. *Qt. Rev. Biol.* 11:387, 1936.

Chapter 13

THE LOCALIZATION OF LESIONS AFFECTING CRANIAL NERVE XII (THE HYPOGLOSSAL NERVE)

Paul W. Brazis

ANATOMY OF CRANIAL NERVE XII
(HYPOGLOSSAL NERVE)

The hypoglossal nerve [1, 3, 7] is the motor nerve of the tongue. Its fibers arise from the *hypoglossal nucleus,* a longitudinal cell column in the medulla that lies beneath the *hypoglossal trigone* of the floor of the fourth ventricle. The column of cells extends from the caudalmost medulla to the medullary-pontine junction. From the hypoglossal nucleus, the nerve fibers travel in a ventrolateral direction through the medullary reticular formation and medial portion of the inferior olive, coursing immediately lateral to the medial longitudinal fasciculus, medial lemniscus, and pyramid.

The fibers of the hypoglossal nerve emerge from the medulla between the olive and the pyramid as 10 to 15 rootlets that are located medial to cranial nerves IX (the glossopharyngeal), X (the vagus), and XI (the spinal accessory). These rootlets unite into two bundles that pass separately through the dura mater and the *hypoglossal canal* of the skull.

After leaving the skull in the hypoglossal canal, the two nerve bundles unite and descend vertically through the neck to the angle of the mandible. During this course, the hypoglossal nerve is quite near the internal carotid artery and the internal jugular vein. In the neck the nerve passes toward the hyoid bone and then turns medially toward the tongue. It courses over the internal and external carotid arteries and eventually lies beneath the digastric, stylohyoid, and mylohoid muscles. The nerve passes between the mylohyoid and hypoglossus muscles and then breaks up into a number of branches (the *muscular* or *lingual branches*), which supply various tongue muscles [7].

From the hypoglossal nerve proper in the neck is given off the *descending hypoglossal ramus,* which courses downward to form the *ansa hypoglossi.* This is formed not by fibers from the hypoglossal nucleus but from fibers from the upper C1 to C3 cervical roots. (The ansa hypoglossi is further discussed in Chapter 2.)

The hypoglossal muscular or lingual branches supply all the intrinsic muscles of the tongue and also the hypoglossus, styloglossus, genioglossus, and geniohyoid muscles (extrinsic muscles of the tongue).

Supranuclear control of the tongue [15] is mediated by corticobulbar fibers that originate mainly within the lower portion of the precentral gyrus (perisylvian) area. The corticobulbar fibers controlling the genioglossus muscles are crossed; the other tongue muscles appear to have bilateral supranuclear control.

CLINICAL EVALUATION OF CRANIAL NERVE XII

The clinical evaluation of cranial nerve XII [3] function consists of observation of the tongue at rest and with protrusion and assessment of the strength and rapidity of tongue movements. Although the hypoglossal nerve does contain some proprioceptive afferents, the nerve is otherwise a purely motor efferent nerve, and thus nerve lesions result in no sensory abnormalities.

Unilateral lesions of the hypoglossal nerve result in paresis, atrophy, furrowing, fibrillations, and fasciculations that affect the corresponding half of the tongue. This unilateral paresis is best demonstrated by voluntary tongue protrusion, during which the tongue deviates to the side of paresis, mainly because of the unopposed action of the normal contralateral genioglossus muscle (assisted by the geniohyoid). With unilateral lesions, dysarthria and dysphagia are minimal, but difficulty with manipulating food in the mouth is often evident.

Bilateral lower motor neuron lesions of the tongue result in bilateral atrophy, weakness, and fibrillations of the tongue. The tongue thus cannot be protruded voluntarily. This bilateral affection results in a marked difficulty with articulation, especially with the pronunciation of d and t phonemes. Dysphagia is prominent, and breathing difficulties may occur when the flaccid tongue falls backward to obstruct the pharynx.

LOCALIZATION OF LESIONS AFFECTING
CRANIAL NERVE XII

Supranuclear Lesions. Lesions of the corticobulbar tract anywhere in its course from the lower precentral gyrus to the hypoglossal nuclei may result in tongue paralysis. Because supranuclear control of the genioglossus muscle originates mainly from the contralateral cortex, a lesion of the corticobulbar fibers above their decussation may result in weakness of the contralateral half of the tongue. Thus, with an internal capsular lesion, the tongue may deviate toward the side of the hemiplegia. A supranuclear lesion is unaccompanied by atrophy or fibrillations of the tongue.

Bilateral upper motor neuron affection of the corticobulbar fibers to the hypoglossal nuclei results in a paretic tongue with no atrophy or signs of denervation. Lateral tongue movements are slow and irregular owing to poor supranuclear control ("spastic tongue"), and a spastic dysarthria is evident.

Nuclear Lesions and Intramedullary Cranial Nerve XII Lesions. Nuclear lesions of cranial nerve XII result in signs and symptoms that are identical to those of the hypoglossal nerve proper (paresis, atrophy, and fibrillations and fasciculations), but because of the close proximity of the two hypoglossal nuclei, dorsal medullary lesions (e.g., multiple sclerosis, syringobulbia) will often result in bilateral lower motor neuron lesions of the tongue. The nuclei may also be affected in motor neuron disease (amyotrophic lateral sclerosis) and in poliomyelitis.

The hypoglossal nerve may be injured, usually unilaterally, anywhere along its course in the medulla. Intramedullary hypoglossal involvement is suggested by the associated affection of the medial lemniscus, pyramid, or other neighboring intramedullary structures. Processes affecting the hypoglossal nerve in its intramedullary course include tumor, demyelinating disease, syringobulbia, and vascular insult. A rare but characteristic syndrome that affects the hypoglossal nerve in its intramedullary course is the *medial medullary syndrome (Dejerine's anterior bulbar syndrome)* [2]. This syndrome results from occlusion of the anterior spinal artery or its parent vertebral artery. The anterior spinal artery supplies the ipsilateral pyramid, medial lemniscus, and hypoglossal nerve; its occlusion thus results in three main signs:

1. Ipsilateral paresis, atrophy, and fibrillations of the tongue (due to affection of cranial nerve XII). The protruded tongue deviates toward the lesion (away from the hemiplegia).
2. Contralateral hemiplegia (due to involvement of the pyramid) with sparing of the face.
3. Contralateral loss of position and vibratory sensation (due to involvement of the medial lemniscus). Because the more dorsolateral spinothalamic tract is unaffected, pain and temperature sensations are spared.

This medial medullary syndrome may occur bilaterally [6], resulting in quadriplegia (with facial sparing), bilateral lower motor neuron lesions of the tongue, and a complete loss of position and vibratory sensation affecting all four extremities.

Because the hypoglossal fibers run somewhat laterally to the medial lemniscus and pyramid, they are occasionally spared in cases of anterior spinal artery occlusion.

Peripheral Lesions of Cranial Nerve XII. Cranial nerve XII has a close spatial relationship with cranial nerves IX (glossopharyngeal), X (vagus), and XI (spinal accessory) in the posterior cranial fossa and as it leaves the skull in the hypoglossal canal. A basilar skull lesion (e.g., tumor or trauma) [4, 8, 9] may involve the twelfth cranial nerve alone, producing an isolated cranial nerve XII lower motor neuron lesion; frequently, the other lower cranial nerves (IX, X, and XI) are variably involved as well. When all four of these nerves are damaged (e.g., by a skull fracture through the hypoglossal canal and jugular foramen), a *Collet-Sicard syndrome* results, consisting of the following signs:

1. Paralysis of the trapezius and sternocleidomastoid muscles (cranial nerve XI)
2. Paralysis of the vocal cord (cranial nerve X) and pharynx (cranial nerve IX)
3. Hemiparalysis of the tongue (cranial nerve XII)
4. Loss of taste on the posterior third of the tongue (cranial nerve IX)
5. Hemianesthesia of the palate, pharynx, and larynx (cranial nerves IX and X)

Other multiple lower cranial nerve palsy syndromes may occur with lesions in the posterior cranial fossa, in the skull, in the retropharyngeal or retrostyloid space, or in the neck (see Chap. 12). With neck lesions, the cervical sympathetic chain may be involved, resulting in an ipsilateral Horner syndrome (meiosis, anhidrosis, and ptosis). These syndromes include the Collet-Sicard, Villaret, Jackson, Tapia, and Garcin syndromes (see Table 12-1).

The hypoglossal nerve may be injured in isolation in the neck or in its more distal course near the tongue. An ipsilateral lower motor neuron type of paresis of half of the tongue results. Causes of this peripheral involvement include carotid aneurysms, local infections, surgical or accidental trauma, and tumors of the retroparotid or retropharyngeal spaces, neck, salivary glands, and base of the tongue.

REFERENCES

1. Brodal, A. *Neurological Anatomy In Relation to Clinical Medicine* (3rd ed.). New York: Oxford University Press, 1981. Pp. 453–457.
2. Davison, C. Syndrome of the anterior spinal artery of the medulla oblongata. *Arch. Neurol. Psychiat.* 37:91, 1937.
3. DeJong, R. N. *The Neurologic Examination Incorporating the Fundamentals of Neuroanatomy and Neurophysiology* (4th Ed.). Hagerstown, Md.: Harper & Row, 1979. Pp. 249–255.
4. Goldenberg, N. A., and Sandler, J. G. Isolated paralysis of the hypoglossal nerve. *Rev. Otoneuroophthal.* 9:429, 1931.
5. Kuypers, H. G. J. M. Corticobulbar connexions to the pons and lower brainstem in man: An anatomical study. *Brain* 81:364, 1958.
6. Meyer, J. S., and Herndon, R. M. Bilateral infarction of the pyramidal tracts in man. *Neurology (Minneap.)* 12:637, 1962.
7. Pearson, A. A. The hypoglossal nerve in human embryos. *J. Comp. Neurol.* 71:21, 1939.
8. Rubenstein, M. K. Cranial neuroneuropathy as the first sign of intracranial metastases. *Ann. Int. Med.* 70:49, 1969.
9. Williams, J. M., and Fox, J. L. Neurinoma of the intracranial portion of the hypoglossal nerve. Review and case report. *J. Neurosurg.* 19:248, 1962.

Chapter 14

THE LOCALIZATION OF LESIONS AFFECTING THE BRAINSTEM

Paul W. Brazis

MEDULLA OBLONGATA

Anatomy of the Medulla. The medulla is the most caudal portion of the brainstem and extends from the caudal border of the pons (limited by a plane passing from the striae medullares dorsally to the caudal pontine fibers ventrally) to a point just rostral to the point of emergence of the first spinal nerve roots. The cross-sectional anatomy at a midmedullary level is illustrated in Figure 14-1. The major clinically relevant medullary structures [2] are as follows:

CRANIAL NERVE NUCLEI AND ROOTS

1. The hypoglossal nucleus (cranial nerve XII)
2. The nucleus ambiguus (cranial nerves IX, X, and bulbar XI)
3. The dorsal motor nucleus of the vagus (cranial nerve X)
4. The medial and spinal vestibular nuclei and the cochlear nuclei (cranial nerve VIII)
5. The nucleus and spinal tract of the trigeminal nerve (cranial nerves V, VII, IX, and X)
6. The nucleus and tractus solitarius (cranial nerves VII, IX, and X)

ASCENDING AND DESCENDING TRACTS AND THEIR NUCLEI

1. The nuclei cuneatus and gracilis, internal arcuate fibers, and medial lemniscus
2. The pyramids (corticospinal tracts)
3. The ventral and dorsal spinocerebellar tracts, the medial and lateral reticulospinal tracts, the medial and lateral vestibulospinal tracts, the rubrospinal tracts, and the spinothalamic tracts
4. The descending sympathetic pathways

OTHER MEDULLARY STRUCTURES

1. The restiform body (inferior cerebellar peduncle)
2. The inferior olivary nucleus

Vascular Supply of the Medulla. The brainstem's large regional arteries [24] have three types of branches:

1. The *paramedian arteries,* penetrating the ventral brainstem surface and supplying midline structures

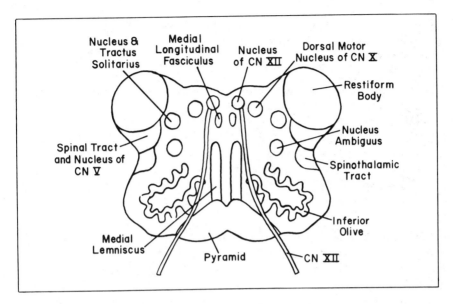

FIG. 14-1. *The medulla.*

2. The *short circumferential arteries,* which transverse laterally on the brainstem and penetrate its ventrolateral lateral surfaces
3. The *long circumferential arteries,* which course around the brainstem and supply its posterior structures and cerebellum

The blood supply to the medulla may be subdivided into two groups:

PARAMEDIAN BULBAR BRANCHES. The paramedian portion of the medulla (the hypoglossal nucleus and emergent nerve fibers, the medial longitudinal fasciculus, the medial lemniscus, the pyramids, and the medial part of the inferior olivary nucleus) is supplied by the *vertebral artery.* At lower medullary levels, the *anterior spinal artery* also contributes to the paramedian zone.

LATERAL BULBAR BRANCHES. The lateral portion of the medulla is supplied by the *vertebral artery* or the *posterior inferior cerebellar artery.* Occasionally, the basilar artery or the anterior inferior cerebellar also contribute.

Medullary Syndromes

MEDIAL MEDULLARY SYNDROME (DEJERINE'S ANTERIOR BULBAR SYNDROME). This syndrome [10] results from occlusion of the anterior spinal artery or its parent vertebral artery. The anterior spinal artery supplies the ipsilateral pyramid, medial lemniscus, and hypoglossal nerve and nucleus. Its occlusion thus results in the following signs:

1. Ipsilateral paresis, atrophy, and fibrillation of the tongue (due to cranial nerve XII affection). The protruded tongue deviates toward the lesion (away from the hemiplegia).
2. Contralateral hemiplegia (due to involvement of the pyramid) with sparing of the face.
3. Contralateral loss of position and vibratory sensation (due to involvement of the medial lemniscus). Because the more dorsolateral spinothalamic tract is unaffected, pain and temperature sensation are spared.

This medial medullary syndrome may occur bilaterally [21], resulting in quadriplegia (with facial sparing), bilateral lower motor neuron lesions of the tongue, and complete loss of position and vibratory sensation affecting all four extremities.

Because the hypoglossal fibers run somewhat laterally to the medial lemniscus and pyramid, they are occasionally spared in cases of anterior spinal artery occlusion. Occasionally, only the pyramid is damaged, resulting in a *pure motor hemiplegia* that spares the face [6].

LATERAL MEDULLARY (WALLENBERG) SYNDROME. This syndrome [7, 8, 16] is most often secondary to brainstem infarction due to vertebral artery or posterior inferior cerebellar artery occlusion. It has also been described with medullary neoplasms (usually metastases), abscess, radionecrosis, and hematoma (secondary to rupture of a vascular malformation).

The characteristic clinical picture results from damage to a wedge-shaped area of the lateral medulla and inferior cerebellum and consists of several signs:

1. Ipsilateral facial hypalgesia and thermoanesthesia (due to trigeminal spinal nucleus and tract involvement)
2. Contralateral trunk and extremity hypalgesia and thermoanesthesia (due to damage to the spinothalamic tract)
3. Ipsilateral palatal, pharyngeal, and vocal cord paralysis with dysphagia and dysarthria (due to involvement of the nucleus ambiguus)
4. Ipsilateral Horner syndrome (due to affection of the descending sympathetic fibers)
5. Vertigo, nausea, and vomiting (due to involvement of the vestibular nuclei)

6. Ipsilateral cerebellar signs and symptoms (due to involvement of the inferior cerebellar peduncle and cerebellum)
7. Occasionally, hiccups (due perhaps to involvement of the medullary respiratory centers) and diplopia (perhaps secondary to involvement of the lower pons)

The motor system (pyramids), tongue movements, and vibration and position sense are typically spared because the corresponding anatomic structures are located in the medial medulla.

Rarely, a *combined syndrome* (medial and lateral medullary syndromes) may occur.

THE LATERAL PONTOMEDULLARY SYNDROME. This syndrome [13] may result from occlusion of an aberrant arterial branch arising from the upper vertebral artery and running superiorly and laterally to the region of exit of cranial nerves VII and VIII from the pons. The clinical findings are those seen in the lateral medullary syndrome plus several pontine findings, including

1. Ipsilateral facial weakness (due to involvement of cranial nerve VII)
2. Ipsilateral tinnitus and occasionally hearing disturbance (due to involvement of cranial nerve VIII)

THE PONS

Anatomy of the Pons. The pons extends from a caudal plane, which passes from the striae medullares through the transverse pontine fibers, to a cephalad plane that passes immediately caudal to the inferior colliculi (dorsally) and to the cerebral peduncles (ventrally). The dorsal part of the pons is referred to as the *tegmentum,* and the ventral portion is referred to as the *basis pontis* or *pontocerebellar* portion (Fig. 14-2). The major pontine structures [2] include the following:

CRANIAL NERVE NUCLEI

1. The cochlear nuclei and the lateral and superior vestibular nuclei (cranial nerve VIII)
2. The motor nucleus of the facial nerve (cranial nerve VII)
3. The abducens nucleus (cranial nerve VI) and the paramedian pontine reticular formation (PPRF, or horizontal gaze "center")

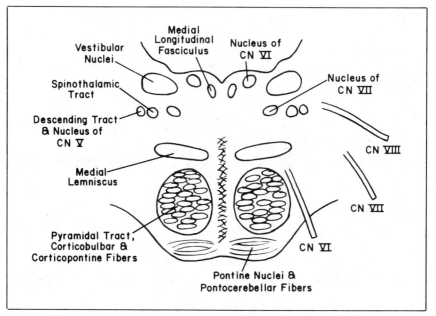

FIG. 14-2. *The pons.*

4. The main motor nucleus and the main sensory nucleus of the trigeminal nerve (cranial nerve V)
5. The superior and inferior salivatory nuclei and the lacrimal nucleus (cranial nerves VII and IX)

ASCENDING AND DESCENDING PONTINE TRACTS

1. The medial longitudinal fasciculus
2. The ventral spinocerebellar, spinothalamic, lateral tectospinal, rubrospinal, corticospinal, corticobulbar, and corticopontocerebellar tracts and the medial lemniscus
3. Auditory connections including the lateral lemniscus, the nucleus of the lateral lemniscus, the trapezoid body, and the superior olivary nuclear complex

OTHER PONTINE STRUCTURES

1. The middle cerebellar peduncle (brachium pontis)
2. The pontine nuclei
3. The locus ceruleus

Vascular Supply of the Pons. The blood supply to the pons [24] may be divided into three groups.

PARAMEDIAN VESSELS. These vessels (4 to 6 in number) arise from the basilar artery and penetrate perpendicularly into the pontine parenchyma. These vessels supply the medial basal pons, including the pontine nuclei, the corticospinal fibers, and the medial lemniscus.

SHORT CIRCUMFERENTIAL ARTERIES. These arteries also arise from the basilar artery and enter the brachium pontis. These vessels supply the ventrolateral basis pontis.

LONG CIRCUMFERENTIAL ARTERIES. These include:

1. *The superior cerebellar artery,* which supplies the dorsolateral pons and brachium pontis, the dorsal reticular formation, and the periaqueductal region (occasionally the ventrolateral pontine tegmentum is also supplied by this vessel).
2. *The anterior inferior cerebellar artery,* which arises from the basilar artery and supplies the lateral tegmentum of the lower two-thirds of the pons and the ventrolateral cerebellum.
3. *The internal auditory artery,* which arises from the anterior interior cerebellar artery (occasionally from the basilar artery) and supplies the auditory and facial cranial nerves.

Pontine Syndromes

VENTRAL PONTINE SYNDROMES

THE MILLARD-GUBLER SYNDROME. A unilateral lesion of the ventrocaudal pons may involve the basis pontis and the fascicles of cranial nerves VI and VII [19]. This involvement results in:

1. Contralateral hemiplegia (sparing the face) due to pyramidal tract involvement).
2. Ipsilateral lateral rectus paresis (cranial nerve VI) with diplopia that is accentuated when the patient "looks toward" the lesion.
3. Ipsilateral peripheral facial paresis (cranial nerve VII).

PURELY MOTOR HEMIPARESIS. Lesions (especially lacunar infarction) involving the corticospinal tracts in the basis pontis may produce a purely motor hemiplegia with or without facial involvement [13, 15, 22]. Other locations of lesions causing purely motor hemiplegia include the posterior limb of the internal capsule, the cerebral peduncle, and the medullary pyramid [6].

DYSARTHRIA–CLUMSY HAND SYNDROME. A lesion in the basis pontis (especially lacunar infarction) [11, 13, 22] at the junction of the upper one-third and lower two-thirds of the pons may result in the dysarthria–clumsy hand syndrome. In this syndrome facial weakness and severe dysarthria and dysphagia occur together with clumsiness and paresis of the hand. Hyperreflexia and a Babinski sign may occur on the same side as the arm paresis, but sensation is spared. A similar clinical presentation may also be seen with lesions in the genu of the internal capsule.

ATAXIC-HEMIPARESIS. A lesion (usually a lacunar infarction) [12, 13, 14, 22] in the basis pontis at the junction of the upper one-third and the lower two-thirds of the pons may result in the ataxic-hemiparesis (homolateral ataxia and crural paresis) syndrome. In this syndrome hemiparesis, which is more severe in the lower extremity, is associated with ipsilateral hemiataxia and occasionally dysarthria, nystagmus, and paresthesias. The lesion is in the contralateral pons. This syndrome has also been described with contralateral thalamocapsular lesions.

THE LOCKED-IN SYNDROME. Bilateral ventral pontine lesions (infarction, tumor, hemorrhage, trauma, or central pontine myelinolysis) may result in the locked-in syndrome (deefferented state) [5, 18, 23]. This syndrome consists of the following signs:

1. Quadriplegia due to bilateral corticospinal tract involvement in the basis pontis
2. Aphonia due to involvement of the corticobulbar fibers destined to the lower cranial nerves
3. Occasionally, impairment of horizontal eye movements due to bilateral involvement of the fascicles of cranial nerve VI

Because the reticular formation is not injured, the patient is fully awake. The supranuclear ocular motor pathways lie dorsally and are thus spared; thus, vertical eye movements and blinking are intact (the patient may actually convey his wishes in Morse code). Deefferentation may also occur with purely peripheral lesions (e.g., polio, polyneuritis, myasthenia gravis).

PRIMARY PONTINE HEMORRHAGE. Pontine hemorrhage [1] usually arises from paramedian arterioles and often begins in the basis pontis. An acute locked-in syndrome may occur, but often these lesions symmetrically dissect the pons, destroying the more dorsal structures. There is usually sudden coma with aphonia, tetraplegia, respiratory abnormalities, pinpoint pupils, ophthalmoplegia, hyperthermia, and progression to death. Ocular bobbing may be present.

DORSAL PONTINE SYNDROMES

FOVILLE SYNDROME. This syndrome [19] is due to lesions involving the dorsal pontine tegmentum in the caudal third of the pons. It consists of

1. Contralateral hemiplegia (with facial sparing) due to interruption of the corticospinal tract
2. Ipsilateral peripheral-type facial palsy due to involvement of the nucleus and fascicles of cranial nerve VII
3. Inability to move the eyes conjugately to the ipsilateral side (gaze is "away from" the lesion) due to involvement of the paramedian pontine reticular formation

RAYMOND-CESTAN SYNDROME. This syndrome is seen with rostral lesions of the dorsal pons. It includes

1. Cerebellar signs (ataxia) with a coarse "rubral" tremor due to involvement of the cerebellum
2. Contralateral reduction of all sensory modalities (face and extremities) due to involvement of the medial lemniscus and the spinothalamic tract
3. With ventral extension, there may be contralateral hemiparesis (due to corticospinal tract involvement) or paralysis of conjugate gaze toward the side of the lesion (due to involvement of the paramedian pontine reticular formation)

LATERAL PONTINE SYNDROMES

MARIE-FOIX SYNDROME. This syndrome is seen with lateral pontine lesions, especially those affecting the brachium pontis. It consists of

1. Ipsilateral cerebellar ataxia due to involvement of cerebellar connections
2. Contralateral hemiparesis due to involvement of the corticospinal tract
3. Variable contralateral hemihypesthesia for pain and temperature due to involvement of the spinothalamic tract

LATERAL TEGMENTAL BRAINSTEM HEMORRHAGE. Lateral tegmental pontomesencephalic hemorrhages result in a clinically uniform syndrome [4] that includes

1. Small reactive pupils with the smaller pupil ipsilateral to the lesion
2. Defects in ocular motility, especially an ipsilateral conjugate gaze

palsy (due to involvement of the paramedian pontine reticular formation), or ipsilateral internuclear ophthalmoplegia (due to involvement of the medial longitudinal fasciculus), or skew deviation
3. Contralateral hemiparesis due to involvement of the corticospinal tract
4. Contralateral hemisensory defects, especially for pain sensation (due to spinothalamic tract involvement)
5. Limb ataxia of the cerebellar type, which is often greater ipsilaterally, due to involvement of cerebellar connections

Other variable findings include altered vertical gaze, decreased hearing, dysarthria, dysphagia, decreased ipsilateral facial sensation or absent corneal reflex, and bilateral ptosis.

THE MESENCEPHALON

Anatomy of the Mesencephalon. The mesencephalon's rostral boundary is the superior colliculi-mammillary bodies plane; the caudal boundary is the plane just caudal to the inferior colliculi. The midbrain (Fig. 14-3) may be divided into the dorsal *tectum* (containing the colliculi), the *tegmentum,* and the *cerebral peduncles.* The major mesencephalic structures [2] include the following:

CRANIAL NERVE NUCLEI

1. The oculomotor nucleus (cranial nerve III)
2. The trochlear nucleus (cranial nerve IV)

MESENCEPHALIC TRACTS

1. The cerebral peduncles
2. The dentatorubrothalamic tract
3. The medial tegmental tract
4. The medial longitudinal fasciculus
5. The posterior commissure
6. The spinothalamic tract
7. The medial lemniscus

OTHER MESENCEPHALIC STRUCTURES

1. The nucleus of Darkschewitsch, the interstitial nucleus of Cajal, and the rostral nucleus of the medial longitudinal fasciculus
2. The superior and inferior colliculi

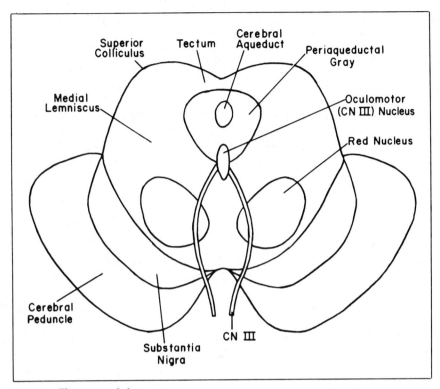

FIG. 14-3. *The mesencephalon.*

3. The red nucleus
4. The substantia nigra

Vascular Supply of the Mesencephalon. The mesencephalon's vascular supply includes paramedian and circumferential vessels.

PARAMEDIAN VESSELS. The *paramedian vessels* (the retromammillary trunk) arise from the origins of the posterior cerebral arteries and include the thalamoperforating arteries (supplying the thalamus) and the peduncular arteries (supplying the medial peduncles and the midbrain tegmentum, including the oculomotor nucleus, the red nucleus, and the substantia nigra).

CIRCUMFERENTIAL ARTERIES. The *circumferential* (peripeduncular) *arteries* include

1. The *quadrigeminal arteries* (arising from the posterior cerebral arteries), which supply the superior and inferior colliculi

2. The *superior cerebellar arteries,* which send branches to the cerebral peduncles and brachium conjunctivum before supplying the superior
cerebellum
3. The *posterior choroidal arteries,* which supply the cerebral peduncles,
the lateral superior colliculi, the thalamus, and the choroid plexus of
the third ventricle
4. The *anterior choroidal arteries* (from the internal carotids or middle cerebral arteries), which in some cases help supply the cerebral peduncles
as well as supramesencephalic structures
5. The *posterior cerebral arteries,* which also give rise to some mesencephalic branches

Mesencephalic Syndromes

THE VENTRAL CRANIAL NERVE III FASCICULAR SYNDROME (WEBER SYNDROME). A lesion affecting the cerebral peduncle, especially the medial peduncle,
may damage pyramidal fibers and the fascicle of cranial nerve III. This
results in the Weber syndrome, which consists of

1. Contralateral hemiplegia (including the lower face) due to corticospinal and corticobulbar tract involvement
2. Ipsilateral oculomotor paresis, including parasympathetic cranial
nerve III paresis (i.e., dilated pupil)

This syndrome may be seen with intrinsic or extrinsic brainstem lesions.
When supranuclear fibers for horizontal gaze are interrupted in the medial peduncle, a supranuclear-type conjugate gaze palsy to the opposite
side may occur *(the midbrain syndrome of Foville).*

DORSAL CRANIAL NERVE III FASCICULAR SYNDROMES (BENEDIKT SYNDROME). A lesion affecting the mesencephalic tegmentum may affect the red nucleus,
the brachium conjunctivum, and the fascicle of cranial nerve III. More
ventral tegmental lesions result in *Benedikt syndrome,* which consists of

1. Ipsilateral oculomotor paresis, usually with a dilated pupil
2. Contralateral involuntary movements, including intention tremor,
hemichorea, or hemiathetosis, due to destruction of the red nucleus

Essentially the same clinical manifestations are noted with more dorsal
midbrain tegmental lesions that injure the dorsal red nucleus and brachium conjunctivum *(Claude syndrome).*

DORSAL MESENCEPHALIC SYNDROMES. Dorsal rostral mesencephalic lesions
produce mainly neuroophthalmologic abnormalities. The dorsal mesen-

cephalic syndrome (also called the Sylvian aqueduct syndrome, the Koeber-Salus-Elschnig syndrome, Parinaud syndrome, and so on) [9, 17] is most often seen with hydrocephalus or tumors of the pineal region. This syndrome includes all or some of the following signs:

1. Paralysis of conjugate upward gaze
2. Pupillary abnormalities (pupils are usually large with light-near dissociation)
3. Convergence-retraction nystagmus on upward gaze (especially elicited by inducing upward saccades by a down-moving optokinetic target)
4. Pathologic lid retraction (Collier's sign)
5. Lid lag

Paralysis of downward gaze may also occur in this syndrome. *Isolated* paralysis of downward gaze may occur with bilateral lesions located dorsal and medial to the red nuclei in the fasciculus retroflexus [20, 25].

TOP OF THE BASILAR SYNDROME. Occlusive vascular disease of the rostral basilar artery frequently results in the "top of the basilar" syndrome [13] due to infarction of the midbrain, thalamus, and portions of the temporal and occipital lobes. This syndrome variably includes

1. *Disorders of eye movements* (unilateral or bilateral paralysis of upward or downward gaze, disordered convergence, convergence-retraction nystagmus, ocular abduction abnormalities, elevation and retraction of the upper eyelids (Collier's sign), skew deviation, and lightning-like eye oscillations)
2. *Pupillary abnormalities* (small and reactive, large or midposition and fixed, corectopia)
3. *Behavioral abnormalities* (somnolence, peduncular hallucinosis, memory difficulties, agitated delirium)
4. *Visual defects* (hemianopia, cortical blindness, Balint syndrome)
5. *Motor and sensory deficits*

REFERENCES

1. Attwater, H. L. Pontine hemorrhages. *Guy's Hosp. Rep.* 65:339, 1911.
2. Brodal, A. *Neurological Anatomy In Relation to Clinical Medicine* (3rd ed.). New York: Oxford University Press, 1981.
3. Caplan, L. R. "Top of the basilar" syndrome. *Neurology* 30:72, 1980.
4. Caplan, L. R., and Goodwin, J. A. Lateral tegmental brainstem hemorrhage. *Neurology* 32:252, 1982.
5. Cherington, M., Stears, J., and Hodges, J. Locked-syndrome caused by a tumor. *Neurology* 26:180, 1976.

6. Chokroverty, S., Rubino, F. A., and Haller, C. Pure motor hemiplegia due to pyramidal infarction. *Arch. Neurol.* 13:30, 1965.
7. Currier, R. D., and DeJong, R. N. The lateral medullary (Wallenberg's) syndrome. *Univ. Mich. Med. Bull.* 28:106, 1962.
8. Currier, R. D., Giles, G. L., and DeJong, R. N. Some comments on Wallenberg's lateral medullary syndrome. *Neurology (Minneap.)* 11:778, 1961.
9. Daroff, R. B., and Hoyt, W. F. Supranuclear Disorders of Ocular Control Systems in Man: Clinical, Anatomical, and Physiological Correlations. *In* Bach-y-Rita, P., Collins, C. C., and Hyde, J. E. (Eds.). *The Control of Eye Movements.* New York: Academic Press, 1971. P. 175.
10. Davison, C. Syndrome of the anterior spinal artery of the medulla oblongata. *Arch. Neurol. Psychiat.* 37:91, 1937.
11. Fisher, C. M. A lacunar stroke: The dysarthria-clumsy hand syndrome. *Neurology* 17:614, 1967.
12. Fisher, C. M. Ataxic hemiparesis: A pathologic study. *Arch. Neurol.* 35:126, 1978.
13. Fisher, C. M. Lacunar strokes and infarcts: A review. *Neurology (N.Y.)* 32:871, 1982.
14. Fisher, C. M., and Cole, M. Homolateral ataxia and crural paresis: A vascular syndrome. *J. Neurol. Neurosurg. Psychiat.* 28:48, 1965.
15. Fisher, C. M., and Curry, H. B. Pure motor hemiplegia of vascular origin. *Arch. Neurol.* 13:30, 1965.
16. Fisher, C. M., Karnes, W. E., and Kubik, C. S. Lateral medullary infarction. The pattern of vascular occlusion. *J. Neuropath. Exp. Neurol.* 20:323, 1961.
17. Hatcher, M. A., and Klintworth, G. K. The sylvian aqueduct syndrome. *Arch. Neurol. Psychiat. (Chic.)* 15:215, 1966.
18. Hawkes, C. H. "Locked-in" syndrome: Report of seven cases. *Br. Med. J.* 4:379, 1974.
19. Hiller, F. The vascular syndromes of the basilar and vertebral arteries and their branches. *J. Neur. Ment. Dis.* 116:988, 1952.
20. Jacobs, L., Anderson, P. J., and Bender, M. B. The lesions producing paralysis of downward but not upward gaze. *Arch. Neurol.* 28:319, 1973.
21. Meyer, J. S., and Herndon, R. M. Bilateral infarction of the pyramidal tracts in man. *Neurology (Minneap.)* 12:637, 1962.
22. Miller, V. T. Lacunar stroke—A reassessment. *Arch. Neurol.* 40:129, 1983.
23. Plum, F., and Posner, J. B. *The Diagnosis of Stupor and Coma* (3rd ed.). Philadelphia: F.A. Davis, 1980. P. 9.
24. Stopford, J. S. B. The arteries of the pons and medulla oblongata. Parts I and II. *J. Anat. Physiol.* 50:131, 255, 1916.
25. Trojanowski, J. Q., and Wray, S. H. Vertical gaze ophthalmoplegia: Selective paralysis of downgaze. *Neurology* 2:397, 1977.

Chapter 15

THE LOCALIZATION OF LESIONS AFFECTING THE CEREBELLUM

José Biller and Paul W. Brazis

ANATOMY OF THE CEREBELLUM

The cerebellum is derived from the somatic afferent portion of the alar plate. It does not initiate motion by itself but rather acts as a monitor or modulator of motor activity "originating" in other brain centers. One of the major cerebellar functions is automatic excitation of antagonist muscles at the end of a movement while simultaneously inhibiting the agonist muscles that initated the movement.

Anatomically, a central portion, the *vermis,* and two lateral portions, the *cerebellar hemispheres,* can be recognized. The vermis is developmentally old and receives mainly spinocerebellar afferents, whereas the hemispheres have more complex fiber connections [20, 27]. The cerebellum consists of three major components—the *anterior* and *posterior lobes* (divided by the primary fissure) and the *flocculonodular lobe* (separated from the posterior lobes by the *posterolateral* or *postnodular fissures*).

From an embryogenetic and phylogenetic standpoint, the cerebellum may also be subdivided into the *archicerebellum,* the *paleocerebellum,* and the *neocerebellum* [3, 25]. The *archicerebellum* corresponds to the flocculonodular lobe and is also called the *vestibulocerebellum* because it has such rich connections with the vestibular system. It also receives input from areas of the brain concerned with eye movements [25, 26, 31, 32]. The *paleocerebellum* consists of the vermis of the anterior lobe, the pyramis, the uvula, and the paraflocculus. It is also known as the *spinocerebellum* because it receives chiefly input from the spinal cord. The *neocerebellum* consists of the middle portion of the vermis and most of the cerebellar hemispheres. Because it receives projections from the pons, it is also termed the *pontocerebellum.* The neocerebellum projects fibers to the cerebral cortex through the thalamus.

Three pairs of nuclei on each side of the midline within the cerebellar core receive input from the cerebellar cortex and incoming afferents. These nuclei are also the main source of cerebellar efferents. From medial to lateral, these nuclei include the *fastigial nuclei,* the *nucleus interpositus (globose and emboliform),* and the *dentate nucleus.* Considering the connections of the nuclei, the cerebellum can be longitudinally subdivided [2, 14, 21] as follows: (1) a *midline zone,* containing cerebellar neurons projecting to the fastigial nucleus; (2) an *intermediate zone,* containing neurons projecting to the nucleus interpositus; and (3) a *lateral zone,* containing neurons projecting to the dentate nucleus.

The cerebellum is connected to the brainstem by three large cerebellar peduncles. The *inferior peduncle (restiform body)* connects the cerebellum to the medulla and carries afferent and efferent fibers. Some afferent fibers of clinical importance include

1. The *dorsal spinocerebellar tract,* originating in the dorsal nucleus of

Clarke (T1–L2), which carries proprioceptive and exteroceptive information mostly from the trunk and ipsilateral lower extremity
2. The *cuneocerebellar tract,* originating in the external arcuate nucleus, which transmits proprioceptive information from the superior extremity and neck
3. The *olivocerebellar tract,* which carries somatosensory information from the contralateral inferior olivary nucleus
4. The *vestibulocerebellar tract,* which transmits information from vestibular receptors on both sides of the body
5. The *reticulocerebellar tract,* arising in the lateral reticular and paramedian nuclei of the medulla

Efferent fibers in the restiform body are mainly cerebellovestibular and constitute the fastigiobulbar tract, which courses in a separate pathway known as the *juxtarestiform body.*

The *middle peduncle (brachium pontis),* the largest of the three peduncles, connects the cerebellum to the pons and carries mainly afferent fibers. Among them is the pontocerebellar tract, which arises in the pontine gray matter and transmits impulses from the cerebral cortex to the intermediate and lateral zones of the cerebellum.

The *superior peduncle (brachium conjunctivum)* connects the cerebellum to the midbrain. It contains mainly cerebellar efferent fibers, although it also contains some *afferent* fibers. These include

1. The *ventral spinocerebellar tract,* which transmits proprioceptive and exteroceptive information from levels below the midthoracic cord
2. The *tectocerebellar tract,* arising in the superior and inferior colliculi, which carries auditory and visual information
3. The *trigeminocerebellar tract,* which carries proprioceptive fibers from the mesencephalic and tactile information from the chief sensory nucleus of the trigeminal nerve

Efferent fibers of the superior peduncle include

1. The *dentatorubral tract,* which carries output to the contralateral red nucleus
2. The *dentatothalamic tract,* which transmits output to the contralateral ventrolateral nucleus of the thalamus
3. The *uncinate bundle of Russel,* which carries output to the vestibular nuclei and reticular formation

VASCULAR SUPPLY OF THE CEREBELLUM
The blood supply to the cerebellum originates from the posterior inferior, the anterior inferior, and the superior cerebellar arteries. These ves-

sels have abundant anastomoses. The upper surface of the cerebellum receives blood from the superior cerebellar artery, the inferior surface is supplied by the anterior inferior and posterior inferior cerebellar arteries, and the anterior surface and flocculus are supplied by the anterior inferior cerebellar artery [11, 12].

CLINICAL MANIFESTATION
OF CEREBELLAR DYSFUNCTION

Cerebellar disease may be the consequence of congenital malformations, inherited cerebellar atrophies, metabolic-endocrine derangements, infectious disease, intoxications, vascular disorders, demyelinating disease, or neoplasms [14, 34]. The classic report of cerebellar symptoms is that of Gordon Holmes [17, 18]. The cardinal features of cerebellar dysfunction will be briefly discussed.

Hypotonia. Hypotonia accompanies acute hemispheric lesions and is seen less often with chronic lesions [4]. It is ipsilateral to the side of the cerebellar lesion and is often more noticeable in the upper limbs, particularly in the proximal musculature. Hypotonic extremities often exhibit pendular reflexes, which may also be diminished. Occasionally cerebellar lesions (e.g., cerebellar hematoma) may be associated with increased tone of the extremity due in part to secondary brainstem (corticospinal tract) compression.

Hypotonia with cerebellar lesions is probably the result of decreased fusimotor activity secondary to cerebellar injury, especially to the dentate nucleus, resulting in a decreased response to stretch in the muscle spindle afferents [13, 16, 36]

Ataxia or Dystaxia. Ataxia refers to a disturbance in the smooth performance of voluntary motor acts [5]. The movements will err in rate, range, force, and duration. In the absence of cerebellar inhibitory and modulating influences, skilled movements originating in the cerebral motor cortex become inaccurate and poorly controlled [34]. Ataxia may affect the limbs, the trunk, or the gait and may be of acute onset (e.g., anticonvulsant intoxication), episodic (e.g., Hartnup's disease), or progressive (e.g., ataxia telangiectasia). Ataxia secondary to cerebellar injury characteristically persists in spite of visual cues (unlike ataxia secondary to posterior column involvement).

The term *ataxia* includes other abnormalities of voluntary movement control such as *asynergia* (lack of synergy of the various muscle components in performing more complex movements, so that the movements are broken up into isolated successive parts—*decompensation of movement*), *dysmetria* (abnormal excursions in movement), *dysdiadochokinesia* (impaired performance of rapidly alternating movements), and past-pointing. Also associated are an *impaired checking response* and an *excessive rebound phenomenon* when an opposed motion is suddenly released.

Typically, patients with cerebellar disease have a wide-based stance and a gait characterized by staggering and impaired tandem walking. Truncal ataxia and titubations suggest a midline cerebellar lesion.

Cerebellar Dysarthria. The dysarthria occurring with cerebellar disease is generally characterized by abnormalities in articulation and prosody [8, 14]. These two abnormalities may occur together or independently. This speech disorder has been described as scanning, slurring, staccato, explosive, hesitant, slow altered accent, and garbled [30]. The dysarthria may be a result of a generalized hypotonia (i.e., a disorder of muscle spindle function) and may affect intonation rather than articulation [23].

In a study of 31 patients with dysarthria in a series of 162 cases of focal cerebellar disease, Lechtenberg and Gilman [28] found that cerebellar hemispheral lesions were associated with speech disorders more often than vermal lesions and that 22 of the 31 patients had predominantly or exclusively left hemispheral lesions. Dysarthria was especially evident with left superior paravermal lesions. Because cerebrocerebellar connections are predominantly contralateral and the nondominant cerebral hemisphere is concerned with prosody of speech [28], the authors concluded that dominance of the left cerebellar hemisphere in the regulation of speech (melody and continuity) may derive from access of this hemisphere to the nondominant cerebral hemisphere.

Tremor. Lesions of the cerebellum, especially those affecting the dentate nucleus, induce a *kinetic (intention) tremor* [6, 9]. A static (postural) tremor may also occur. Lesions of the dentate nucleus may result in tremor because the lesion interrupts a rubroolivocerebellocircuit [24].

Ocular Motor Dysfunction. Nystagmus is frequently observed in association with cerebellar disorders. Gaze-evoked nystagmus, rebound nystagmus, and abnormal optokinetic nystagmus may be seen with midline cerebellar lesions [10, 14, 19]. These abnormalities may also occur with hemispheral disorders. Positional nystagmus, mimicking positional nystagmus of the benign paroxysmal type, may occur with posterior fossa tumors. Ocular dysmetria [7], a conjugate overshoot and undershoot of a target with voluntary saccades, may occur with midline [31] or lateral

[32] cerebellar lesions. Other ocular signs seen with cerebellar disorders include irregular tracking, ocular flutter, opsoclonus, ocular bobbing, paresis of conjugate gaze, and skew deviation [15, 22, 33]. Because most of the disorders that give rise to these abnormalities affect brainstem structures also, the cerebellar role in their genesis has not been defined. Overall, most "cerebellar" eye signs cannot be localized to specific areas of the cerebellum.

Cerebellar disease may also be associated with generalized asthenia, megalographia, catalepsy, and "cerebellar fits." These latter events do not represent seizures but are episodes of decerebrate rigidity that are usually seen with large midline cerebellar masses [34, 39]. Other signs seen with cerebellar disorders may reflect increased intracranial pressure (headache, nausea, vomiting, obscuration of vision, papilledema) or regional involvement due to extension of the primary process (e.g., deafness, tinnitus, dizziness, and facial numbness in the cerebellopontine angle syndrome).

CEREBELLAR SYNDROMES

Generally speaking, precise clinical localization is difficult with lesions of the cerebellum. The cerebellar syndromes may be divided as follows:

1. The rostral vermis syndrome (anterior lobe)
2. The caudal vermis syndrome (flocculonodular and posterior lobe)
3. The hemispheric syndrome (posterior lobe, variably anterior lobe)
4. The pancerebellar syndrome (all lobes)

Rostral Vermis Syndrome. The clinical characteristics of this syndrome include

1. A wide-based stance and gait
2. Ataxia of gait, with proportionally little ataxia on a heel-to-shin maneuver with the patient lying down
3. Normal or only slightly impaired arm cooordination
4. Infrequent presence of hypotonia, nystagmus, and dysarthria

This syndrome is best exemplified by the restricted form of cerebellar cortical degeneration that occurs in alcoholic patients [37]. The pathologic changes in this condition affect the anterior and superior vermis. In advanced cases they may spread to involve the anterior part of the anterior lobes.

Caudal Vermis Syndrome. The clinical characteristics of this syndrome include

1. Axial disequilibrium and staggering gait
2. Little or no limb ataxia
3. Sometimes spontaneous nystagmus and rotated postures of the head

This syndrome is typically seen with disease processes that damage the flocculonodular lobe, especially medulloblastoma in children [1]. As these tumors grow, a hemispheric cerebellar syndrome may be superimposed due to neocerebellar involvement.

Cerebellar Hemispheric Syndrome. Patients with this syndrome typically show incoordination of ipsilateral appendicular movements, particularly when they require fine motor coordination. Thus, this incoordination affects mainly muscles that are closely controlled by the precentral cortex, such as those involved in speech and finger movements. The most likely etiologies include infarcts, neoplasms, and abscesses [14].

Pancerebellar Syndrome. This syndrome is a combination of all the other cerebellar syndromes and is characterized by bilateral signs of cerebellar dysfunction affecting the trunk, limbs, and cranial musculature. It is seen with infections and peri-infectious processes, hypoglycemia, hyperthermia, and other toxic-metabolic disorders [35, 38].

REFERENCES

1. Baily, P., and Cushing, H. Medulloblastoma cerebelli: A common type of midcerebellar glioma of childhood. *Arch. Neurol. Psychiat. (Chic.)* 14:192, 1925.
2. Brodal, A. Cerebrocerebellar pathways. Anatomical data and some functional implications. *Acta Neurol.* (Suppl.) 51:153, 1972.
3. Brodal, A. *Neurologic Anatomy In Relation to Clinical Medicine* (3rd ed.). New York: Oxford University Press, 1981, Pp. 294–298.
4. Brown, J. R. Localizing cerebellar syndromes. *J.A.M.A.* 141:518, 1949.
5. Brown, J. R. Diseases of the Cerebellum. *In* Baker, A. B., and Baker, L. H. (Eds.). *Clinical Neurology.* Philadelphia: Harper & Row, 1955.
6. Carrea, R. M. E., and Mettler, F. A. Function of the primate brachium conjunctivum and related structures. *J. Comp. Neurol.* 102:151, 1955.
7. Cogan, D. G. Ocular dysmetria: Flutter-like oscillations of the eyes and opsoclonus. *Arch. Ophthalmol.* 51:318, 1954.
8. Cole, M. Dysprosody due to posterior fossa lesions. *Trans. Am. Neurol. Assoc.* 96:151, 1971.
9. Dow, R. S., and Moruzzi, G. *The Physiology and Pathology of the Cerebellum.* Minneapolis: University of Minnesota Press, 1958.

10. Ellenberger, C., Keltner, J. L., and Stroud, M. H. Ocular dyskinesia in cerebellar disease. *Brain* 95:685, 1972.
11. Gillilan, L. A. Arteries of primate cerebellum. *J. Neurol. Neurosurg. Psychiat.* 28:295, 1969.
12. Gillilan, L. A. Anatomy and Embryology of the Arterial System of the Brainstem and Cerebellum. *In* Vinken, P. J., and Bruyn, G. W. (Eds.). *Handbook of Clinical Neurology.* New York: American Elsevier Publishing Co., 1972.
13. Gilman, S. Fusimotor fiber responses in the decerebellate cat. *Brain Res.* 14:218, 1969.
14. Gilman, S., Bloedel, J. R., and Lechtenberg, R. *Disorders of the Cerebellum.* Philadelphia: F. A. Davis, 1981.
15. Glaser, J. S. *Neuro-ophthalmology.* Hagerstown, Md.: Harper & Row, 1978. Pp. 212–213 and 221–240.
16. Granit, R., Holmgren, B., and Merton, P. A. The two routes for excitation of muscle and their subservience to the cerebellum. *J. Physiol. (Lond.)* 130:312, 1955.
17. Holmes, G. The clinical symptoms of cerebellar disease and their interpretation. *Lancet* 1:1177, 1922.
18. Holmes, G. The cerebellum of man. *Brain* 62:1, 1939.
19. Hood, J. D., Kayan, A., and Leech, J. Rebound nystagmus. *Brain* 96:507, 1973.
20. Ingram, W. R. *A Review of Anatomical Neurology.* Baltimore: University Park Press, 1976. Pp. 195–237.
21. Jansen, J., and Brodal, A. Experimental studies on the intrinsic fibers of the cerebellum. II. The corticonuclear projection. *J. Comp. Neurol.* 73:267, 1940.
22. Keane, J. R. Ocular skew deviation. *Arch. Neurol.* 32:185, 1975.
23. Kent, R., and Netrell, R. A case study of an ataxic dysarthria: Cineradiographic and spectrographic observations. *J. Speech Hearing Disorders* 40:115, 1975.
24. Larochelle, L., et al. The rubro-olivo-cerebello-rubral loop and postural tremor in the monkey. *J. Neurol. Sci.* 11:53, 1970.
25. Larsell, O. The cerebellum: A review and interpretation. *Arch. Neurol. Psychiat.* 38:580, 1937.
26. Larsell, O. The development of the cerebellum in man in relation to its comparative anatomy. *J. Comp. Neurol.* 87:85, 1947.
27. Larsell, O., and Jansen, J. *The Comparative Anatomy and Histology of the Cerebellum: The Human Cerebellum, Cerebellar Connections, and Cerebellar Cortex.* Minneapolis: University of Minnesota Press, 1972.
28. Lechtenberg, R., and Gilman, S. Speech disorders in cerebellar disease. *Ann. Neurol.* 3:285, 1978.
29. Ross, E. D. The aprosodias – Functional anatomic organization of the affective components of language in the right hemisphere. *Arch. Neurol.* 38:571, 1981.
30. Ross, E. D., and Mesulam, M. Dominant language functions of the right hemisphere? Prosody and emotional gesturing. *Arch. Neurol.* 36:144, 1979.
31. Selhorst, J. B., et al. Disorders in cerebellar ocular motor control. I. Saccadic overshoot dysmetria. An oculographic, control system, and clinico-anatomical analysis. *Brain* 99:497, 1976.
32. Selhorst, J. B., et al. Disorders in cerebellar ocular motor control. II. Macrosaccadic oscillation. *Brain* 99:509, 1976.

33. Smith, J. L., David, N. J., and Klintworth, G. Skew deviation. *Neurology* 14:96, 1964.
34. Stewart, T. G., and Holmes, G. Symptomatology of cerebellar tumors. A study of forty cases. *Brain* 27:522, 1904.
35. Valsamis, M. P., and Mancall, E. Toxic cerebellar degeneration. *Hum. Pathol.* 4:513, 1973.
36. Van der Meulen, S. P., and Gilman, S. Recovery of muscle spindle activity in cats after cerebellar ablation. *J. Neurophysiol.* 28:943, 1965.
37. Victor, M., Adams, R. D., and Mancall, E. L. A restricted form of cerebellar cortical degeneration occurring in alcoholic patients. *Arch. Neurol. (Chic.)* 1:579, 1959.
38. Victor, M., and Ferrendelli, J. A. The Nutritional and Metabolic Diseases of the Cerebellum: Clinical and Pathological Aspects. *In* Fields, W. S., and Willis, W. D. (Eds.). *The Cerebellum in Health and Disease.* St. Louis: W.H. Green, 1970.
39. Weisenburg, T. H. Cerebellar localization and its symptomatology. *Brain* 50:357, 1927.

Chapter 16

THE LOCALIZATION OF LESIONS OF THE HYPOTHALAMUS AND PITUITARY GLAND

Joseph C. Masdeu

ANATOMY OF THE REGION

The hypothalamus [4, 5, 10] constitutes the lateral wall of the third ventricle. It is separated from the thalamus by the hypothalamic sulcus. The two walls of the third ventricle merge anteriorly to form the lamina terminalis, which is related superiorly to the anterior commissure and inferiorly to the optic chiasm. Lateroposteriorly, the hypothalamus borders on the globus pallidus, internal capsule, subthalamic region, and crus cerebri. An inferior prolongation of the floor of the third ventricle, the pituitary stalk or infundibulum, joins the hypothalamus with the pituitary gland or hypophysis. Each pillar of the fornix, descending rostrocaudally to end in the mammillary body, divides the hypothalamus into a medial and a lateral region (Figs. 16-1 and 16-2).

Main Hypothalamic Nuclear Groups. The location of the hypothalamic nuclei can be appreciated by visualizing the hypothalamus as divided by (1) a coronal plane through the infundibular stalk and (2) an angled parasagittal plane containing the fornix [14]. By this means, there are four regions—anterior, posterior, medial, and lateral. The positions of the hypothalamic nuclei in these regions are indicated in Figure 16-1 and in the diagram that follows.

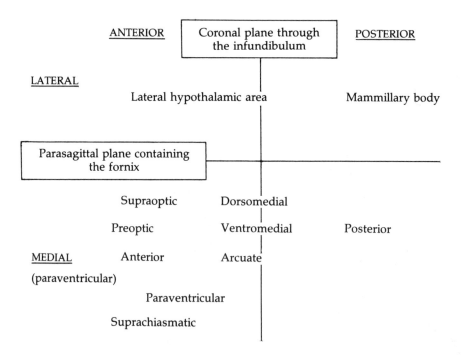

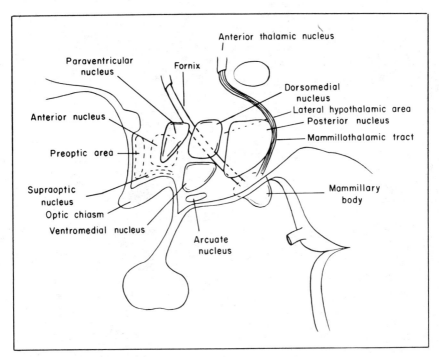

FIG. 16-1. *Hypothalamic nuclei.*

Connections of the Hypothalamus. The origin, pathways, and termination of the main afferent and efferent hypothalamic connections are listed in Table 16-1. In summary, the hypothalamus has strong to and fro connections with (1) the midbrain and posterior tegmentum, which play an important role in alertness; (2) the limbic system, through the medial temporal cortex, anteromedial thalamic region, and amygdala, which play an important role in emotion and memory; and (3) the "autonomic" nuclei of the brainstem and spinal cord, such as the dorsal nucleus of the vagus and the nucleus tractus solitarius. Although direct connections have been traced to the ipsilateral intermediolateral cell column of the spinal cord, much of the influence of the hypothalamus on the autonomic centers of the cord is probably exerted through the brainstem reticular formation [4, 5]. Pathways from the retina and olfactory system convey to the hypothalamus information needed for the circadian control of vegetative functions and for feeding and reproductive behavior.

Hypothalamic control of vegetative functions is exerted to a great extent through the pituitary gland. The hormonal secretions of the anterior pituitary are regulated by the hypothalamic releasing factors or, as they are currently termed, the *hypophysiotropic hormones,* which are released

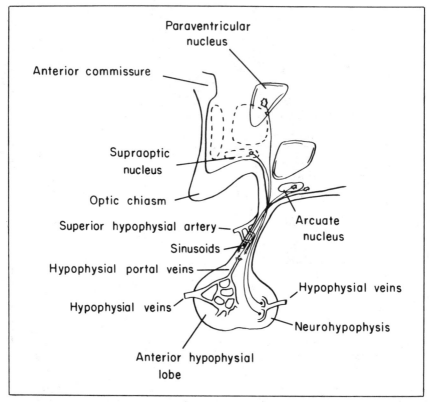

FIG. 16-2. *Hypothalamic–pituitary connections.*

into the infundibular portal system (Fig. 16-2). The infundibulum also contains the important supraopticohypophyseal tract, constituted by axons from neurons in the supraoptic and paraventricular nuclei. These axons terminate in a rich capillary network in the posterior lobe of the pituitary (neurohypophysis), where they secrete oxytocin and antidiuretic hormone.

LOCALIZATION OF THE
CLINICAL MANIFESTATIONS OF
HYPOTHALAMIC-PITUITARY DYSFUNCTION

Before discussing the most likely location of a lesion causing such symptoms or signs as are attributable to the hypothalamic-pituitary region (Table 16-2), several points should be noted.

1. Because these structures are small, several portions may be involved simultaneously.

TABLE 16-1. *Connections of the Hypothalamus*[a]

Origin	Tract	Termination and Neurotransmitter (when known)
AFFERENT HYPOTHALAMIC CONNECTIONS		
Medial temporal cortex	Fornix	Mammillary body
Midbrain tegmental nuclei	Mammillary peduncle	Mammillary body
Amygdala	Stria terminalis	Ventromedial nucleus Arcuate nucleus
Periaqueductal gray	Dorsal longitudinal fasciculus	Posterior nucleus
Raphe nuclei		Arcuate nucleus (serotonin)
Nucleus locus coeruleus		Arcuate nucleus (noradrenaline)
Nucleus tractus solitarius		Paraventricular nucleus Dorsomedial nucleus Arcuate nucleus
Retina		Suprachiasmatic nucleus Arcuate nucleus
Olfactory nerve	Medial forebrain bundle	Lateral area
Septal nuclei	Medial forebrain bundle, fornix	Mammillary body
Dorsomedial thalamic nucleus		Lateral area
Orbitofrontal cortex		Lateral area
EFFERENT HYPOTHALAMIC CONNECTIONS		
Paraventricular nucleus	Supraopticohypophysial	Neurohypophysis [posterior pituitary] (oxytocin, antidiuretic hormone)
Arcuate nucleus	Tuberoinfundibular	Hypophysial portal system (hypophysiotrophic hormones [and dopamine])
Mammillary body	Mammillothalamic	Anterior thalamic nucleus
Mammillary body	Mammillotegmental	Dorsal and ventral tegmental nuclei
Lateral area	Medial forebrain bundle	Septum
Medial nuclei	Dorsal longitudinal fasciculus	Periaqueductal gray
Ventromedial nucleus		Raphe nuclei Nucleus locus coeruleus
Several nuclei	Several pathways (uncrossed)	Dorsal nucleus of the vagus Nucleus of the solitary tract Nucleus ambiguus Intermediolateral cell column of the spinal cord

[a]Anatomically larger connections are listed first.

TABLE 16-2. *Clinical Manifestations of Hypothalamic or Pituitary Dysfunction*

Disturbances of temperature regulation
  Hypothermia
  Hyperthermia
  Poikilothermia
Disturbances of alertness and sleep
  Hypersomnia
  Insomnia
Autonomic disturbances
  Cardiac
  Pulmonary
  Gastrointestinal
  "Diencephalic epilepsy"
Disturbances of water balance
  Diabetes insipidus
  Essential hypernatremia
  Inappropriate secretion of ADH
  Primary hyperdipsia
Disturbances of caloric balance
  Obesity
  Emaciation
Disturbances of reproductive functions
  Hypogonadotropic hypogonadism
  Nonpuerperal galactorrhea
  Precocious puberty
  Uncontrollable sexual behavior
Other endocrine disturbances
Disturbances of memory
Disturbances of emotional behavior and affect
  Rage and fear
  Apathy
Headache
Impaired visual acuity, visual field defects
Diplopia

2. Lesions that progress rapidly cause a more florid clinical symptomatology than those that proceed slowly. For instance, a surgical or vascular lesion in the posterior hypothalamus will render the patient comatose, whereas a slowly growing tumor affecting the same structures will cause only apathy.
3. Unilateral lesions are seldom symptomatic.
4. The changes of hypothalamic function with age are reflected in the disparity of syndromes caused in different age groups by similarly located lesions [18].

Disturbances of Temperature Regulation. The hypothalamic "thermostat" for normal temperature regulation is located in the anterior preoptic hypothalamic area. Neurons located in this area alter their firing rate in response to a warm or cold environment. However, central control of the physiologic mechanisms for heating (decreased sweating, central pooling of blood, shivering, and so on) and cooling (increased sweating, peripheral vasodilation, panting, decreased motor behavior) is located in the posterior hypothalamus, which receives thermal information from the anterior "thermostat" through cholinergic pathways traversing the medial forebrain bundle, as well as from brainstem thermoreceptors. The posterior hypothalamus integrates this information and generates signals that put the appropriate physiologic, affective, and behavioral responses into effect [18].

PHYSIOLOGIC RHYTHMS

1. Diurnal variation. Body temperature peaks in early evening and reaches the lowest point in early morning [15].
2. Menstrual cycle. Body temperature increases at the time of ovulation.

HYPOTHERMIA

CHRONIC. Most often the lesion involves the posterior or the entire hypothalamus. When discomfort is also present, the lesion may be in the anterior hypothalamus [7]. The most common causes include Wernicke's encephalopathy, head trauma, craniopharyngioma, glioblastoma multiforme, surgery, hydrocephalus, infarction, and sarcoidosis [15].

PAROXYSMAL. *Spontaneous Periodic Hyperthermia; "Diencephalic Epilepsy."* Fewer than 20 patients have been reported to have episodic decrease of body temperature. The onset is abrupt, with sweating and vasodilatation leading to hypothermia (as low as 30 degrees), which is accompanied by nausea, vomiting, hypotension, bradycardia, cardiac arrhythmias, ataxia, asterixis, and mental dullness. The episodes last from minutes to days; they may recur only after decades, or they may recur more often, even daily. Responsible lesions may involve the arcuate nucleus and premammillary area. This hypothalamic disturbance is often associated with agenesis of the corpus callosum [18].

HYPERTHERMIA

PYROGEN-INDUCED. Pyrogens are the most common cause of hyperthermia. Cases labeled as *hypothalamic hyperthermia* often have an infectious source of pyrogens. This type of hyperthermia is mediated by the anterior hypothalamus and prostaglandin E1 (which can be blocked by aspirin and butazolidine) [15].

SUSTAINED HYPERTHERMIA. Sustained hyperthermia occurs only as a consequence of an acute process (craniotomy, trauma, bleeding) and lasts for less than 2 weeks. The lesion affects the anterior hypothalamus. Cardiovascular changes, normally present with fever, are disproportionately small with hyperthermia due to hypothalamic lesions [18].

PAROXYSMAL HYPERTHERMIA. Fewer than 10 cases of paroxysmal hyperthermia have been reported. Involvement of the ventromedial hypothalamus has been suspected in such instances. One case responded to phenytoin administration [18].

POIKILOTHERMIA. Poikilothermia is the fluctuation in body temperature of more than 2°C with changes in ambient temperature. It is the most common central neurogenic abnormality of heat regulation in humans. Such patients are unaware of their condition and show no sign of discomfort or behavioral regulation with thermal stress. Poikilothermia results from posterior hypothalamic lesions [18].

Disturbances of Alertness and Sleep

COMA, HYPERSOMNIA, OR AKINETIC MUTISM. These are occasionally related to posterior hypothalamic or larger lesions. The most common reported causes have been tumors and Wernicke's encephalopathy. Hypersomnia and coma result from midbrain lesions more often than from hypothalamic lesions.

INSOMNIA. Fewer than 10 cases have been reported implicating the anterior hypothalamus [18].

Autonomic Disturbances. Sympathetic areas tend to be ventromedial and posterior. Stimulation of these areas causes an expression of rage or fear associated with hypertension, pupillary dilation, tachycardia, vasoconstriction of vascular beds, vasodilation of muscular beds, increased cardiac output, and increased cardiac contractility.

Parasympathetic areas tend to be paraventricular or lateral and anterior. Stimulation of these areas causes pupillary constriction. Stimulation of the anterior parasympathetic areas causes hypotension and bradycardia, whereas stimulation of the posterior parasympathetic areas causes only increased blood flow through the bowel and decreased blood flow in skeletal muscle [18].

CARDIAC MANIFESTATIONS. Hypertension, cardiac arrhythmias, electrocardiographic (EKG) abnormalities simulating myocardial infarction, or even myocardial infarction in a nonvascular pattern may follow subarachnoid or intraventricular hemorrhages, particularly those due to a ruptured anterior communicating artery aneurysm. Outpouring of catecholamines with the acute event causes these autonomic changes. Not only the hypothalamus but also other brain structures with an autonomic role (such as the medulla) may be responsible for the altered circulatory physiology.

RESPIRATORY ABNORMALITIES. Pulmonary edema and hemorrhage can result from acute hypothalamic damage (hemorrhages, head trauma). Sudden dysfunction of the parasympathetic region in the anterior hypothalamus with consequent hypertension, left heart strain, and loss of pulmonary surfactant may explain the clinical picture [15, 18].

GASTROINTESTINAL ABNORMALITIES. Acute hypothalamic lesions (trauma, encephalitis, acute multiple sclerosis, hemorrhage, infarction, abscess, meningitis) can cause gastrointestinal ulceration. Neurogenic ulcers are most specifically located in the lower esophagus, which is otherwise an uncommon site for ulceration. However, neurogenic ulcers may be caused by acute lesions anywhere in the neuraxis, from the anterior hypothalamic region to the dorsal nucleus of the vagus or even in the spinal cord [17].

DIENCEPHALIC EPILEPSY. This term refers to episodes of hypertension, tachycardia, flushing, salivation, sweating, and oscillations in temperature in association with preserved alertness but also with the behavioral and affective responses appropriate to the altered autonomic response [18]. The electroencephalogram may be abnormal in half the cases, showing slowing but seldom the paroxysmal dysrhythmias characteristic of most forms of epilepsy. About half the patients respond to anticonvulsants. Although autonomic disturbances are common in many types of seizures, the clinical picture described here has been found with third ventricular tumors or third ventricular dilation caused by hydrocephalus [15, 18].

Disturbances of Water Balance. Hypothalamic osmoreceptors are in or near the supraoptic and paraventricular nuclei. It has been postulated that intracellular dehydration, manifested by increased intracellular sodium concentration, or extracellular dehydration, manifested by increased angiotensin II concentration in the hypothalamic blood, may stimulate these osmoreceptors, which in turn elicit the release of antidiuretic hormone (ADH) by the large cells of the supraoptic and paraventricular nuclei. By contrast, when the intravascular volume increases, peripheral volume receptors in the large veins and left atrium mediate inhibition of ADH secretion [18].

The lateral hypothalamus, classically considered the drinking center, contains osmoreceptors but may also influence drinking behavior by causing general excitability of the region. In experimental animals, destructive lesions of the lateral hypothalamus cause some degree of adipsia (reduced water intake) but not enough to result in dehydration. By contrast, destructive lesions of the ventromedial nuclei may cause hyperdipsia.

DIABETES INSIPIDUS (DECREASED ADH RELEASE BUT NORMAL THIRST). Although lack of ADH prevents water reabsorption in the distal tubule with consequent excretion of a large volume of dilute urine, an intact thirst mechanism induces water intake, thereby preventing hypernatremia. Diabetes insipidus [15, 18] results from destruction of at least 90 percent of the large neurons in the supraoptic and paraventricular nuclei. Except for the familial variety, the lesion often involves the supraopticohypophysial tract rather than the neuronal bodies themselves. In such cases the disorder is often transient.

Diabetes insipidus may be either familial or caused by granulomas (sarcoidosis, meningovascular syphilis, histiocytosis), vascular lesions, trauma, or meningitis. Anxiety, alcohol, phenytoin, and anticholinergic agents reduce the secretion of ADH.

ESSENTIAL HYPERNATREMIA (DECREASED ADH RELEASE WITH ABSENCE OF THIRST). Diagnosis of this rare syndrome [15, 18] requires evidence of (1) hypernatremia unaccompanied by a corresponding fluid deficiency, (2) preserved renal responsiveness to ADH, (3) impaired secretion of ADH with hypernatremia, and (4) absence of thirst despite preserved conscious behavior. Some patients with the syndrome have a remarkable tolerance for hypernatremia, to the point of developing water intoxication when the condition is treated. Sodium levels that reach 170 mEq/L, however, are attended by muscle cramping, tenderness and weakness, fever, anorexia, paranoia, and lethargy. Lesions causing this syndrome have affected the tuberal region or the entire hypothalamus.

INAPPROPRIATE SECRETION OF ADH (SIADH) (ELEVATED ADH RELEASE WITH NORMAL THIRST). This syndrome [15, 18] is characterized by (1) serum hyposmolarity and hyponatremia, (2) normal renal excretion of sodium, and (3) inappropriately high urine osmolality without body fluid depletion.

Serum levels of ADH are elevated. The patient has anorexia, nausea, vomiting, and irritability that may progress to paranoid delusions and generalized seizures when the serum sodium level falls below 110 mEq/L. Partial damage of the supraoptic and paraventricular nuclei or neighboring areas may cause the syndrome. Such damage may be due to trauma, subarachnoid hemorrhage, hydrocephalus, tumors, meningitis, encephalitis, or drugs, particularly vincristine, chlorpropamide, cyclophosphamide, carbamazepine, and chlorpromazine. Production of ADH by a tumor or inflammatory tissue outside the hypothalamus may also cause the syndrome, which has been also linked to myxedema, cardiac failure, and nonneoplastic pulmonary disease, as well as to porphyria and other peripheral neuropathies. Impairment of peripheral afferent inhibitory pathways carrying information from the volume receptors to the hypothalamus has been invoked to explain SIADH with polyneuropathies [18].

PRIMARY POLYDIPSIA OR HYPERDIPSIA (EXCESSIVE WATER DRINKING IN THE ABSENCE OF HYPOVOLEMIA OR HYPONATREMIA. Patients with this disturbance [18] may drink in response to (1) conditioned behavior ("beer drinker's hyponatremia," "tea party epilepsy") or other psychogenic factors, (2) hyperangiotensinemia, found in renal patients with thirst despite a normal electrolyte balance maintained with hemodialysis, and (3) rarely, hypothalamic disease [8]. In the last case, drinking often compensates for mild diabetes insipidus.

Disturbances of Caloric Balance and Feeding Behavior

OBESITY. Lesions in the ventromedial portion of the hypothalamus may cause obesity [1, 21]. Characteristically, such patients have hyperphagia until a higher body weight is reached, at which point they maintain a stable body weight unless the lesion progresses. The feeding behavior of patients with hypothalamic lesions resembles that of obese individuals with no demonstrable lesions; they (1) eat only a slight excess of food each day; (2) are less active; (3) eat fewer meals each day; (4) eat more at each meal; (5) eat more quickly; (6) eat more of a good-tasting food; (7) eat less of a bad-tasting food; (8) eat more when food is easily accessible; and (9) react more emotionally and are appeased by food intake [15]. Obesity after ventromedial lesions may result from affection of the catecholaminergic pathways coursing in this region rather than from destruction of the nuclei themselves. Most frequent lesions include craniopharyngioma, pituitary adenoma, surgery for the removal of these tumors, other types of trauma, encephalitis, and vascular lesions of the base of the brain [3]. Compulsive eating may be caused by rather nonspecific brain lesions. It may be occasionally responsive to anticonvulsant therapy [9]. The following syndromes are thought to be due to hypothalamic dysfunction:

KLEINE-LEVIN SYNDROME. Kleine-Levin syndrome is a rare variety of compulsive eating behavior in adolescent males, characterized by episodes of hyperphagia, with or without excess appetite (bulimia), hypersomnolence, hyperactivity when awake, and behavioral disturbances, particularly hypersexuality. Although traditionally considered a hypothalamic derangement, a recent report described medial thalamic pathology in one case [6]. A viral illness precedes the onset of the syndrome in some cases. The disorder usually disappears during the third decade.

BABINSKI-FRÖHLICH SYNDROME. Babinski-Fröhlich syndrome comprises obesity and hypogenitalism [18]. Obesity results from damage to the ventromedial region, whereas gonadotropin deficiency follows destruction of the adjacent infundibulum.

PRADER-LABHART-WILLI SYNDROME. Prader-Labhart-Willi syndrome comprises obesity, hypogenitalism, short stature, and a tendency to develop diabetes mellitus [10]. Affected infants tend to be somnolent and eat little, but between 6 months and 2 years of age they begin to eat in excess and become obese. Morphologic changes in the hypothalamus have not been found.

LAURENCE-MOON-BARNET-BIEDL SYNDROME. Laurence-Moon-Barnet-Biedl syndrome comprises obesity, hypogonadism, mental deficiency, tapetoretinal degeneration, and polydactyly [18]. The condition is transmitted as an autosomal dominant trait. Hypothalamic lesions have not been found.

EMACIATION

DIENCEPHALIC SYNDROME OF INFANCY. This syndrome [15, 18] is characterized by emaciation, with loss of subcutaneous fat, nystagmus, and an inappropriately jovial behavior. Progressive emaciation occurs despite normal food intake. Growth hormone levels may be high. The syndrome usually appears in boys aged 3 to 12 months and is caused by a slow-growing astrocytoma of the anterior hypothalamus or optic nerve. Children who survive beyond their second year become obese and irritable.

LATERAL HYPOTHALAMIC SYNDROME. Fewer than 5 case reports deal with lateral hypothalamic lesions causing aphagia [18]. Multiple sclerosis [13], tumors, and trauma have been implicated.

ANOREXIA NERVOSA. Anorexia nervosa is characterized by anorexia, weight loss, and amenorrhea in an otherwise endocrinologically normal young woman [15]. Although the syndrome suggests hypothalamic dysfunction, in most cases no morphologic changes have been found in the hypothalamus [16].

Disturbances of Reproductive Functions

HYPOGONADOTROPIC HYPOGONADISM. This type of hypogonadism may follow any hypothalamic or pituitary lesion. It is manifested by amenorrhea or male gonadal dysfunction.

NONPUERPERAL GALACTORRHEA

PROLACTIN-SECRETING PITUITARY TUMORS. About one-third of chromophobe adenomas secrete prolactin.

STRUCTURAL DAMAGE TO THE INFUNDIBULUM OR HYPOTHALAMUS. Such damage may interrupt the dopaminergic pathway that inhibits prolactin secretion by the pituitary. This pathway originates in the arcuate nucleus [15].

OTHER CAUSES. Other causes of this disorder include irritative lesions of the anterior chest wall, thoracic spinal cord lesions, neuroleptic and contraceptive drugs, and hypothyroidism [15].

PRECOCIOUS PUBERTY. Although generally idiopathic, precocious puberty may be due to hypothalamic disease or pineal tumors, some of the latter affecting also the floor of the third ventricle [20].

EXCESSIVE OR UNCONTROLLABLE SEXUAL BEHAVIOR. Occasionally this behavior may be a consequence of lesions of the caudal hypothalamus [19].

Other Endocrine Disturbances.
Disorders such as panhypopituitarism, hypothalamic hypothyroidism, acromegaly, and Cushing's syndrome are reviewed in standard endocrinology textbooks.

Disturbances of Memory.
The mammillary bodies are frequently involved in Korsakoff's psychosis, characterized by an impairment in the acquisition of new items of information (recent memory loss). However, lesions in the mammillary bodies [24] or fornix [8] may be unaccompanied by memory loss. Because memory loss occurs following lesions of the ventromedial region of the hypothalamus, it has been postulated that this area is crucial for the storage of information [1, 21]. Its deafferentation by lesions of both the fornical projection and the amygdalofugal pathway coursing in the lateral hypothalamus may also cause amnesia [18].

TABLE 16-3. *Presenting Complaints in 1,000 Cases of Pituitary Adenoma*

Complaints	Number of cases
Visual disturbances	421
Headache	137
Acromegaly	136
Related to hypopituitarism	95
Amenorrhea	48
Diplopia	7
Others	156

Source: Hollenhorst, R. W., and Younge, B. R. Ocular manifestations produced by adenomas of the pituitary gland: Analysis of 1000 cases. *In* Kohler, P. O., and Ross, G. T. (Eds.). *Diagnosis and Treatment of Pituitary Tumors.* Amsterdam: Excerpta Medica, 1973.

Disturbances of Emotional Behavior and Affect

RAGE AND FEAR. When caused by hypothalamic lesions, rage and fear occur in episodic outbursts, usually triggered by a threatening stimulus (such as restraint or a delay in feeding) and are part of a fully coordinated behavioral response with an intense autonomic component [18]. Between the outbursts, the behavior is normal and the patient may realize the inappropriateness of such behavior and apologize for it. Attacks of rage may also result from lesions of the orbitofrontal cortex or temporal lobe. When the hypothalamus is responsible, the ventromedial region is usually involved. By contrast, stimulation of the posterior "sympathetic" area elicits responses of fear and horror.

APATHY. Apathy may follow lesions of the posterior or lateral hypothalamus.

Headache.

In 1 of 7 patients with a pituitary tumor the presenting complaint is headache. It is usually bitemporal or bifrontal, behind the eyes, and is thought to be due to compression of the diaphragma sellae [15].

Impaired Visual Acuity; Visual Field Defects.

About half the patients with pituitary adenoma present with visual complaints, and about 15 percent or more have decreased visual acuity or field defects on formal testing (Table 16-3) [11]. Bitemporal defects, related to compression of the inferior aspect of the chiasm, are most common. However, asymmetrical tumor growth may cause preferential involvement of one eye, with unilateral blindness, or of the optic tract, with consequent homonymous hemianopia. The position of the chiasm in relation to the sella also determines the pattern of the visual field defect. The chiasm lies over the sella

TABLE 16-4. *Clinical Findings with Lesions in the Different Regions of the Hypothalamus or in the Pituitary Gland*

Anterior Hypothalamus ("parasympathetic area")
  Hyperthermia
  Insomnia
  Diabetes insipidus
  Emaciation
Posterior Hypothalamus ("sympathetic area")
  Hypothermia
  Poikilothermia
  Hypersomnia, coma
  Apathy
Medial Hypothalamus
  Hyperdipsia (excessive water intake)
  Diabetes insipidus
  Syndrome of inappropriate ADH secretion
  Obesity
  Amnesia
  Rage
  Dwarfism
Arcuate Nucleus and Infundibulum
  Hypopituitarism
Lateral Hypothalamus
  Adipsia (reduced water intake)
  Emaciation
  Apathy
Pituitary Gland
  Visual field defects
  Headache
  Decreased hormonal action
    Dwarfism
    Hypogonadism
    Hypothyroidism
    Glucocorticoid deficiency (usually with panhypopituitarism)
  Excessive hormonal secretion (adenomas)
    Cushing's syndrome
    Gigantism (child), acromegaly (adult)
    Hyperprolactinemia

in 80 percent of brains, over the tuberculum sellae in 9 percent of brains (prefixed chiasm), and over the dorsum sellae in 11 percent of brains (postfixed chiasm) [2]. About 6 percent of the patients have central or temporal scotomas, which may pass unnoticed if only the periphery of the visual field is tested.

Optic glioma of childhood is accompanied by signs of hypothalamic dysfunction in about one-third of the cases [12]. These patients present with impaired visual acuity, which may remain stable, and optic disc pallor.

Diplopia. Diplopia with hypothalamic-pituitary tumors is rare unless (1) the tumor is large, (2) it becomes suddenly enlarged by hemorrhage into it (pituitary apoplexy) [23], or (3) it involves primarily the cavernous sinus (carotid aneurysm, metastatic tumors). Tumors extending laterally from the sella tend to cause dysfunction of the oculomotor nerve, which is expressed by ptosis and adduction weakness.

CLINICAL FINDINGS RESULTING FROM LESIONS IN THE DIFFERENT AREAS OF THE HYPOTHALAMUS AND IN THE PITUITARY GLAND

In the previous section the presenting complaints were discussed as means of localizing the lesion. In Table 16-4, the reverse path is followed: given the site of the lesion, the most likely clinical findings are listed.

REFERENCES

1. Beal, M. F., et al. Gangliocytoma of third ventricle: Hyperphagia, somnolence, and dementia. *Neurology* (N.Y.) 31:1224, 1981.
2. Bergland, R. M., Ray, B. S., and Torack, R. M. Anatomical variations in the pituitary gland and adjacent structures in 225 human autopsy cases. *J. Neurosurg.* 28:93, 1968.
3. Bray, G. A., and Gallagher, T. F., Jr. Manifestations of hypothalamic obesity in man: A comprehensive investigation of eight patients and a review of the literature. *Medicine* 54:301, 1975.
4. Brodal, A. *Neurological Anatomy in Relation to Clinical Medicine* (3rd ed.). New York: Oxford University Press, 1981. Pp. 726–754.
5. Carpenter, M. B. *Human Neuroanatomy* (7th ed.). Baltimore: The Williams & Wilkins Co., 1976. Pp. 478–495.
6. Carpenter, S., Yassa, R., and Ochs, R. A pathologic basis for Kleine-Levin syndrome. *Arch. Neurol.* 39:25, 1982.
7. Fox, R. H., et al. Hypothermia in a young man with an anterior hypothalamic lesion. *Lancet* 2:185, 1970.
8. Garcia-Bengochea, F., et al. The section of the fornix in the surgical treatment of certain epilepsies. *Trans. Am. Neurol. Assoc.* 79:176, 1954.
9. Green, R. S., and Rau, J. H. Treatment of compulsive eating disturbances with anticonvulsant medication. *Am. J. Psychiat.* 131:428, 1974.
10. Haymaker, W., Anderson, E., and Nauta, W. J. *The Hypothalamus.* Springfield, Ill.: Charles C Thomas, 1969.
11. Hollenhorst, R. W., and Younge, B. R. Ocular Manifestations Produced by Adenomas of the Pituitary Gland: Analysis of 1000 Cases. *In* Kohler, P. O., and Ross, G. T. (Eds.). *Diagnosis and Treatment of Pituitary Tumors.* Amsterdam: Excerpta Medica, 1973.

12. Hoyt, W. F., and Baghdassarian, S. A. Optic glioma of childhood. *Br. J. Ophthalmol.* 53:793, 1969.
13. Kamalian, N., Keesey, R. E., and ZuRhein, G. M. Lateral hypothalamic demyelination and cachexia in a case of "malignant" multiple sclerosis. *Neurology* (Minn.) 25:25, 1975.
14. Langevin, H., and Iversen, L. L. A new method for the microdissection of the human hypothalamus, with mapping of cholinergic GABA and catecholamine systems in twelve nuclei and areas. *Brain* 103:623, 1980.
15. Martin, J. B., Reichlin, S., and Brown, G. M. *Clinical Neuroendocrinology.* Philadelphia: F. A. Davis, 1977.
16. Mecklenburg, R. S., et al. Hypothalamic dysfunction in patients with anorexia nervosa. *Medicine* 53:147, 1974.
16a. Morgane, P. J., and Panksepp, J. *Handbook of the Hypothalamus* (3 vol.). New York: Marcel Dekker, 1981.
17. Pernet, G. E. Stress ulcers and the neurosurgeon. *J. Iowa Med. Soc.* 54:583, 1964.
18. Plum, F., and Van Uitert, R. Nonendocrine Diseases and Disorders of the Hypothalamus. *In* Reichlin, S., Baldessarini, R. J., and Martin, J. B. *The Hypothalamus.* New York, Raven Press, 1978. Pp. 415–473.
19. Poeck, K., and Pilleri, G. Release of hypersexual behavior due to lesion in the limbic system. *Acta Neurol. Scand.* 41:233, 1965.
20. Puschett, J. B., and Goldberg, M. Endocrinopathy associated with pineal tumor. *Ann. Intern. Med.* 69:203, 1968.
21. Reeves, A. G., and Plum, F. Hyperphagia, rage, and dementia accompanying a ventromedial hypothalamic neoplasm. *Arch. Neurol.* 20:616, 1969.
22. Stuart, C. A., Neelon, F. A., and Lebovitz, H. E. Disordered control of thirst in hypothalamic-pituitary sarcoidosis. *N. Engl. J. Med.* 303:1078, 1980.
23. Symonds, C. Ocular palsy as the presenting symptom of pituitary adenoma. *Bull. Johns Hopkins Hosp.* 111:72, 1962.
24. Victor, M., Adams, R. D., and Collins, G. H. *The Wernicke-Korsakoff Syndrome.* Philadelphia: F.A. Davis, 1971, Pp. 166–170.

Chapter 17

THE ANATOMIC LOCALIZATION OF LESIONS IN THE THALAMUS

Joseph C. Masdeu

FUNCTIONAL ANATOMY OF THE THALAMUS

The paired thalamic nuclei are egg-shaped structures of gray matter located on both sides of the third ventricle. They represent the largest portion of the diencephalon; other diencephalic structures are the epithalamus (pineal and habenular complex), the subthalamic nucleus, and the hypothalamus. Anatomically and functionally, four regions can be distinguished in the thalamus—anterior, posterior, medial, and lateral, partially separated from each other by white matter laminae that are visible to the naked eye [6, 10, 53, 61]. In the core of the thalamus, a fifth region is encased by these laminae—the intralaminar nuclei. Finally, the lateral aspect of the thalamus is covered by a thin layer of cells—the reticular nucleus of the thalamus. A simplified account of the thalamic nuclei and their connections, pertinent to clinical localization, is given in Table 17-1. Characteristically, thalamic connections are reciprocal, that is, the target of the axonal projection of any given thalamic nucleus sends back fibers to that nucleus. Nevertheless, thalamocortical projections are often larger than their corticothalamic counterparts (e.g., the geniculocalcarine projection). Figure 17-1 illustrates the position and main cortical projections of the thalamic nuclei.

From a diagnostic standpoint, the complex thalamic anatomy can be considered in four main regions:

1. The midline, intralaminar, reticular, and ventral anterior nuclei mediate general cortical alerting responses and are termed *nonspecific* thalamic nuclei. By contrast, *specific* thalamic nuclei receive sensory information from the body, process it, and project the pertinent output to specific areas of the cortex, such as the somatosensory area and visual cortex. The nonspecific thalamic nuclei receive strong projections from the midbrain reticular formation and fibers from the spinothalamic tract as well as from other sensory pathways. Some stimuli (e.g., auditory, pain) excite this alerting system more easily than others (e.g., visual). These nuclei project back to the midbrain and to the specific thalamic nuclei. Lesions that involve these structures bilaterally cause impairment of alertness.

2. The medial (dorsomedial) and anterior thalamic nuclear groups play an important role in memory and emotions. They are connected with the hypothalamus, the "limbic lobe" (cingulate gyrus, medial temporal region, insula), and the frontal lobe. Even unilateral lesions of these structures may cause recent memory loss [12]. It has been postulated that the medial thalamic nucleus may mediate acquisition of new information [28]. This nucleus receives afferents from the temporal lobe and projects to the orbital cortex of the frontal lobe.

3. The ventral lateral and basal nuclear groups are concerned with elaboration and relay to the cortex of sensory information and with sen-

sorimotor control. Elaboration and relay to the cortex of sensory information concerns mainly three structures, as follows:

A. The ventral posterior nuclear group, in which taste and somatosensory information is elaborated and projected to the somatosensory cortex of the parietal lobe. Within the thalamus, lateral inhibition increases sharpness in spatial localization. Information from receptors in the head reaches the ventral posterior medial nucleus through the trigeminothalamic pathways. The ventral lateral nucleus processes somatosensory information conveyed by the spinothalamic tract and medial lemniscus.
B. The medial geniculate body, in which auditory information from the inferior colliculus passes on to the transverse temporal gyrus, buried in the depth of the Sylvian fissure.
C. The lateral geniculate body, which is the relay station for the visual pathway that receives from the retinal neurons the axons that form the optic tract and originates the axons that through the optic radiations project to the calcarine cortex. Lesions of this thalamic nucleus are discussed in Chapter 6.

Sensorimotor control is carried out by the more anterior of the ventrolateral nuclei (ventral lateral and ventral anterior) and perhaps by the intralaminar nuclei. The ventrolateral nucleus integrates input from the cerebellum, basal ganglia, and mechanoreceptors from the musculoskeletal system; it projects to the precentral cortex or primary motor cortex (area 4). This nucleus coordinates predominantly the finer, distal, motor movements. The ventral anterior nucleus may play a role in voluntary attention. It has strong connections with the pallidum, medial thalamic nuclei, and frontal cortex.

Anatomically, the thalamus constitutes the keystone for two large sensorimotor control loops: (1) the cerebello-rubro-thalamo-cortico-ponto-cerebellar loop, and (2) the cortico-striato-pallido-thalamo-cortical loop. Although the physiologic role of each loop is far from clear, it is known that lesions in each loop cause different syndromes. Obviously, the anatomy allows ample possibilities for lesions to affect both loops. Symptoms and signs derived from cerebellar lesions are discussed in Chapter 15. Those derived from basal-ganglia lesions are discussed in Chapter 18. Motor findings that point to the thalamus as the site of the lesion will be given preferential attention here.

4. The fourth main region of the thalamus comprises the dorsolateral and posterior nuclear groups, particularly the pulvinar, which seem to modulate cortical attention needed for the accurate production of lan-

270

TABLE 17-1. *Source and Destination of the Thalamic Connections**

Thalamic Regions and Nuclei	Afferent Connections	Efferent Connections
Anterior		
Anterior nucleus	Mammillary bodies (mammillothalamic tract)	Cingulate gyrus
	Hippocampus (fornix)	
Medial		
Medial (or dorsal medial) nucleus	Frontal lobe	Frontal lobe
	Amygdala	Lateral hypothalamus
	Inferior temporal cortex	Ventral anterior thalamic nucleus
	Centromedian thalamic nucleus	
	Zona incerta	
Midline nuclei	Hypothalamus	Hypothalamus
		Dorsal medial thalamic nucleus
Lateral		
Dorsal		
Lateral dorsal nucleus	Posteromedial temporal region (fornix)	Cingulate gyrus, posterior part
		Mesial parietal cortex
Ventral		
Ventral anterior nucleus	Pallidum	Orbitofrontal cortex
	Substantia nigra	Intralaminar thalamic nuclei
	Dorsal medial thalamic nucleus	Dorsal medial thalamic nucleus
Ventral lateral nucleus	Pallidum (lenticular fasciculus; ansa lenticularis)	Paracentral cortex, areas 4 and 3a [30]
	Contralateral cerebellum (dentatorubrothalamic tract; thalamic fasciculus)	
Ventral posterior lateral nucleus	*Contralateral* receptors for joint position, vibration, epicritic touch (medial lemniscus)	Postcentral gyrus, areas 3b, 1, and 2 [30]
	Contralateral receptors for touch, heat and cold, painful stimuli (spinothalamic tract)	
	Dorsal medial thalamic nucleus	
	Septal region	
	Frontal lobe (medial forebrain bundle)	
	Somatosensory cortex	

*In parentheses is the name of the white matter bundles that correspond to each connection.

TABLE 17-1 (continued)

Thalamic Regions and Nuclei	Afferent Connections	Efferent Connections
Ventral posterior medial nucleus	*Contralateral* spinal trigeminal nucleus [face, painful stimuli] *Contralateral* main trigeminal nucleus [touch, propioception] Mesencephalic trigeminal nucleus [bite mechanoreceptors]	Postcentral gyrus; lower lateral, "face" region
Posterior		
Dorsal		
Lateral posterior nucleus	Pulvinar	Superior and inferior parietal lobules
Pulvinar		
Medial	Medial geniculate body	Superior and inferior parietal lobules
Lateral	Lateral geniculate body	
Inferior	Ventral lateral thalamic nucleus	Posterior temporal region Peristriate occipital cortex
Ventral		
Posterior thalamic zone	*Bilateral* receptors of noxious stimuli	Other thalamic nuclei
Medial geniculate body	Bilateral hearing (brachium of the inferior colliculus)	Transverse temporal gyrus of Heschl
Lateral geniculate body	Contralateral visual field (optic tract)	Calcarine cortex
Intralaminar		
Centromedian and parafascicular nuclei	Pallidum Frontal lobe, areas 4 and 6	Striatum: caudate, puta- Ventral lateral thalamic nuclei
Smaller intralaminar nuclei	Brainstem reticular formation; spinothalamic tract	Ventral anterior thalamic nuclei Orbital cortex
Reticular nucleus	Thalamocortical projection	Thalamic nuclei

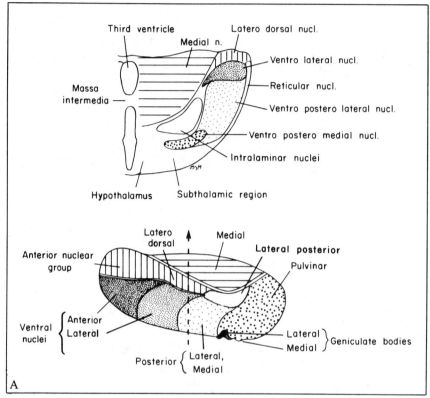

FIG. 17-1. (A) *Thalamic nuclei. Top, Frontal section of the thalamus at the level of the dashed line on the figure at the bottom. Bottom, Laterodorsal view of the thalamus, showing the position of the thalamic nuclei.* **(B)** *Afferents and cerebral cortical projections of the thalamic nuclei. Top, Main sources of afferents to the different thalamic nuclei and their cortical projections. Bottom, Main cortical representation of the different thalamic nuclei, illustrated on the lateral and medial aspects of the cerebral hemispheres. (Both A and B modified from M. B. Carpenter [10].)*

guage-related tasks in the left hemisphere and visuospatial tasks in the right [40]. This area is much better developed in humans than in lower mammals. During ontogenesis, it is the last region to reach adult morphology [61].

VASCULAR SUPPLY OF THE THALAMUS

Cerebrovascular disease is the most common cause of discrete thalamic pathology resulting in signs and symptoms of localizing value. Infarcts are more common than hemorrhages. Therefore, some knowledge of the vascular supply of the thalamic nuclei helps greatly to understand

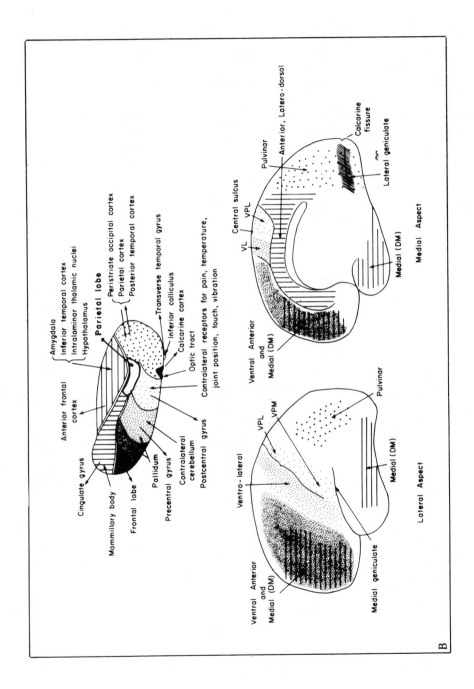

B

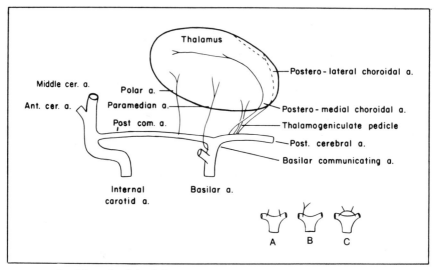

FIG. 17-2. *Arterial supply of the thalamus. Insert: Variations in the origin of the paramedian arteries, which may arise from each basilar communicating artery* **(A)**, *from a single pedicle originating in one basilar communicating artery* **(B)**, *or from a vascular arcade connecting both basilar communicating arteries* **(C)**. *(Modified from P. Castaigne et al. [12].)*

the so-called thalamic syndromes and the localization of thalamic lesions.

The thalamic arteries arise from the posterior communicating arteries and from the perimesencephalic segment of the posterior cerebral arteries [12, 32]. The origin and territory of supply of the different thalamic vessels differ in each person [43, 44, 45]. For instance, when the posterior communicating artery is small or absent, arterial twigs from the posterior cerebral artery supply the thalamic territory that is otherwise supplied by branches of the posterior communicating artery. Table 17-2 summarizes the more common vascular patterns (Fig. 17-2). For this account, the segment of the posterior cerebral artery proximal to the ostium of the posterior communicating artery has been termed the *basilar communicating artery* [12, 44].

LOCALIZATION OF ISCHEMIC THALAMIC LESIONS

In localizing ischemic lesions of the thalamus, several points should be kept in mind:

1. The whole arterial supply for the thalamus arises from the vertebrobasilar system, with a small or absent contribution from the posterior communicating artery [12].

TABLE 17-2. *Vascular Supply of the Thalamus*

Name of Vessel	Origin	Distribution
Polar arteries	Posterior communicating artery	Thalamic nuclei Reticular Ventral anterior Medial (anterior portion)
Paramedian thalamo-mesencephalic arteries	Basilar communicating artery (portion of posterior cerebral artery proximal to ostium of posterior communicating artery)	Thalamic nuclei Reticular Ventrolateral Medial Midline (paraventricular) Centromedian Other structures Red nucleus (superior-medial portion) Interpeduncular nucleus Decussation of the superior cerebellar peduncle Third nerve nucleus
Thalamogeniculate pedicle	Posterior cerebral artery, proximal to geniculate body level	Ventral caudal nuclei
Posteromedial choroidal arteries	Posterior cerebral artery, just distal to ostium of posterior communicating artery	Thalamic nuclei Centromedian Ventral posterior medial Medial geniculate body Pulvinar Medial (posterior portion) Anterior Other structures Crus cerebri Subthalamic nucleus Substantia nigra Red nucleus (lateral)
Posterolateral choroidal arteries	Posterior cerebral artery (between lateral geniculate body and dorsal pulvinar level)	Thalamic nuclei Lateral geniculate body Pulvinar (inferolateral portion) Laterodorsal Other structures Hippocampus Choroid plexus

2. The middle cerebral and anterior choroidal arteries do not supply the thalamus to such an extent that thalamic infarction would result from occlusion of these vessels [45]. Some internal capsular dysfunction, however, may result from occlusion of thalamic vessels [37]. In rare cases the anterior cerebral artery may contribute to the supply of the posterolateral thalamus through a posterior pericallosal vessel, which is anastomotic with the posterolateral choroidal artery [32].
3. The paramedian thalamic vessels often arise from a single pedicle that originates in one of the basilar communicating arteries (Fig. 17-2). Thus unilateral posterior cerebral artery occlusions may result in bilateral paramedian thalamic infarcts [12].

The *arterial territory* responsible for a thalamic ischemic infarct may be inferred from the clinical findings, as follows:

Paramedian Territory. These infarcts tend to involve also the paramedian region of the midbrain. The following findings result [12]:

Recent memory loss
Behavioral changes
Impaired level of consciousness
Oculomotor paresis
Contralateral hemiataxia
Delayed action tremor on the contralateral limbs

This syndrome is often due to occlusion of the top of the basilar artery [7, 18].

Thalamogeniculate (Lateral Thalamic) Territory. Ischemia in this territory causes the classic thalamic syndrome, described by Dejerine and Roussy [62]:
Transient slight hemiparesis
Hemianesthesia
Paroxysmal pain (thalamic pain)
Hemiataxia
Choreoathetoid movements
Athetoid posture ("thalamic hand")
Homonymous hemianopsia (often due to simultaneous medial occipital infarction)

All these findings occur on the side of the body contralateral to the lesioned thalamus. The more severe forms of the syndrome accompany proximal occlusion of the posterior cerebral artery. Partial forms result from lacunar infarction restricted to one of the larger thalamogeniculate vessels [38]. Disease of such small perforating arteries often accompanies diabetes and chronic hypertension.

CLINICAL MANIFESTATIONS OF LESIONS IN THE THALAMUS

The following considerations facilitate the understanding of the clinical manifestations of thalamic lesions:

1. Due to the smallness of the thalamus, *several of the nuclei* and even several of the different functional regions outlined above are usually affected simultaneously even by discrete lesions such as infarcts. Because arteriolar vascular territories cross the nuclear boundaries, as a rule ischemic disease affects several nuclei, often partially [12]. Even more important for lesion localization is the understanding that most thalamic lesions involve in addition the *neighboring areas.* Paramedian thalamic vascular lesions tend to affect the midbrain as well, with a resultant decrease in the level of alertness to the point of coma [12]. Thus, other motor or sensory findings that would point to thalamic involvement cannot be elicited. Laterally located lesions may disrupt the internal capsule, thereby causing motor and sensory deficits [25] that will mask those deficits characteristically present with thalamic involvement. For instance, the tendency to avoid using an otherwise strong limb contralateral to a lesioned ventral lateral thalamic area ("thalamic neglect") will not be manifest if capsular involvement has resulted in a hemiparesis. Lesions extending inferiorly may yield hemiballismus, for which the subthalamic lesion is probably primarily responsible.
2. Except for sensory deficits, unilateral thalamic lesions result in transient deficits. By contrast, bilateral lesions or unilateral lesions, such as hemorrhages or tumors, that press against the contralateral thalamus or impinge upon the midbrain may render the patient comatose or akinetic and mute.
3. Timing has a particular impact on the clinical expression of thalamic lesions. As the effects of an acute lesion recede, neglect may disappear, inability to walk may yield to mild ataxia, and hemisensory loss diminishes. Other findings, however, particularly the so-called "positive symptoms" (tremor, pain), usually become more pronounced within a few weeks after the injury.

Disturbances of Alertness. Sudden bilateral paramedian thalamic lesions such as infarcts may cause a decreased level of alertness ranging from somnolence to coma [12], generally transient. Prolonged coma may result if the lesion extends into the midbrain tegmentum. These patients often have oculomotor paresis [12]. By contrast, patients with pure thalamic involvement have very small reactive pupils ("diencephalic pupil"), and their extraocular movements, elicited by the doll's-eye maneuver, are full [47]. Akinetic mutism, discussed in Chapter 21, may follow bilateral paramedian thalamic lesions [3, 12, 50]. Other reported disturbances include inversion of the nycthemeral rhythm [18] and dissociation of sleep stages, detected by electroencephalography, between the two hemispheres [31]. The hemisphere affected by a thalamic tumor showed earlier onset of deeper sleep stages. The intralaminar, reticular, and ventral anterior nuclei seem to play the greatest role in mediating normal alertness [6]. Lesions in the region of the intralaminar nuclei cause drowsiness [26]. Electrical stimulation of this region induces arousal from sleep [60].

Disturbances of Mood and Affect. Apathy and lack of drive for motor expression can be considered minor forms of akinetic mutism. Both have been reported with lesions of the paramedian region of the thalamus. Less often, such lesions may cause agitation or dysphoria and even undue joviality, accompanied by confabulation [12]. Kleine-Levin syndrome, which is characterized by episodes of somnolence, hyperphagia, impaired recent memory, and hypersexual behavior and is traditionally believed to be related to hypothalamic disease, may be due to paramedian thalamic lesions [11]. Failure of goal-directed regulation of behavior has been observed with a lesion affecting the right anteroventral thalamic region [39]. Impaired "activation" of the frontal cortex by the ventral anterior nucleus may be the cause of such a deficit.

Memory Disturbances. Recent memory may be transiently or permanently impaired by lesions of the medial thalamic nuclear region [12, 28, 56]. This deficit appears most consistently with bilateral lesions but may be associated with even unilateral lesions of either thalamus [12]. Some patients seem to be aware of their deficit [51, 63], and others do not [56]. Whether this can be accounted for by differences in the site of the lesion remains to be determined.

Storage of new information is most severely impaired with medial thalamic lesions. Patients who are alert and active perform adequately in tests, such as digit span, which are intended to test the so-called immediate memory. Although amnesia is most profound for events taking place after the injury (recent memory loss), it often includes some information acquired days or months previously [36, 63].

In regard to the content of recall, a patient with bilateral medial thalamic lesions was described who recognized by their voices relatives whom he had failed to identify visually (prosopagnosia) [36]. Isolated disorientation in time results from discrete lesions in the medial thalamic region [51]. It has been suggested that lesions involving the left thalamus affect mainly verbal memory, whereas those in the nondominant paramedian thalamic region impair memory related to visual-spatial tasks [52, 58].

Sensory Disturbances. Thalamic lesions may cause sensory loss, often accompanied by paresthesias and pain.

PARESTHESIAS AND PAIN. Clinically, small lesions in the ventral posterior lateral nucleus of the thalamus may yield only contralateral paresthesias that lack "objective" sensory loss when tested at the bedside [20]. Such paresthesias tend to occur on one side of the face, particularly around the mouth, and in the distal portion of the limbs. These areas of the body have the largest representation in the thalamic sensory nuclei. When the trunk is also numb, the subjective feeling of numbness may stop abruptly in the midline, although on objective testing the sensory loss often fades toward the midline [37]. Such a "thalamic midline split," which is absent with parietal lesions, has been thought to have some clinical value in identifying the site of the lesion [38]. The numb areas of the body may feel swollen, enlarged, shortened, twisted, or torn, or they may tingle. Objects held with the limb contralateral to the lesion may feel abnormally heavy. Finally, the patient may be unaware of a profound sensory loss.

Pain referred to as *thalamic pain* is perhaps the best known component of Dejerine and Roussy's "thalamic syndrome," described above [62]. The unpleasant or excruciatingly painful sensation on the side of the body contralateral to a thalamic lesion (an infarct is most common) may appear at the time of the injury [20] or when the sensory loss begins to improve. The pain feels localized to the skin. Cutaneous stimuli trigger paroxysmal exacerbations of the pain, which persists after the stimulus has been removed. The latency between the stimulus and pain perception is prolonged, suggesting that the pathways conveying it are polysynaptic. Because the perception of epicritic pain, such as that induced with a pinprick, is reduced on the painful areas, this symptom has been termed *anesthesia dolorosa* or painful anesthesia; a similar symptom may follow damage of the posterior root ganglia (herpes zoster) or trigeminal nerve or nucleus (trigeminal neuralgia with anesthesia). Such pain remains despite conventional analgesics but responds to carbamazepine or some neuroleptics (amitriptyline and perphenazine). Involvement of the posterior ventrobasal region of the thalamus has been regarded as critical in the genesis of thalamic pain [6].

Thalamic pain seldom occurs with tumors. It has been described most often with vascular lesions, some of which involve not only the thalamus but also the deep parietal white matter [1]. Besides, delayed pain may follow cortical parietal infarcts, particularly those in the bank of the Sylvian fissure (pseudo-thalamic syndrome) [4].

LOSS OF SENSORY MODALITIES. All sensory modalities are processed in the ventral posterior nucleus of the thalamus contralateral to the side of the body where they are perceived. Within the nucleus there is a definite topographic distribution: the head is represented anteroinferomedially, whereas the leg is represented posterosuperolaterally; the arm is represented in an intermediate position. A larger volume of the nucleus is dedicated to the mouth, tongue, and distal portion of the extremities; their thalamic representation is almost completely crossed. The large oral thalamic and cortical representation in humans may well be related to language functions [13]. The face, proximal portion of the limbs, and trunk are represented in a smaller volume of thalamic tissue, mainly contralateral but partially ipsilateral [6]. Thalamic sensory loss tends to occur maximally in the distal portion of the limbs and often spares the face. Such sparing may be related to the different vascular supply of this portion of the ventroposterior region (paramedian territory) or to the bilateral thalamic representation of the face.

In regard to the thalamic topography of the different sensory modalities, physiologic experimental studies have shown that cells concerned with deep pressure and movements of the limbs are preferentially located in the rostral and caudal ends of the ventral posterior lateral nucleus. The central part of the nucleus contains neurons that respond to cutaneous stimuli. In humans, however, lesions large enough to produce any sensory loss most often involve several modalities. No extant clinicopathologic studies allow precise identification of thalamic areas for touch versus joint position or vibration. Pain sensation has been obtained by stimulation of the basal part of the nucleus [6].

Because perceptions of a pinprick, temperature, touch, and vibration are altered more after thalamic than after cortical lesions, these sensory modalities have been termed *primary* or *thalamic*. By contrast, conscious joint position identification, two-point discrimination, stereognosis, and graphesthesia tend to be more impaired after cortical parietal lesions, and are thus termed *secondary* or *cortical* sensory modalities. Nevertheless, parietal lesions often cause some impairment of thalamic modalities and vice versa. Occasionally, a lesion in the thalamus may disturb mainly the so-called cortical sensory modalities [57, case 1;33].

Anesthesia and impaired temperature perception tend to occur with basal lesions near the medial geniculate body [6]. Because vibration sense remains unaltered after surgical removal of the parietal cortex, it has been assumed that hemispheric lesions causing loss of vibratory sense necessarily implicate the thalamus or the thalamocortical projections [49].

Disturbances of visual acuity and hearing are discussed in Chapters 6 and 10. Visual field defects caused by thalamic lesions frequently involve the superior quadrant bilaterally. In one patient an intolerance to light ("central dazzle") was ascribed to a thalamic lesion [15].

Motor Disturbances. Just as the sensory disturbances described in the previous section can be related to lesions in the ventral posterior nucleus of the thalamus, motor disturbances can be related to lesions of the ventral lateral nucleus and the adjacent subthalamic region.

Following an acute thalamic lesion, even a unilateral lesion, the patient may be transiently unable to stand or even sit, despite normal strength of the limbs when tested against resistance [25, 34a, 55]. *Neglect* to use the limbs contralateral to the lesion (thalamic neglect) may convey to the examiner the false impression that the patient is hemiplegic [14, 58]. Certainly large infarcts, lacunes [38], hematomas [57], and tumors may involve the neighboring internal capsule, causing a more or less profound hemiplegia. However, purely thalamic involvement does not result in hemiparesis. Lesions in the ventral lateral nucleus of the thalamus cause contralateral hypotonia, reduction of emotional expression, and transient neglect [26]. This syndrome may occur even with lesions that are discrete enough to spare all sensory modalities and the early (thalamic) components of the somatosensory evoked response. Such lesions, which are circumscribed to the ventral lateral nucleus, would spare the ventral posterior nucleus. Because the late components of the somatosensory evoked response are abolished, it has been postulated that the ventral lateral nucleus plays a key role in the activation of the parietal cortex. Bilateral thalamic or subthalamic lesions cause *akinesia* as a result of a peculiar form of sensory inattention [55].

Damage to the dentatorubrothalamic projection to the ventral lateral nucleus by a lesion rostral to the decussation of the superior cerebellar peduncle results in *hemiataxia* of the contralateral limbs. Some weeks after the injury (which is most often ischemic) *tremor* at a rate of between 3 and 5 cycles per second may appear in the affected extremities. It is mainly distal and increases greatly during the performance of any movement. This tremor may be abolished by a surgical lesion of the ventral lateral nucleus of the thalamus. If the central tegmental tract is also involved, tremor with a similar rate may affect the eyelids, eyes, or palate ("palatal myoclonus"). Such ischemic lesions occupy the territory of the thalamopeduncular paramedian vessels and are often related to occlusion of the top of the basilar artery [12].

Lesions that are slightly more rostral, involving the subthalamic region and the pallidothalamic projections to the ventral lateral nucleus, may cause transient contralateral *hemiballismus*. After some days or weeks the amplitude of the movement decreases and either disappears or adopts a choreic or athetotic pattern. *Chorea* or *athetosis* may also appear sometime after an infarct of this region in a patient who initially was free of adventitious movements [12]. Although they are most common after lesions of the subthalamic nucleus, such abnormal movements may occur with pallidostriatal or purely thalamic lesions, more often when the latter are bilateral [9, 14, 24]. It has been postulated that the critical lesion required to produce athetosis would destroy the pallidothalamic projection to the cortex while sparing the corticospinal tract [17].

Abnormal posturing of the hand, often termed *thalamic hand,* may appear 2 or more weeks after the occurrence of a vascular lesion of the same region. The hand assumes a posture that is commonly seen in patients with athetosis—flexion at the wrist and metacarpophalangeal joints, whereas the interphalangeal joints are hyperextended. Flexion of the metacarpophalangeal joints increases from the second digit, which may be actually extended to the fifth digit, which is markedly flexed. The fingers may be forcibly abducted. The thumb is either abducted or pushed against the palm [33].

Other abnormal movements described with thalamic lesions include action *myoclonus* [2] and *asterixis* [16]. *Imitation synkineses,* also called mirror movements, are common after thalamic lesions [22]. In such cases the distal portion of the limb contralateral to the thalamic lesion tends to imitate the movement performed by the healthy side. When the patient forcibly makes a fist with the sound hand, the fingers of the other hand curl up into the palm, and the patient ends by making a fist with both hands. Loss of position sense or loss of cortical activation by the thalamus may underlie these abnormal movements, which can be decreased, like the choreic movements described above, when the patient concentrates his attention on avoiding them.

A decreased corneal reflex may be present in patients with hemiparesis and hemisensory loss due to a cerebral hemispheric lesion [21]. Loss of parietal excitatory influence on the lower brainstem seems to be responsible for this finding [42]. Pure thalamic lesions, even those that cause a marked hemisensory loss, do not depress the corneal reflex [41].

Disturbances of Ocular Motility. Lesions restricted to the thalamus cause only subtle changes in ocular motility. Visual information from the superior colliculus, relayed by the pulvinar to the parietal lobe ("second visual system"), contributes to the detection and localization of visual events in space and to the production of saccadic eye movements that allow the "first" (geniculostriate) visual system to identify such events. Lesions in the pulvinar have been said to cause (1) a decrease in the critical flicker frequency and neglect of visual objects in the periphery of the contralateral visual field, (2) prolonged latency of visually evoked saccadic eye movements, and (3) a paucity of spontaneous eye movements directed toward the contralateral hemifield [64].

Much more striking, and more obvious at the bedside, are eye movement abnormalities that occur when a lesion includes the midbrain and thalamus; this often happens with paramedian thalamopeduncular infarcts [12]. In such cases, impairment of oculomotor function results in abnormal pupils, ptosis, and restriction of vertical eye movements and of adduction. Large thalamic hemorrhages may impinge on the midbrain or impair its function by causing raised intracranial pressure [23]. Rather typical eye findings ensue: The eyes become tonically deviated down and slightly adducted, as if peering at the tip of the nose [57].

In some instances the eyes may be tonically deviated to the side of the hemiparesis, opposite the thalamic bleed ("wrong-way eyes") [19, 57]. Although this is more frequent with thalamic hemorrhage, such a finding has been reported to occur with extrathalamic supratentorial lesions [46].

Depression of the reticular activating system (most often metabolic in nature) or involvement of both thalami results in small pupils (1 mm in diameter) that react well to light (diencephalic pupils) [47].

Disturbances of Symbolic Behavior. The thalamus modulates the association cortex involved in the processing of language and other "higher" cortical functions. Although compared with large cortical lesions, unilateral thalamic lesions do not impair these functions as much, the pattern of impairment has some localizing value. Mention has already been made of the contralateral motor neglect caused by lesions in the ventral lateral nucleus of the thalamus and of the contralateral visual inattention that results from lesions in the pulvinar.

Patients with right thalamic lesions may have constructional apraxia and display marked neglect of the left hemifield [58, 59]. Thalamic lesions may play a role in the production of pure alexia in humans [27].

Dominant-hemisphere thalamic lesions (hemorrhage has been reported most often) may cause a *transient* language disturbance characterized by (1) reduced spontaneous speech with paraphasic errors and perseveration, (2) varying degrees of auditory comprehension impairment, (3) preserved repetition and reading, (4) defective spontaneous writing

and writing to dictation but normal copying, (5) word-production anomia but spared word selection and word symbolism, and (6) distractibility. This deficit tends to resolve itself in a few weeks [1a, 8, 29]. Electrical
stimulation of the ventrolateral thalamus produces an acceleration of
speaking. The patient feels urged to speak faster [26]. Stimulation also
enhances later recall of objects presented to the patient. The left thalamus is involved in attention mechanisms that gate storage and retrieval
of both long-term and short-term verbal memory [40]. Derangement of a
specific cortical attention mechanism because of the thalamic lesion
would result in a lack of drive to speak and perseveration of apparently
unrelated verbal material [48]. Such language impairment resembles the
language impairment that results from left medial frontal lesions [5, 34,
35].

TOPOGRAPHIC LOCALIZATION
OF THALAMIC LESIONS

ANTERIOR THALAMIC REGION. Discrete lesions may be silent or cause language
disturbances when they affect the dominant hemisphere, or inattention,
which results more often when the right hemisphere is involved. Bilateral
lesions may cause akinesia and attentional disturbances. Lesions extending to the subthalamic area may cause athetosis, chorea, or postural
abnormalities (thalamic hand).

MEDIAL THALAMIC REGION. Lesions in this location may pass unnoticed
when they are small and unilateral. Large or bilateral lesions cause impairment of recent memory, apathy or agitation, attentional derangements, and somnolence or coma. Lesions that extend to the midbrain-
diencephalic junction may cause contralateral tremor and vertical gaze
palsy, affecting particularly downward gaze.

VENTROLATERAL THALAMIC REGION. Sensory loss, paroxysmal pains, and
hemiataxia in the contralateral side of the body are the most striking se-
quelae of lesions in this region. Hemineglect and language disturbances
may appear transiently.

POSTERIOR REGION. Basal lesions in this region may cause hemianesthesia,
"thalamic pain," and visual field defects. Dorsal lesions give rise to attentional disorders of the ipsilateral hemisphere, resulting in transient
aphasia when the dominant hemisphere is involved.

REFERENCES
1. Agnew, D. C., et al. In Bonica, J. J., et al (Eds.). Advances in Pain Research
   and Therapy, Vol. 5. New York: Raven Press, 1983. P. 941.

1a. Alexander, M. P., and LoVerme, S. R., Jr. Aphasia after left hemispheric intracerebral hemorrhage. *Neurology* (N.Y.) 30:1193, 1980.

2. Avanzini, G., Broggi, G., and Caraceni, T. Intention and action myoclonus from thalamic angioma. *Eur. Neurol.* 15:194, 1977.

3. Barraquer-Bordas, L., et al. Sur une nécrose thalamique avec méningo-épendymite subaiguë. *Acta Neurol. Belg.* 67:8, 1967.

4. Biemond, A. The conduction of pain above the level of the thalamus opticus. *Arch. Neurol. Psychiat.* (Chic.) 75:231, 1956.

5. Botez, M. I., and Barbeau, A. Role of subcortical structures, and particularly of the thalamus, in the mechanisms of speech and language. *Int. J. Neurol.* 8:300, 1971.

6. Brodal, A. *Neurological Anatomy in Relation to Clinical Medicine* (3rd ed.). New York: Oxford University Press, 1981. Pp. 94, 144, 230, 289, 361, 427, 656, 665, 668, 823, 836.

7. Caplan, L. R. "Top of the basilar" syndrome. *Neurology* 30:72, 1980.

8. Cappa, S. F., and Vignolo, L. A. "Transcortical" features of aphasia following left thalamic hemorrhage. *Cortex* 15:121, 1979.

9. Carpenter, M. B. Athetosis and the basal ganglia. *Arch. Neurol. Psychiat.* (Chic.) 63:875, 1950.

10. Carpenter, M. B. *Human Neuroanatomy* (7th ed.). Baltimore: The Williams & Wilkins Co., 1976. Pp. 435–477.

11. Carpenter, S., Yassa, R., and Ochs, R. A pathologic basis for Kleine-Levin syndrome. *Arch. Neurol.* 39:25, 1982.

12. Castaigne, P., et al. Paramedian thalamic and midbrain infarcts: Clinical and neuropathological study. *Ann. Neurol.* 10:127, 1981.

13. Celesia, G. G. Somatosensory evoked potentials recorded directly from human thalamus and sm I cortical area. *Arch. Neurol.* 36:399, 1979.

14. Cooper, I. S. *Parkinsonism. Its Medical and Surgical Therapy.* Springfield, Ill.: Charles C Thomas, 1961.

15. Cummings, G. L., and Gittinger, J. W., Jr. Central dazzle: A thalamic syndrome? *Arch. Neurol.* 38:372, 1981.

16. Donat, J. R. Unilateral asterixis due to thalamic hemorrhage. *Neurology* 30:83, 1980.

17. Dooling, E. C., and Adams, R. D. The pathological anatomy of posthemiplegic athetosis. *Brain* 98:29, 1975.

18. Façon, E., Steriade, M., and Wertheim, N. Hypersomnie prolongée engendrée par des lésions bilatérales du système activateur médial. Le syndrome thrombotique de la bifurcation du tronc basilaire. *Rev. Neurol.* 98:117, 1958.

19. Fisher, C. M. Some neuro-opthalmological observations. *J. Neurol. Neurosurg. Psychiat.* 30:383, 1967.

20. Fisher, C. M. Thalamic pure sensory stroke. A pathologic study. *Neurology* 28:1141, 1978.

21. Fisher, M. A., Shahani, B. T., and Young, R. R. Assessing segmental excitability after acute rostral lesions: II. The blink reflex. *Neurology* 29:45, 1979.

22. Foix, C., and Hillemand, P. Les syndromes de la region thalamique. *La Presse Med.* 33:113, 1925.

23. Gilner, L. L., and Avin, B. A reversible ocular manifestation of thalamic hemorrhage. *Arch. Neurol.* 34:715, 1977.

24. Goldblatt, D., Markesbery, W., and Reeves, A. G. Recurrent hemichorea following striatal lesions. *Arch. Neurol.* 31:51, 1974.

25. Groothuis, D. R., Duncan, G. W., and Fisher, C. M. The human thalamo-

cortical sensory path in the internal capsule: evidence from a small capsular hemorrhage causing a pure sensory stroke. *Ann. Neurol.* 2:328, 1977.

26. Hassler, R. Thalamic Regulation of Muscle Tone and the Speed of Movements. *In* Purpura, D. P., and Yahr, M. D. (Eds.). *The Thalamus.* New York: Columbia University Press, 1966. Pp. 419–438.

27. Henderson, V. W., Alexander, M. P., and Naeser, M. A. Right thalamic injury, impaired visuospatial perception, and alexia. *Neurology* (N.Y.) 32:235, 1982.

28. Horel, J. A. The neuroanatomy of amnesia. A critique of the hippocampal memory hypothesis. *Brain* 101:403, 1978.

29. Jenkyn, L. R., Alberti, A. R., and Peters, J. D. Language dysfunction, somasthetic hemi-inattention, and thalamic hemorrhage in the dominant hemisphere. *Neurology* (N.Y.) 31:1202, 1981.

30. Jones, E. G., Wise, S. P., and Coulter, J. D. Differential thalamic relationships of sensory-motor and parietal cortical fields in monkeys. *J. Comp. Neurol.* 183:833, 1979.

31. Kanno, O., Hosaka, H., and Yamaguchi, T. Dissociation of sleep stages between the two hemispheres in a case with unilateral thalamic tumor. *Folia Psychiatr. Neurol. Jpn.* 31:69, 1977.

32. Margolis, M. T., Newton, T. H., and Hoyt, W. F. The Posterior Cerebral Artery: Section II, Gross and Roentgenographic Anatomy. *In* Newton, T. H., and Potts, D. G. (Eds.). *Radiology of the Skull and Brain.* Vol. 2, Book 2, *Angiography.* St. Louis: C.V. Mosby, 1974. Pp. 1551–1566.

33. Martin, J. J. Thalamic Syndromes. *In* Vinken, P. J., and Bruyn, G. W. (Eds.). *Handbook of Clinical Neurology,* Vol. 2. New York: American Elsevier, 1969. Pp. 469–496.

34. Masdeu, J. Aphasia after infarction of the left supplementary motor area. *Neurology* 30:359, 1980.

34a. Masdeu, J. C., and Gorelick, P. Inability to stand due to unilateral thalamic lesions. *Neurology* 33(2):145, 1983.

35. Masdeu, J. C., Shoene, W. C., and Funkenstein, H. Aphasia following infarction of the left supplementary motor area. *Neurology* 28:1220, 1978.

36. McEntee, W. J., et al. Diencephalic amnesia: A reappraisal. *J. Neurol. Neurosurg. Psychiat.* 39:436, 1976.

37. Mohr, J. P., et al. Sensorimotor stroke due to thalamocapsular ischemia. *Arch. Neurol.* 34:739, 1977.

38. Mohr, J. P. Lacunes. *Stroke* 13:3, 1982.

39. Newlin, D. B., and Tramontana, M. G. Neuropsychological findings in a hyperactive adolescent with subcortical brain pathology. *Clin. Neuropsych.* 2:178, 1981.

40. Ojemann, G. A. Asymmetric function of the thalamus in man. *Ann. N.Y. Acad. Sci.* 299:380, 1977.

41. Ongerboer de Visser, B. W., and Moffie, D. Effects of brain-stem and thalamic lesions on the corneal reflex: An electrophysiological and anatomical study. *Brain* 102:595, 1979.

42. Ongerboer de Visser, B. W. Corneal reflex latency in lesions of the lower postcentral region. *Neurology* (N.Y.) 31:701, 1981.

43. Percheron, G. Les artères du thalamus humain. Artère et territoire thalamiques polaires de l'artère communicante postérieure. Rev. Neurol. (Paris) 132:297, 1976.

44. Percheron, G. Les artères du thalamus humain. Artères et territoires thalamiques paramedians de l'artere basilaire communicante. *Rev. Neurol.* (Paris) 132:309, 1976.
45. Percheron, G. Les artères du thalamus humain. Les artères choroïdiennes. *Rev. Neurol.* (Paris) 133:533, 1977.
46. Pessin, M. S., et al. "Wrong-way eyes" in supratentorial hemorrhage. *Ann. Neurol.* 9:79, 1981.
47. Plum, F., and Posner, J. B. *The Diagnosis of Stupor and Coma* (3rd ed.). Philadelphia: F. A. Davis, 1980.
48. Reynolds, A. F., et al. Left thalamic hemorrhage with dysphasia: A report of five cases. *Brain Lang.* 7:62, 1979.
49. Roland, P. E., and Nielsen, V. K. Vibratory thresholds in the hands. Comparison of patients with suprathalamic lesions with normal subjects. *Arch. Neurol.* 37:775, 1980.
50. Segarra, J. M. Cerebral vascular disease and behaviour. I. The syndrome of the mesencephalic artery (basilar artery bifurcation). *Arch. Neurol.* 22:408, 1970.
51. Spiegel, E. A., et al. The thalamus and temporal orientation. *Science:* 121:771, 1955.
52. Squire, L. R., and Moore, R. Y. Dorsal thalamic lesion in a noted case of human memory dysfunction. *Ann. Neurol.* 6:503, 1979.
53. Van Buren, J. M., and Borke, R. C. *Variations and Connections of the Human Thalamus.* New York: Springer-Verlag, 1972.
54. Van Buren, J. M., and Borke, R. C. Nucleus dorsalis superficialis (lateralis dorsalis) of the thalamus and the limbic system in man. *J. Neurol. Neurosurg. Psychiat.* 37:765, 1974.
55. Velasco, F., and Velasco, M. A reticulothalamic system mediating proprioceptive attention and tremor in man. *Neurosurgery* 4:30, 1979.
56. Victor, M., Adams, R. D., and Collins, G. H. *The Wernicke-Korsakoff Syndrome.* Philadelphia: F.A. Davis, 1971.
57. Walshe, T. M., Davis, K. R., and Fisher, C. M. Thalamic hemorrhage: A computed tomographic-clinical correlation. *Neurology* 27:217, 1977.
58. Watson, R. T., and Heilman, K. M. Thalamic neglect. *Neurology* 29:690, 1979.
59. Watson, R. T., Valenstein, E., and Heilman, K. M. Thalamic neglect. Possible role of the medial thalamus and nucleus reticularis in behavior. *Arch. Neurol.* 38:501, 1981.
60. Westmoreland, B. F., Groover, R. V., and Klass, D. W. Spontaneous sleep and induced arousal. *J. Neurol. Sci.* 28:353, 1976.
61. Yakovlev, P. I. Development of the Nuclei of the Dorsal Thalamus and of the Cerebral Cortex. Morphogenetic and Tectogenetic Correlation. *In* Locke, S. (Ed.). *Modern Neurology. Papers in Tribute to Derek Denny-Brown.* Boston: Little, Brown, 1969.
62. Wilkins, R. H., and Brody, I. A. The thalamic syndrome. *Arch. Neurol.* 20:559, 1969.
63. Ziegler, D. K., Kaufman, A., and Marshall, H. E. Abrupt memory loss associated with thalamic tumor. *Arch. Neurol.* 34:545, 1977.
64. Zihl, J., and Von Cramon, D. The contribution of the "second" visual system to directed visual attention in man. *Brain* 102:835, 1979.

Chapter 18

THE LOCALIZATION OF LESIONS AFFECTING THE BASAL GANGLIA

José Biller and Paul W. Brazis

ANATOMY OF THE BASAL GANGLIA

There is no generally accepted definition of the structures included in the term *basal ganglia*. In this chapter, the basal ganglia are considered to include

1. The *corpus striatum* (or *neostriatum*), made up of the putamen and caudate nucleus
2. The *claustrum* (sometimes included as part of the corpus striatum)
3. The *substantia nigra*, made up of a *pars compacta* and a *pars reticularis*
4. The *globus pallidus*, with its *internal* and *external* portions (also representing the *palaeostriatum*)
5. The *subthalamic nucleus of Luys*

Other nuclei, including the amygdala and the nucleus accumbens, are occasionally included as ventral striatal structures.

The basal ganglia play a major role in the control of posture and movement. Marsden [38] proposes that "the basal ganglia are responsible for the automatic execution of learned motor plans"; that is, they subconsciously run a sequence of motor programs to achieve a motor plan that has been "laid down by practice."

The major anatomic connections of the basal ganglia [10, 16] are complex (see Fig. 18-1) and include several "closed circuits" of connections. Some of the main connections will now be discussed.

Inputs into the Striatum (the Caudate and Putamen)

CORTICAL PROJECTIONS TO THE NEOSTRIATUM. All parts of the cerebral cortex give rise to efferent fibers to the caudate and putamen. These projections terminate mainly ipsilaterally in a topographic pattern (e.g., the frontal cortex projects fibers to the ventral head of the caudate and rostral putamen). The cortex also sends fibers to the substantia nigra, subthalamic nucleus, and claustrum.

THALAMOSTRIATAL PROJECTIONS. The intralaminar nuclei of the thalamus, especially the center median (CM) nucleus, send fibers to the striatum.

NIGROSTRIATAL PROJECTIONS. Fibers originating in the pars compacta of the substantia nigra project to the striatum.

RAPHE NUCLEI–STRIATAL PROJECTIONS. The brainstem raphe nuclei send ascending fibers to the striatum.

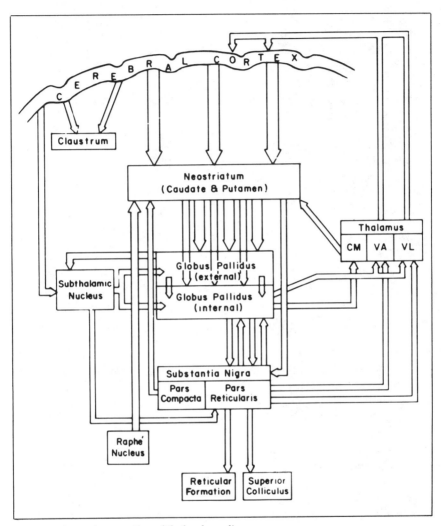

FIG. 18-1. *Anatomic connections of the basal ganglia.*

Striatal Efferents. The majority of striatal efferents project to the globus pallidus (to both the internal and external segments). Other striatal efferents go to the substantia nigra.

Pallidal Afferents and Efferents. The globus pallidus receives ascending afferent fibers from the substantia nigra and subthalamus (mainly to the medial or internal pallidum). Both the external and internal globus pallidus also receive afferents from the striatum.

The major outflow from the globus pallidus arises from the internal portion and projects to the ventral anterior (VA) and ventral lateral (VL) nuclei of the thalamus. These thalamic nuclei also receive afferents from the pars reticularis of the substantia nigra. Because the VL thalamic nucleus projects to the motor cortex and the VA thalamic nucleus projects to the premotor cortex, the major basal ganglia efferents thus influence the motor system.

Efferents from the internal globus pallidus also project to the center median thalamic nuclei, which in turn project to the putamen. A closed circuit is thus formed: putamen–internal pallidum–center median nucleus–putamen. The internal globus pallidus also sends fibers to the lateral habenular nucleus.

The external portion of the pallidum sends fibers to the internal pallidum and to the subthalamic nucleus. The subthalamic nucleus in turn sends fibers to both the internal and external pallidum. Thus, another closed circuit is formed: external globus pallidus–subthalamus–external and internal globus pallidus.

Other pallidal efferents also project to the substantia nigra, red nucleus, inferior olive, hypothalamus, and mesencephalic reticular formation.

Nigral Afferents and Efferents. The pars reticularis of the substantia nigra receives fibers from the cerebral cortex, the striatum, the globus pallidus, and the subthalamic nucleus.

The majority of the nigral efferents arise from the pars reticularis and project in an ascending direction to the medial (internal) segment of the globus pallidus. Other nigral (pars reticularis) efferents project to the VA and VL thalamic nuclei (thus exerting control over the motor system) and to the reticular formation and superior colliculus.

The pars compacta of the substantia nigra sends fibers to the striatum. It can thus be seen that the basal ganglia exert their influence mainly by way of the cerebral cortex (i.e., they do not send fibers that connect directly with brainstem and spinal cord structures). They provide a subcortical network by which the entire cerebral cortex can influence the motor system (motor and premotor cortex) mainly by the following circuit: diffuse cerebral cortex–neostriatum–globus pallidus and substantia nigra–VA and VL thalamic nuclei–motor and premotor cortex.

LESIONS OF THE BASAL GANGLIA

Basal ganglia lesions are rarely discrete. Pathologic processes affecting the basal ganglia are often diffuse. When discrete, they usually also affect neighboring structures such as the internal capsule, the hypothalamus, and the white matter of the cerebral hemispheres. Therefore, except for contralateral hemiballismus with subthalamic nuclear damage, correlation between basal ganglia lesions and clinical motor dysfunction tends to be obscure.

The literature concerning behavioral effects of lesions of the basal ganglia in experimental animals is often conflicting, and these lesions rarely produce models of human movement disorders. Therefore, these studies will not be reviewed. In general, stimulation and destructive lesions of the caudate, putamen, and globus pallidus produce inhibition of movement or contralateral body turning [42].

Some disorders in *humans* associated with lesions of the basal ganglia follow:

1. Lesions of the *subthalamic nucleus* produce contralateral hemiballismus [14].
2. Small unilateral lesions of the anteroventral *caudate* may cause choreoathetosis [35].
3. Lesions affecting the *Guillain-Mollaret triangle* (red nucleus-inferior olive-dentate nucleus) may produce palatal myoclonus [24].
4. Bilateral pallidal lesions result in akinesia, and lesions of the substantia nigra result in parkinsonism.

MOVEMENT DISORDERS

Chorea. Chorea [8, 20, 23, 43, 51, 52] is characterized by sudden, brief, spontaneous, involuntary, continuous, irregular, arrhythmic, and unpredictable jerks of the appendicular, facial, or truncal musculature. The muscles involved vary somewhat depending on the underlying disease process (e.g., truncal involvement is predominant in Huntington's chorea and distal appendicular involvement is predominant in Sydenham's chorea). The involuntary movements may be unilateral *(hemichorea)* or bilateral, occur at rest or during volitional acts, cease during sleep, intensify during stress, and are often camouflaged by the patient through a superimposed purposeful act.

Chorea is often associated with altered muscle tone (e.g., hypotonia in Sydenham's chorea, rigidity and hypokinesis in the Westphal type of Huntington's disease, and dystonia in the juvenile variant of Huntington's disease). Choreic patients have a tendency to pronate the upper extremity when they attempt to maintain an extended posture, and they are often unable to sustain a tight hand grip *(milk-maid's grip)* [19]. The tongue cannot be maintained in a protruded position and darts in and out irregularly *(trombone tongue)*.

The pathogenesis of choreiform movements is essentially unknown, although in most associated disease processes there is damage to the striatum. The evidence linking these abnormal movements specifically to the caudate and putamen is by no means convincing, because most associated disease processes (e.g., Huntington's disease) show diffuse or multiple lesions that affect other neural structures.

Unilateral chorea (*hemichorea*) is customarily seen with lesions of the contralateral corpus Luysii or its connections, although it has also been known to occur with lesions of the thalamus or caudate nucleus. The choreic movements may involve the entire half of the body or may spare the face [36]. It is often unfruitful and nonpragmatic to distinguish hemichorea from hemiballismus; in fact, the two disorders probably represent opposite ends of a spectrum of hyperkinesias. Hemichorea is usually seen with infarction or hemorrhage but may occur as a complication of thalamotomy or, rarely, secondary to neoplasm.

Ballismus. Ballismus [27, 28, 34, 55] is a hyperkinesia that is usually confined to one-half of the body (*hemiballismus*) but may involve a single extremity (*monoballismus*) or, exceptionally, both halves of the body (*paraballismus*). Hemiballismus is characterized by the abrupt onset of flail-like, usually irregular, arrhythmic, violent movements that are often of great amplitude. These abnormal movements are often continuous during wakefulness and cease with sleep. Hemiballismus is often associated with decreased muscle tone in the involved extremities.

The principal etiologies for hemiballismus are vascular lesions (infarct and hemorrhage) that affect the contralateral subthalamic nucleus (of Luysii) [14] or disrupt the afferent or efferent connections of this structure. The involved vascular supply to the subthalamic nucleus comes from branches of the posterior cerebral, posterior choroidal, and posterior communicating arteries. Rarely, this nucleus may be involved by encephalitis, tumor, or demyelinating disease.

Athetosis. Athetosis [13] is characterized by slow, uncoordinated, writhing, involuntary movements of wide amplitude. These movements predominantly affect the distal appendicular musculature, especially in the upper extremities, although facial and axial muscles may also be involved.

Athetoid movements may be unilateral (*hemiathetosis*) or bilateral and may interfere considerably with activities of daily living. These movements are often associated with episodic muscular hypertonia affecting the axial and appendicular muscles. The differentiation of athetosis from chorea and dystonia may at times be difficult or artificial because it is not uncommon to see patients with "mixed" dyskinesias (i.e., *choreoathetosis*).

Athetosis is usually noted with degenerative disorders [15] (e.g., Wilson's disease, status marmoratus, perinatal anoxia) involving widespread cerebral structures, including the globus pallidus, subthalamus, red nucleus, and midbrain tegmentum. A focal lesion (vascular or neoplasm) that damages the cortex and striatum but spares the motor cortex and its efferents may rarely cause athetosis. Paroxysmal choreoathetosis has been reported with head injury [47] and as a familial disorder termed *paroxysmal dystonic choreoathetosis* [31].

Athetoid movements must be differentiated from "pseudoathetoid" movements, which are noted on attempts to maintain posture (e.g., extending the arms) and are due to faulty proprioception (as in lesions affecting the large peripheral nerve fibers, the posterior columns and their connections, and the parietal lobe).

Dystonia. Dystonia is characterized by slow, long-sustained, contorting movements and postures involving mainly the proximal appendicular and axial muscles. The dystonic movements are typically slow and "wrapping," although sporadically patients may demonstrate superimposed, rapid involuntary jerks termed *dystonic spasms.* The dystonic posturing results in abnormal attitudes of the affected body parts (e.g., torticollis, tortipelvis, lordotic or scoliotic postures, inversion of the hands and forearms, equinovarus deformity) [29].

There is no consistent underlying structural abnormality. Dystonia may be idiopathic (dystonia musculorum deformans) or symptomatic (drug-induced, Wilson's disease) and *generalized,* or it may be idiopathic (spasmodic torticollis, writer's cramp, musician's cramp, spasmodic dysphonia, blepharospasm, orofacial dyskinesia) or symptomatic (posthemiplegic dystonia) and *segmental.*

TORTICOLLIS. Torticollis (wry-neck) [4, 9, 22, 30] is a hyperkinesia characterized by tonic or clonic spasm of the neck musculature, especially the sternocleidomastoid and trapezius muscles. This affection results in a more or less stereotyped deviation of the head into an anomalous position with the chin twisted to one side or the head displaced backward *(retrocollis)* or forward *(antecollis).* This condition is usually unilateral and may be congenital, secondary to acquired abnormalities of the cervical spine (e.g., spondylosis) or due to an extrapyramidal disorder of unknown etiology and pathologic substrate *(spasmodic torticollis).*

WRITER'S CRAMP. Writer's cramp [50] is a segmental dystonia characterized by spasms, cramps, aches, and occasional tremors of the hand muscles induced by writing. Examination reveals no evidence of oromandibular, axial, or appendicular dystonia, blepharospasm, or torticollis. The etiology and pathologic substrate are unknown.

BLEPHAROSPASM. Blepharospasm is characterized by spontaneous forceful eye closure that may render the patient functionally blind. These movements may occur in patients with parkinsonism or torsion dystonia or as a side effect of neuroleptic drugs. Blepharospasm may also occur with oromandibular dystonia, as in Meige's syndrome (idiopathic blepharospasmoromandibular dystonia) [5, 37, 54], a condition probably related to dopaminergic predominance in the striatum.

OROFACIAL DYSKINESIA. Orofacial dyskinesias [2] are abnormal involuntary movements of the facial musculature, lips, and tongue that may appear spontaneously, especially in elderly edentulous patients, or in Huntington's disease, Sydenham's chorea, or Wilson's disease. Their occurrence after prolonged neuroleptic therapy [25] favors an etiology involving denervation supersensitivity of the striatum.

SPASMODIC DYSPHONIA. Spasmodic dysphonia [3, 18] is a disorder of unknown etiology characterized by a tremulous, forced voice with a low tone and volume and often associated with facial grimacing.

Myoclonus. Myoclonus [1, 53] is a movement disorder characterized by brisk, shocklike, involuntary, repetitive, synchronous or asynchronous contractions of a muscle or group of axial or appendicular muscles. These involuntary movements may be sufficiently forceful to displace the affected part or the entire body.

Myoclonus may be segmental or generalized, may occur spontaneously or on attempted movement (action myoclonus) [32], and may be precipitated by cutaneous, auditory, visual, or muscular (e.g., sudden muscle stretch) stimuli. This movement disorder may occur with structural or metabolic lesions of the spinal cord, brainstem, cerebellum, and cerebral cortex and may occur in normal individuals as well (e.g., "sleep starts").

Palatal myoclonus [24, 41] is a rhythmic contraction (60–180 per minute) affecting the palatal and pharyngeal structures that may be associated with synergistic movements of the ocular muscles and head. Palatal myoclonus persists in sleep and is associated with lesions (usually vascular or demyelinating) that interrupt the connections between the red nucleus, the inferior olivary nucleus, and the dentate nucleus (the *Guillain-Mollaret triangle*).

Tics. Tics are abnormal movements that are sudden, rapid, usually stereotyped, and predominantly clonic. They may be willfully suppressed for short periods of time and disappear in sleep. These movements usually start around the eyes or mouth but may spread to the neck or shoulders or become generalized.

Tics may occur secondary to drugs (L-dopa, neuroleptics) or striatal disorders (e.g., encephalitis lethargica) and may also occur in the *syndrome of Gilles de la Tourette* [11, 46, 49]. In this syndrome, tics are often associated with vocalizations (grunting, barking, throat clearing, spitting, coughing) or occasionally with more complicated motor activity such as echopraxia (imitations of acts), jumping, or kicking. Coprolalia (obscene language) occurs in less than one-third of affected individuals.

Tremor. Tremor [26, 39, 45, 48] is characterized by involuntary, *rhythmic,* oscillatory movements resulting from alternating contractions of antagonist muscles. Tremor usually affects the distal extremities and, less often, the head and neck.

Tremor may be classified as normal *(physiologic)* or abnormal. *Abnormal tremors* may be classified as:

1. *Resting tremor* (3–7 Hz), which is seen in the relaxed extremities. This type is usually noted with diseases affecting the basal ganglia (e.g., Parkinson's disease).
2. *Postural tremor* (6–11 Hz), which is most noticeable in extremities that maintain an antigravity posture (e.g., essential tremor).
3. *Intention tremor* (3–7 Hz), which is most prominent in goal-directed movement (e.g., finger-to-nose testing) and often increases in amplitude as the target is reached. Intention tremor is usually associated with cerebellar disease.

Parkinsonism. Bradykinesia, rigidity, resting tremor, and disorders of postural reflexes are the cardinal features of Parkinson's disease [12, 21]. This disorder is probably due to loss of dopaminergic cells (in the substantia nigra) that project to the striatum, resulting in an imbalance between cholinergic and dopaminergic transmitters [6, 7].

Bradykinesia is a disorder of voluntary movement that leads to disability characterized by delay in the initiation and execution of willed movements and a general reduction of associated automatic movements. Bradykinesia explains (at least partially) the facial hypomimia, reduced blinking, impaired ocular convergence, monotonous and low-volume speech (bradylalia, eventually leading to anarthria) [17], drooling of saliva, micrographia, and slow shuffling gait with reduced associated movements that occur in parkinsonism.

Rigidity is characterized by a resistance to passive movements that affects both agonist and antagonist muscles (e.g., flexors and extensors;

pronators and supinators) to a similar extent and that is constant throughout the entire range of movement. The phenomenon of *cogwheel rigidity* is characterized by periodic modifications of muscle tone that can be seen and felt when passively moving the extremity.

Parkinsonism *tremor* is characteristically present at rest, increased by anxiety, absent in sleep, and decreased by volitional activity. This tremor typically affects mainly the distal appendicular muscles, leading to flexion-extension movements of the metacarpophalangeal and interphalangeal joints of the fingers, adduction-abduction movements of the thumbs ("pill rolling"), and pronation-supination movements of the wrists. It usually begins in one hand and may be present initially only in the thumb or a single finger. The tremor then typically spreads to the ipsilateral lower extremity ("hemi-parkinsonism") before involving the opposite half of the body.

In addition to a tremor at rest (4–6 Hz), an action tremor (7–12 Hz) may occasionally occur [33]. Tremor of the protruded tongue is not uncommon, whereas tremors of the head, lips, and jaw are less frequent.

Disorders of postural fixation may affect the head, trunk, or limbs or the entire body, resulting in forward displacement of the head, forward or backward instability of the trunk, and difficulty in maintaining an erect posture when being slightly pushed [40].

Patients with parkinsonism may demonstrate a "simian posture" (forward flexion of the trunk, flexion of the elbows, and partial flexion of the knees), the "parkinsonian hand" (mild dorsiflexion of the wrist, flexion of the metacarpophalangeal joints, extension and adduction of the fingers and slight ulnar deviation), and the dystonic foot posture [44] (extension of the great toe, flexion of the toes, arching of the sole, and inversion of the foot). Other features include constipation, bladder dysfunction, seborrhea, hyperhydrosis, sleep abnormalities, exaggerated nasopalpebral reflex (glabellar tap or Meyerson's sign), blepharospasm, blepharoclonus, and oculogyric crisis.

REFERENCES

1. Aigner, B. R., and Mulder, D. W. Myoclonus. Clinical significance and an approach to classification. *Arch. Neurol.* 2:600, 1960.
2. Altrocchi, P. H. Spontaneous oral-facial dyskinesia. *Arch. Neurol.* 36:506, 1972.
3. Aminoff, M. J., Dedo, H. H., and Izdebski, K. Clinical aspects of spasmodic dysphonia. *J. Neurol. Neurosurg. Psychiat.* 41:361, 1978.
4. Ansari, K. A., and Webster, D. D. Quantitative measurements in spasmodic torticollis. *Dis. Nerv. Syst.* 35:33, 1974.
5. Ashizawa, T., Patten, B. M., and Jankovic, J. Meige syndrome. *South. Med. J.* 73:863, 1980.
6. Barbeau, A. The pathogenesis of Parkinson's disease. A new hypothesis. *Can. Med. Assoc. J.* 87:802, 1962.

7. Barbeau, A. Parkinson's Disease: Etiological Considerations. *In* Yahr, M. D. (Ed.). *The Basal Ganglia*. New York: Raven Press, 1967. Pp. 281–292.
8. Bird, M., Palkes, I., and Prensky, A. L. A follow-up study of Sydenham's chorea. *Neurology* (Minn.) 26:601, 1976.
9. Boisen, E. Torticollis caused by an infratentorial tumor: Three cases. *Br. J. Psych.* 134:306, 1979.
10. Brodal, A. N. *Neurological Anatomy In Relation to Clinical Medicine* (3rd ed.). New York: Oxford University Press, 1981. Pp. 211–226.
11. Bruun, R. D., and Shapiro, A. K. Differential diagnosis of Gilles de la Tourette's syndrome. *J. Nerv. Ment. Dis.* 155:328, 1972.
12. Calne, D. B. Current view on Parkinson's disease. *Can. J. Neurol. Sci.* 10:11, 1983.
13. Carpenter, M. B. Athetosis and basal ganglia. Review of literature and study of forty-two cases. *Arch. Neurol. Psychiat.* 63:875, 1950.
14. Carpenter, M. B. Ballism associated with partial destruction of the subthalamic nucleus of Luys. *Neurology* 5:479, 1955.
15. Carpenter, M. B. Status marmoratus of the thalamus and striatum associated with athetosis and dystonia. *Neurology* (Minn.) 15:139, 1955.
16. Carpenter, M. B. Anatomical Organization of the Corpus Striatum and Related Nuclei. *In* Yahr, M.D. (Ed.). *The Basal Ganglia*. New York: Raven Press, 1976.
17. Critchley, E. Speech disorders in parkinsonism: A review. *J. Neurol. Neurosurg. Psychiat.* 49:751, 1981.
18. Critchley, M. Spastic dysphonia ("inspiratory speech"). *Brain* 62:96, 1939.
19. Dejong, R. N. *The Neurologic Examination* (4th ed.). Hagerstown, Md.: Harper & Row, 1979. Pp. 292–303.
20. Duvoisin, R. Clinical diagnosis of the dyskinesias. *Med. Clin. North Am.* 56:1321, 1972.
21. Fields, W. S. *Pathogenesis and Treatment of Parkinsonism*. Springfield, Ill.: Charles C Thomas, 1958.
22. Gilbert, G. J. Familial spasmodic torticollis. *Neurology* 27:11, 1977.
23. Heathfield, K. W. G. Huntington's chorea: A centenary review. *Postgrad. Med. J.* 49:32, 1973.
24. Herrman, J., and Brown, J. W. Palatal myoclonus: A reappraisal. *J. Neurol. Sci.* 5:473, 1967.
25. Jankovic, J. Drug-induced and other orofacial-cervical dyskinesias. *Ann. Intern. Med.* 94:788, 1981.
26. Jankovic, J., and Fahn, S. Physiologic and pathologic tremors. Diagnosis, mechanism, and management. *Ann. Intern. Med.* 93:460, 1980.
27. Kellman, H. Hemiballismus: A clinicopathologic study of two cases. *J. Nerv. Ment. Dis.* 101:363, 1945.
28. Klawans, H. L., et al. Treatment and prognosis of hemiballismus. *N. Engl. J. Med.* 295:1348, 1976.
29. Korczyn, A. D., et al. Torsion dystonia in Israel. *Ann. Neurol.* 8:387, 1980.
30. Lal, S. Pathophysiology and pharmacotherapy of spasmodic torticollis: A review. *Canad. J. Neurol. Sci.* 6:427, 1979.
31. Lance, J. W. Familial paroxysmal dystonic choreoathetosis and its differentiation from related syndromes. *Ann. Neurol.* 2:285, 1977.
32. Lance, J. W., and Adams, R. D. The syndrome of intention or action myoclonus as a sequel to hypoxic encephalopathy. *Brain* 86:11, 1963.
33. Lance, J. W., Schwab, R. S., and Peterson, E. A. Action tremor and the cogwheel phenomenon in Parkinson's disease. *Brain* 86:95, 1963.

34. Lea-Plaza, H., and Viberall, E. Hemiballismo. *Rev. Med. Chil.* 73:938, 1945.
35. Liles, S. L., and Davis, G. D. Athetoid and choreiform hyperkinesias produced by caudate lesions in the cat. *Science* 164:195, 1969.
36. Lloyd, J. H., and Winkelmann, N. W. A case of acute posthemiplegic choreiform movements on the unparalyzed side. *Am. J. Med. Sci.* 169:247, 1925.
37. Marsden, C. D. Blepharospasm–oromandibular dystonia syndrome (Brueghel's syndrome): A variant of adult onset torsion dystonia? *J. Neurol. Neurosurg. Psychiat.* 39:1204, 1976.
38. Marsden, C. D. The mysterious motor function of the basal ganglia: The Robert Wartenberg Lecture. *Neurology* (N.Y.) 32:514, 1982.
39. Marshall, J. Observations on essential tremor. *J. Neurol. Neurosurg. Psychiat.* 25:122, 1962.
40. Martin, J. P., Hurwitz, L. J., and Finlayson, M. N. The negative symptoms of basal gangliar disease. *Lancet* 1:1, 1962.
41. Matsuo, F., and Ajax, E. T. Palatal myoclonus and denervation supersensitivity in the central nervous system. *Ann. Neurol.* 5:72, 1979.
42. McDowell, F. H., Lee, J. E., and Sweet, R. D. Extrapyramidal Disease. *In* Baker, A. B., and Baker, L. H. *Clinical Neurology.* Philadelphia: Harper & Row, 1982.
43. Nausieda, P. A., et al. Sydenham's chorea: An update. *Neurology* (Minn.) 30:331, 1980.
44. Nausieda, P. A., Klawans, H. L., and Weiner, W. J. The dystonic foot response of parkinsonism. *Neurology* 27:403, 1977.
45. Poirier, L. J. Recent reviews of tremors and their treatment. *Modern Trends in Neurology* 5:80, 1970.
46. Rappaport, J. Maladie des tics in children. *Am. J. Psychol.* 116:177, 1959.
47. Robin, J. J. Paroxysmal choreoathetosis following head injury. *Ann. Neurol.* 2:447, 1977.
48. Shahani, B. T., and Young, R. R. Physiological and pharmacological aids in the differential diagnosis of tremor. *J. Neurol. Neurosurg. Psychiat.* 39:772, 1976.
49. Shapiro, A. K., Shapiro, E., and Wayne, H. L. The symptomatology and diagnosis of Gilles de la Tourette's syndrome. *J. Am. Acad. Child Psychiat.* 12:702, 1973.
50. Sheehy, M. P., and Marsden, C. D. Writer's cramp–A focal dystonia. *Brain* 105:461, 1982.
51. Shoulson, I., and Chase, T. N. Huntington's disease. *Ann. Rev. Med.* 26:419, 1975.
52. Shoulson, I. Pharmacotherapy of chorea. *Neurol. Neurosurg. Update* 3(39):1, 1982.
53. Swanson, P. D., Luttrell, C. N., and Magladery, J. W. Myoclonus–A report of 67 cases and review of the literature. *Medicine* 41:339, 1962.
54. Tolosa, E. S., and Chin-Wan, L. A. Meige disease: Striatal dopaminergic preponderance. *Neurology* (Minn.) 29:1126, 1979.
55. Winfield, M. E. Transient hemiballism. *Ann. Intern. Med.* 53:822, 1960.

Chapter 19

THE LOCALIZATION OF LESIONS AFFECTING THE CEREBRAL HEMISPHERES

Joseph C. Masdeu

ANATOMY OF THE CEREBRAL HEMISPHERES

The paired cerebral hemispheres derive from the telencephalic cerebral vesicles, in the most rostral part of the neuraxis [17, 25]. They are in continuity with the diencephalon and are interconnected by three white matter commissures, a larger one or corpus callosum and two smaller ones—the anterior commissure and the commissure of the fornix. In the adult the cerebral hemispheres, shaped like a cap, cover the midbrain-diencephalic structures. A midline sagittal slit, the longitudinal fissure, separates the two hemispheres. Thus, each hemisphere has a larger *lateral aspect* and smaller *medial* and *inferior aspects*. Folds (gyri) and furrows (sulci) pattern the surface of the cerebral hemispheres. The larger sulci (fissures) serve as anatomic landmarks separating different regions of the cerebral hemispheres.

On the *lateral aspect* of each hemisphere, two large sulci separate three regions: one *(the temporal lobe)* that is inferior to the Sylvian or transverse sulcus and two that are superior to it, one *(the frontal lobe)* anterior to the rolandic or central sulcus and another *(the parietal lobe)* posterior to the rolandic sulcus (Fig. 19-1A). The *insula* lies buried in the depth of the Sylvian sulcus. The most posterior portion of the lateral aspect corresponds to the *occipital* lobe. An imaginary line, drawn from the superior extent of the parietooccipital sulcus in the medial aspect of the hemisphere to a notch in the inferior aspect (preoccipital notch), constitutes the lateral boundary between the occipital lobe and the parietal and temporal lobes.

Two sulci running anteroposteriorly divide the frontal lobe into *superior, middle,* and *inferior* frontal gyri. Perpendicular to these, and separated from them by the precentral sulcus, lies the *precentral* gyrus, which is just anterior to the central sulcus. Similarly, two transverse sulci divide the temporal lobe into *superior, middle,* and *inferior* temporal gyri. On the inferior bank of the Sylvian sulcus, the *transverse* gyrus (Heschl's) runs anterolaterally over the superior aspect of the first temporal gyrus. It constitutes the primary auditory area and the anterior limit of the planum temporale or supratemporal plane, which, in the average right-handed person, is one-third larger in the left hemisphere (Fig. 19-2) [45]. A similar but less pronounced asymmetry exists between the posterior part of the third frontal gyrus (triangular and opercular portions) of both hemispheres [35, 37]. Dorsal to the rolandic sulcus lies the *postcentral* gyrus, separated from the rest of the parietal convexity by the postcentral sulcus. A transverse sulcus divides the rest of the parietal lobe into *superior* and *inferior* parietal lobules. The latter curves anteriorly around the posterior extent of the Sylvian sulcus *(supramarginal* gyrus) and posteriorly around the posterior extent of the superior temporal sulcus *(angular* gyrus).

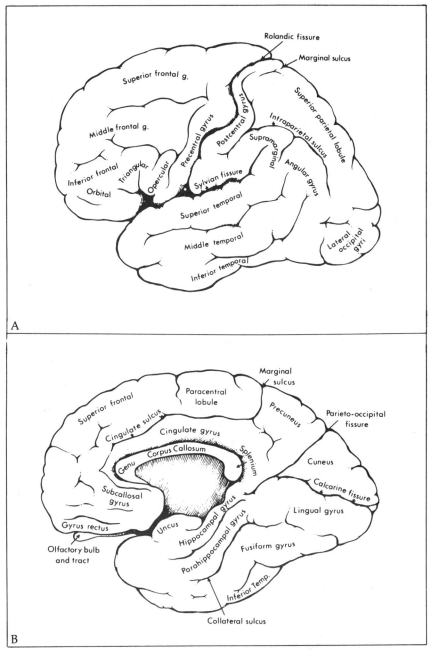

FIG. 19-1. *Lateral **(A)** and inferomedial **(B)** views of the cerebral hemispheres. The orbital aspect of the frontal lobes can be seen only in a direct inferior view, but the entire temporal and occipital lobes can be appreciated in this figure.*

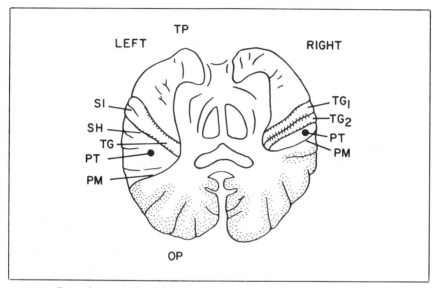

FIG. 19-2. *Exposed upper surfaces of the temporal lobes, shown in a horizontal section of the brain. The area (planum temporale, PT) limited anteriorly by the transverse temporal gyrus of Heschl (TG) and posteriorly by the posterior extent of the horizontal portion of the temporal operculum (PM) tends to be larger on the left side. Other abbreviations: TP = temporal pole; OP = occipital pole. (Reproduced with permission N. Geschwind and W. Levitsky [45]. Copyright © 1969 by the American Association for the Advancement of Science.)*

The *medial* or *mesial aspect* of the cerebral hemisphere sweeps around the corpus callosum and, posteroinferiorly, blends rather smoothly with the inferior aspect of the hemisphere (Fig. 19-1B). Among the major sulci in the medial aspect, three run radially and one runs parallel to the corpus callosum. The latter, called the cingulate sulcus, separates the *cingulate gyrus*, centripetal to it, from the mesial aspect of the first frontal and paracentral gyri. The mesial aspect of the frontal and parietal paracentral gyri *(paracentral lobule)* is well demarcated from the rest of the mesial parietal lobe *(precuneus)* by one of the three radial sulci mentioned above — the marginal sulcus, which arises in the cingulate sulcus. The other two radial sulci are more dorsal. The large parietooccipital sulcus separates the parietal precuneus from a mesial wedge of occipital lobe *(cuneus)*, limited inferiorly by the calcarine sulcus. These two sulci meet anteriorly to join the posterior extent of the cingulate sulcus, which limits dorsally the isthmus of the cingulate gyrus, as it sweeps around the posterior end (splenium) of the corpus callosum. As the cingulate gyrus becomes more anterior, traversing the inferior aspect of the splenium, it blends with the *parahippocampal* gyrus in the medial aspect of the temporal lobe. Hidden in the recess between the medial aspect of the temporal lobe and the lateral aspect of the midbrain, the *hippocampal* gyrus courses anteriorly next to the parahippocampal gyrus, separated from it by the hippocampal sulcus. Anteriorly, they converge into a small nub (the *uncus*), near the amygdalar nuclear complex.

The *inferior aspect* of the hemisphere is constituted by the orbital surface of the frontal lobe and the inferomedial aspect of the occipital and temporal lobes (Fig. 19-1B). A few irregular orbital gyri and a medially located straight gyrus (gyrus rectus), which lies medial to the olfactory bulb and tract, make up the orbitofrontal surface. The demarcation between the temporal and the occipital lobes is indistinct on their inferior aspect. A *fusiform or occipitotemporal* gyrus, anterolaterally, and a *lingual* gyrus, posteromedially, can be distinguished on the swath that lies between the collateral sulcus (lateral to the parahippocampal gyrus) and the third temporal gyrus.

In addition to the temporal and frontal lobe asymmetries mentioned above, the right frontal lobe is often larger than the left, and the left occipital lobe is larger than the right [100]. Such anatomic asymmetries may reflect the different functional specialization of each cerebral hemisphere in regard to language and other functions.

The convoluted pattern on the surface of the cerebral hemispheres emerges during ontogenesis, to accommodate into the smallest volume the large expansion of cortical gray matter (cortex) that characterizes the human brain. Six layers of cells (neurons) can be distinguished in most of the cortex (neocortex) (Fig. 19-3). From surface to depth they have been termed (1) the molecular layer, rich in fibers; (2) the external granular layer, composed of small round or star-shaped neurons; (3) the external pyramidal layer, containing medium-sized pyramidal neurons, their larger apical dendrites oriented toward the surface; (4) the internal granular layer, which, in addition to small, round neurons, contains a thick plexus of horizontally directed fibers; (5) the internal pyramidal or ganglionic layer, constituted by the larger pyramidal neurons; and (6) the multiform layer, made up of spindle-shaped neurons. Two small areas in the inferomesial aspect of the hemispheres have a simpler cortex: the olfactory area (paleocortex) and the hippocampal formation (archicortex). Except for the primary visual cortex in binocular primates, in which this number is doubled, the number of neurons in a column (Fig. 19-3) through the depth of the neocortex is the same in different cortical areas and mammalian species [86]. In humans, the cortex is thicker to accommodate the same number of neurons that are further spread apart by the richer network of connections.

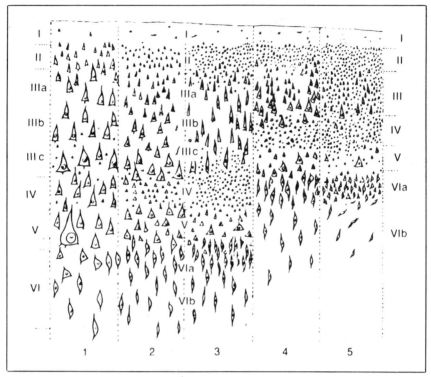

FIG. 19-3. *The histologic appearance of the five fundamental types of neocortex, according to von Economo [34]: 1, agranular (pyramidal); 2, frontal; 3, parietal; 4, polar; 5, granular (koniocortex).*

Although it is six-layered throughout, the neocortex is not homogeneous. In areas that receive a heavy sensory projection, the granular layers are much bulkier than the pyramidal layers (granular cortex or koniocortex, Fig. 19-3). The opposite holds true for the areas in which the larger motor projections to the brain stem and spinal cord originate (agranular or pyramidal cortex). Actually, the cortex may be parcellated according to the cellular composition (cytoarchitecture) of the different cortical areas. Brodmann's cytoarchitectural map (Fig. 19-4) depicts 50 different areas.

The cerebral hemispheres process intraindividual and extraindividual information. Most of the latter input reaches the primary cortical areas through the thalamus. Information concerning the interior homeostasis travels from the brainstem and hypothalamus through the medial thalamus, reaching mainly the pericallosal, mesial temporal, insular, and orbital cortex (limbic lobe). In order to act, both of these systems need to be "activated" by the brainstem reticular formation.

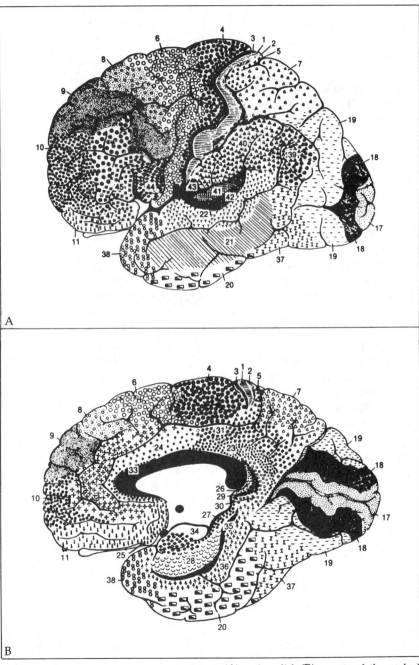

FIG. 19-4. *Brodmann's parcellation of the lateral* **(A)** *and medial* **(B)** *aspects of the cerebral hemispheres according to the specific cytoarchitecture of the different areas [18].*

Shifts away from the physiologic condition of the organism prompt a motor reply to correct such an imbalance. This is accomplished through inherited programs, common to the species (i.e., innate programs, such as instincts), and programs learned through the individual's life. Such programs may concern the performance of the motor act itself (skills, which are mediated mainly by the parietal and frontal lobes) or the relation of new information to old information within the framework of time (data-based learning, which is mainly mediated by the temporal and prefrontal cortex). Information of particular relevance to the survival of the individual or the species is stored with greater ease and firmness.

The main anatomic connections of the cortex are listed in Table 19-1. As a summary, the retrorolandic portion of the cerebral hemispheres is chiefly involved in the processing of sensory information about the outside world and about the motor acts being performed by the individual. Both of these, but particularly the latter, require the integration of sensory information of different modalities (visual, somatosensory, and so on). Lesions in the "primary" sensory areas cause loss of a specific sensory modality. These primary areas are listed in Table 19-1 (Fig. 19-5). The cortex surrounding the primary sensory areas processes the modality-specific information and integrates it with information from other sense organs and information about the physiologic milieu of the individual.

Simply stated, the cortex adjacent to the primary sensory areas (secondary sensory areas) processes unimodal sensory information, often keeping a somatotopic organization, whereas the cortex lying between the different secondary sensory areas (tertiary sensory cortex) integrates multimodal sensory information. For instance, somatosensory information reaches somatotopically the postcentral gyrus (Fig. 19-6), which projects somatotopically to the superior (arm and leg) and inferior (head) parietal lobules. Somatotopic information is integrated with auditory and visual information in the inferoposterior portions of the inferior parietal lobule (angular gyrus) and with visual and vegetative information in the posteromedial portions of the parietal lobe (cuneus) [80]. Lesions of the primary somatosensory area result in sensory loss, whereas lesions in the multimodal association areas result in motor performances that show the lack of multimodal integration. For instance, bilateral lesions of the posterior portion of the superior parietal lobule give rise to impairment of hand movements under visual guidance [26].

The prerolandic portion of the hemispheres contains programs concerned with planning, initiation, and execution of movements. The mesial frontal cortex (cingulate gyrus, supplementary motor area) is closely linked with the reticular activating system and the limbic lobe. It appears to mediate the drive to move in a meaningful direction (cortical

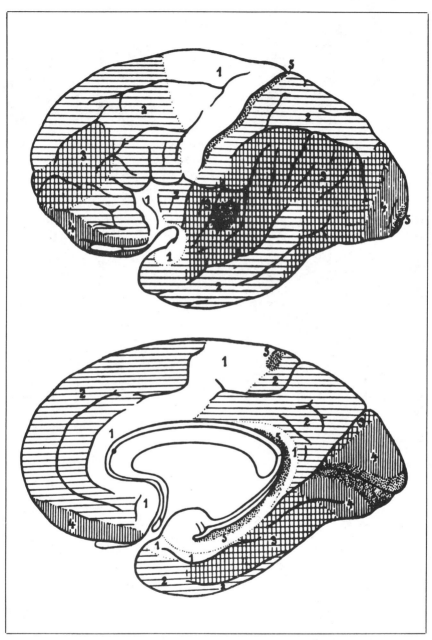

FIG. 19-5. *Distribution of the five fundamental types of cortex depicted in Fig. 19-3. Note that the primary sensory, auditory (transverse temporal gyrus of Heschl), visual (calcarine cortex), and somesthetic (postcentral gyrus) areas have granular cortex. Association cortex sprawls among them.*

TABLE 19-1. *Cerebral Hemispheric Connections*

Function Type	Origin	Cortical Area	Destination
SENSORY AREAS			
Smell	Olfactory bulb	Piriform lobe (temporal uncus and surrounding cortex, area 28)	Hippocampus Amygdala
Taste	Ventroposteromedial thalamic nucleus	Parainsular portion of parietal operculum	
Vision			
Primary visual area	Lateral geniculate body	Lips of calcarine sulcus (striate area, area 17)	Parastriate cortex (area 18) Peristriate cortex (area 19) Pulvinar Superior colliculus
Secondary visual areas	Striate area Lateral geniculate body Pulvinar	Parastriate cortex (area 18) Peristriate cortex (area 19)	Middle frontal gyrus (area 8) Inferior parietal lobule Temporal lobe
Auditory			
Primary auditory area	Medial geniculate body	Transverse temporal gyrus (Heschl's), area 41 (higher frequencies located more medially)	Planum temporale Foot of middle frontal gyrus (area 8a)
Secondary auditory areas	Area 41	Superior temporal gyrus (area 22)	Posterior portion of superior temporal gyrus (Wernicke's area)
	Area 8a	Parastriate cortex (area 9)	Inferior parietal lobe

Somatosensory

Primary somatosensory areas (receptors on contralateral side of the body or bilateral)	Ventral posterior thalamic nuclei	Postcentral gyrus, first somatosensory area (somatotopically organized, see Fig. 19-6)	Areas 2 and 5 Precentral gyrus (motor cortex, area 4) Supplementary motor area Second somatosensory area
Muscle spindles		Area 3a	
Cutaneous receptors for "texture"		Areas 3b, 1	
Deep tissue (joints, aponeuroses), "shape" discrimination		Area 2	
Painful stimuli?	Thalamus (ventrobasal nuclear complex?)		Postcentral gyrus Supplementary motor area
Second somatotosensory areas	Areas 2 and 5 Superior portion (leg, trunk, arm) Inferior portion (neck, head)	Second somatosensory area (upper bank of Sylvian fissure, adjacent to the insula)	
		Superior parietal lobule	Precuneus (mesial parietal cortex)
		Supramarginal gyrus	Angular gyrus
Tertiary somatosensory areas (cortical sensory convergence zones)	Precuneus	Angular gyrus Posterior cingulate gyrus (area 23) Peristriate belt (area 19) Precuneus	Mesial temporal cortex Orbitofrontal cortex Frontal association cortex
	Angular gyrus	Peristriate belt (area 19) Posterior portion of superior and middle temporal gyri Inferomedial temporal cortex	Supplementary motor area

TABLE 19-1 (continued)

Function Type	Origin	Cortical Area	Destination
MOTOR AREAS			
Primary motor area	Thalamus (VL) (from cerebellum and basal ganglia) Somatosensory areas Supplementary motor area (mesial frontal) "Premotor" cortex	Precentral gyrus (area 4), somatotopically organized (see Fig. 19-5)	Striatum Brainstem Spinal cord
Supplementary motor area	Precentral gyrus (area 4) First and second primary somatosensory areas Cingulate gyrus	Supplementary motor area	Precentral gyrus Striatum (caudate) Pontine nuclei
Frontal eye fields	Peristriate cortex (area 19)	Foot of the middle frontal gyrus (area 8)	Midbrain and pontine reticular formation Cervical cord
Secondary association motor areas	Multimodal parietooccipitotemporal areas (angular gyrus, precuneus) "Prefrontal" areas, orbitofrontal cortex Anterior cingulate gyrus (area 24)	"Premotor" frontal cortex (areas 6, 8, 9, 44, 45)	Primary motor areas Secondary sensory areas Striatum Thalamus Brainstem
Tertiary association motor areas	Anteromedial thalamus Temporal pole Anterior portion of cingulate gyrus (area 24) Angular gyrus Precuneus	"Prefrontal cortex" (areas 9, 10, 11)	Same as origin
AREAS INVOLVED IN MNESTIC PROCESSES	Association motor and sensory areas Medial thalamus Medial hypothalamus	Temporal lobe	Same as origin

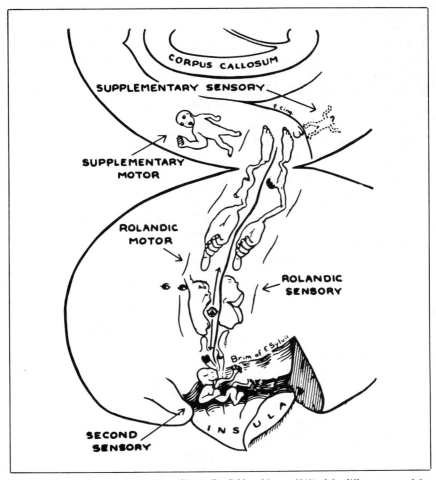

FIG. 19-6. *Cortical representation (according to Penfield and Jasper [81]) of the different parts of the body in the perirolandic motor and sensory areas. The frontal pole of the brain is represented in the left portion of the figure.*

attention). Although seemingly alert, patients with large bilateral lesions in this region remain motionless and mute (akinetic mutism). From the limbic system, information about past events and their bearing on the well-being of the individual reaches the anterior portions of the frontal lobe, where it is integrated with sensory information from the thalamus and from the multimodal association areas of the hemisphere. Thus, the best course of action within a temporal framework is delineated. The frontal cortex rostral to the precentral gyrus mediates complex motor programs, which are elicited under the "command" of the mesial frontal region and executed by way of the subcortical nuclei (basal ganglia, brainstem nuclei) and primary motor cortex. The cerebellum and the sensory nuclei of the brainstem, including the vestibular complex, provide the motor system with essential feedback information.

This brief introduction has attempted to highlight the main framework of the incredibly complex structure of the cerebral hemispheres, which is still far from clear. Some understanding of the anatomic structure facilitates the identification of the most likely location of a cerebral hemispheric lesion based on its clinical consequences.

SYMPTOMS AND SIGNS CAUSED BY CEREBRAL HEMISPHERIC LESIONS

Lesions of the phylogenetically most recent part of the central nervous system differ in their manifestations from those that affect more primitive levels. Thus,

1. The greater plasticity of the hemispheres, probably mediated by the large number of cortical neurons, results in *less pronounced deficits* with lesions that, had they affected a similar volume of the brainstem or spinal cord, would have caused a major motor or sensory disturbance.
2. This plasticity also results in a *more complete recovery* from elementary neurologic deficits, such as weakness or numbness, although more complex motor or sensory deficits may remain. At the bedside or in a quick office visit these are *more difficult to detect* than elementary deficits, even though they may be very disruptive to the patient's professional and family life. Functional recovery following lesions of the association cortex of the hemispheres is probably mediated by functional reorganization of the cortex, where a sound cortical area assumes the functions formerly subserved by the lesioned area [31a].
3. Because this plasticity is mediated by extensive multisynaptic arrays, which are *susceptible to metabolic disturbances* that interfere with the elaboration and processing of neurotransmitters, toxic-metabolic insults affecting the whole brain impair particularly the functions newly acquired in the process of "repair" of a focal lesion [35a]. Thus, they may bring about again a clinical deficit that had been well compensated. For instance, a patient with a mild residual difficulty in naming objects following a large lesion of the dominant temporal lobe, which initially caused a severe sensory aphasia, may again become unable to understand conversational speech when he suffers a bout of pneumonia.

4. When obtaining the history pertinent to a cerebral hemispheric lesion, the examiner must realize that the *patient is often unaware of the extent of the deficit,* particularly when it involves complex (multimodal) behavior (aphasia, apraxia). Patients with right-hemispheric lesions tend to be impervious to their deficit more often than patients with left-hemispheric lesions. Anton syndrome, in which the patient denies an otherwise obvious blindness that is related to a cortical parietooccipital lesion, is only one instance of such lack of insight. Something similar occurs with other hemispheric-related sensory deficits. Their extension and quality are less precise than when the sensory loss is caused by lesions in more elementary structures of the nervous system, such as the brainstem or a sensory peripheral nerve. Most patients with an ulnar neuropathy can outline a precise area of numbness in the medial aspect of their hand. By contrast, a patient with a hemispheric lesion, even affecting the primary somatosensory cortex of the postcentral gyrus, may have a difficult time localizing the area of sensory loss. This characteristic of hemispheric lesions, combined with the difficulty of eliciting all of the deficits in a short interview, make it often necessary to obtain information from people who know the patient well in order to localize a cerebral hemispheric lesion correctly.

5. The neurologic deficit caused by cerebral hemispheric lesions tends to be *more inconsistent* than deficits related to lesions in the lower echelons of the nervous system. Reduced attention, which may be related to the time of the day, a noisy environment, or lack of adequate stimuli, is only one of the many factors that can influence the outcome of a given neurologic examination. Repeated interviews minimize this problem and allow the examiner to arrive at a much more accurate picture of the nature (and therefore the localization) of the patient's disturbance. Of course, the luxury of repeated examinations is unaffordable when a quick decision has to be reached in an emergency management situation, but it should be available when planning the long-term management and rehabilitation of these patients.

6. For adequate localization, *global deficits,* such as alexia, *must be analyzed.* The patient may be unable to understand written material because his saccades to the left side are incomplete, leading him to miss the beginning of words and sentences (right frontoparietal lesion), or because he cannot grasp the meaning of an array of strokes that make up a written word (left occipital lesion). It behooves the examiner to go beyond the obvious disturbance and try to understand its structure and the primary defect responsible for it.

7. The same function is represented in different areas of the cortex or even in contralateral hemispheres in different patients. This *individual variability* makes the localization of hemispheric disease particularly taxing [77, 78]. The most common anatomic correlations of clinical signs and symptoms are described below, but any attempt to pinpoint the exact square centimeter of the cortex that accounts for a deficit in a particular patient is a futile endeavor [31a]. Likewise, identification of the area of the cerebral hemispheres most likely to be injured in the context of a set of symptoms and signs does not mean that the function lost "is localized" in that area of the brain.

8. For the sake of rationalization, the complex and fluid clinical picture displayed by patients with cerebral lesions has been compartmentalized into different syndromes. It should be realized, however, that often the *difference between syndromes is merely one of degree.* A similar amount of tissue loss underlies the global aphasia that is present a few weeks after infarction and the Broca's (motor) aphasia that develops some months later [61]. Also, initially the localization of the deficit is compounded not only by edema and metabolic abnormalities at the site of the lesion but also by dysfunction (diaschisis) of areas of the brain away from the primarily damaged region, particularly those heavily interconnected with it, such as the homologous area of the contralateral hemisphere [35a].

9. Lesions that affect the same portion of the cerebral hemispheres may present very different clinical pictures depending on the *tempo and nature of the damage.* Sudden, "through" lesions, such as infarcts that destroy all the neurons in a portion of the cortex, tend to cause a more severe deficit than tumors that infiltrate slowly the same area of the brain. For instance, small infarcts often cause aphasia, but tumors have to be quite large before they cause an aphasic syndrome. Weakness may be rather profound after a small infarct, but a tumor will seldom cause severe weakness until it has extensively involved a cerebral hemisphere. Thus, localization for diffuse lesions is less accurate. However, due to the plasticity of the hemispheres, as time elapses after an acute, through lesion, its clinical manifestations may resemble those of an infiltrative lesion of the same area. Rather than being restricted to a lobe or gyrus, many pathologic processes (Alzheimer's disease, encephalitis, arteriosclerotic vascular disease) affect the hemispheres in a diffuse or disseminated fashion. A combination of deficits, which are predominantly manifestations of bilateral damage to the multimodal association cortex, then constitutes the clinical presentation.

10. Lesions that affect the cortex selectively (e.g., hypoxic laminar necrosis) give rise to a clinical picture that differs from lesions circum-

scribed to the white matter (e.g., multiple sclerosis). Characteristic of cortical lesions are (1) seizures, and (2) multimodal motor and sensory deficits such as aphasia and apraxia. Although subcortical lesions may cause aphasic symptoms, these are seldom as pronounced or lasting as they are with cortical lesions.

Characteristic of white matter lesions are (1) weakness, (2) spasticity, (3) visual field deficits, (4) "pure" motor syndromes, and (5) urinary incontinence. Lesions that involve the white matter of the hemispheres cause symptoms that are referable to the cortical region originating the white matter tract involved. Lesions in the internal capsule are often vascular and tend to spare a parathalamic rim of the capsule where the sensory tracts are located. As a result, they often cause "pure" motor syndromes. The face and bulbar muscles are most affected with lesions in the genu or anterior part of the posterior limb, whereas more posteriorly located lesions cause arm weakness, and those in the most posterior part of the posterior limb give rise to leg weakness and visual field defects.

11. More than any other portion of the nervous system, the cerebral hemispheres are amenable to lesion localization provided by *computed tomography* (CT) and *nuclear magnetic resonance* (NMR). Positron emission tomography will probably continue to be confined to research centers. Although it has been available for only a short period of time, NMR has great potential for lesion localization. CT has been extremely useful not only for defining the anatomy of cerebral damage in a particular patient but also for reaching a better understanding of the clinical picture caused by lesions in the different areas of the brain [30, 60a]. However, CT allows much better visualization of the subcortical structures than of the cortex, which is often obscured by some degree of bone artefact, a defect that is particularly prominent in the older scanners. As a result, the role of subcortical structures in the production of different syndromes can be overemphasized. The clinical evaluation of a patient with a cerebral hemispheric lesion is still paramount for a lucid management plan. Lesions as common as brain infarcts may remain invisible on CT scan for some time after the ictus or may pass unnoticed altogether if they are restricted to the cortex or cause coagulative necrosis. Tumors are easily detected on CT scan, but diseases such as Alzheimer's senile dementia cause only indirect signs on CT. The degree and distribution of atrophy only partially suggest the nature of the deficit. Likewise, longstanding cortical lesions that give rise to focal epilepsy often remain uncovered by CT scan. Finally, a good understanding of the anatomic correlation of behavioral symptoms allows the clinician to correlate the CT findings with the presenting complaints, thus avoid-

ing the mistake of managing as an active lesion one that bears no relation to the present illness (such as hydrocephalus in a patient with Alzheimer's disease) or of having a false sense of security when a negative CT scan fails to disclose an active lesion (such as a recent infarct).

Because the output of the brain is ultimately a motor output, no matter where in the cerebral hemispheres a lesion has occurred, the physician will become aware of it by observing the patient's motor performance. Such a motor performance depends on (1) the patient's level of alertness, mediated by the ascending reticular activating system, (2) the ability to concentrate on a task (cortical attention), (3) the perception of sensory stimuli and of their relation to past experiences, and (4) the ability to carry out the sequence of movements that makes up the motor act itself, whether it be a handshake or an oral account of the patient's illness. Hemispheric lesions can disturb any or several of the last three steps. The resulting disorders will be considered successively (Table 19-2).

Disturbances of Attention. Attention may be defined as the waking state in which sensory or amnestic information is selectively perceived, allowing the coherent performance of planned motor behavior. This selectivity is associated with unawareness of a great deal of irrelevant stimuli and memories [56]. It results from active neural facilitatory and inhibitory processes taking place at various levels of the nervous system from the peripheral sense organs to the cortex. Although attention requires a certain level of alertness, alertness is not always associated with attention. Such is the case of the akinetic mute state, in which the patient appears alert, yet lies immobile and mute, while his eyes dart in the direction of any novel stimulus. Alertness, which precedes attention, can be nonspecific (such as in the alerting reaction that occurs when a person adopts an exploratory attitude to the immediate environment, becoming receptive to a great deal of stimuli) or specific (when the meaning of the most significant stimulus is recognized and alertness is specifically and steadily directed toward it). The latter may be properly called attention. Concerning its origin, attention may be "passive" (involuntarily triggered by external stimuli and basic drives) or "active" (voluntarily generated and directed); it is the latter that is most impaired by cortical lesions. Disorders of attention due to hemispheric lesions may affect the patient's behavior toward events on one hemispace (hemiinattention) or globally.

UNILATERAL INATTENTION. Unilateral inattention or neglect is characterized by the patient's lack of orienting responses to unilateral novel stimuli in the absence of a primary sensory or motor deficit that could explain such behavior [51, 54]. This deficit may be primarily sensory or motor.

SENSORY INATTENTION. Sensory inattention can be *unimodal* (e.g., visual inattention), in which case stimuli of a specific sensory modality are less well perceived on one side. Most commonly these patients have *extinction* on double simultaneous stimulation, failing to report stimuli delivered to the side contralateral to the lesion. Lesions affecting areas 18 and 19, in the parietooccipital region, cause visual extinction, whereas lesions in the anterior association areas of the parietal lobe cause contralateral extinction of double tactile stimuli.

The other variety of unilateral sensory inattention is *multimodal*. These patients neglect the hemispace contralateral to the lesion when performing complex tasks such as dressing, in which they may fail to cover the neglected side (dressing apraxia), or drawing, in which the different elements of a picture may be placed in an abnormal spatial relationship to one another (constructional apraxia). Lesions of the right inferior parietal lobule are most apt to cause this syndrome.

HEMIAKINESIA. Hemiakinesia is the expression of unilateral motor neglect. The patient may not look toward one side of the space, even though he readily reacts to sensory stimuli coming from that space, or he may not move the limbs contralateral to the lesion unless specifically asked to do so, showing then good strength. Lesions in areas 6 and 8 of the medial and lateral "premotor area" of the right frontal lobe may cause this syndrome, which is rarer and less pronounced with lesions of the left hemisphere [28]. As discussed in Chapter 17, thalamic lesions may also cause unilateral inattention. All of these disorders appear more readily and profoundly with lesions of the right hemisphere, which is nondominant for language. Electrophysiologic studies have indicated that the nondominant hemisphere mediates attentional mechanisms directed to both hemifields, whereas the left hemisphere is mainly concerned with the right hemispace [63].

GLOBAL INATTENTION. Global inattention is manifest by inability to concentrate on a task, with consequent motor and verbal *impersistence*. For instance, upon instruction the patient cannot keep his arms up and the eyes closed for more than a few seconds. Simultaneously there is heightened distractibility, and the patient attends to all kinds of irrelevant stimuli, often returning to a previous motor or verbal performance *(perseveration)*. In the verbal sphere, these patients are laconic or even mute and may tend to repeat sentences spoken to them or near them (echolalia), and even to imitate gestures (echopraxia). Such disturbances are most often seen in patients with senile dementia, who have diffuse corti-

TABLE 19-2. *Clinical Manifestations of Cerebral Hemispheric Lesions*

I. *Attentional Disturbances*
   A. Unilateral inattention
      1. Sensory (sensory hemineglect)
         a. Unimodal
         b. Multimodal
      2. Motor (hemiakinesia)
   B. Global inattention
      1. Motor impersistence
      2. Motor perseveration
      3. Echolalia, echopraxia
      4. Akinetic mutism

II. *Emotional Disturbances*
   A. Due to diencephalic or brainstem lesions (accompanying somnolence, rage or fear of hypothalamic origin, or amnesia)
   B. Distorted perception of noxious stimuli
      1. Blunted (cingulate gyrus, temporal tip)
      2. Heightened (septal region?)
   C. Distorted perception of other sensory stimuli
      1. Blunted
         a. Wernicke's aphasia
         b. Sensory aprosodia
      2. Heightened
         a. Delusions
         b. Perception without object (hallucinations)
   D. Distorted perception of social nuances
      1. Blunted (frontal)
      2. Heightened (temporal)
   E. Distorted motor expression of emotions
      1. Hypokinesia (frontal, right hemisphere)
      2. Hyperkinesia (mesial temporooccipital)
      3. Uninhibited emotional expression. Pathologic laughter and crying (bilateral corticobulbar tract)

III. *Memory Disturbances*

IV. *Sensory Disturbances*
   A. Smell
   B. Taste
   C. Vision (calcarine cortex, visual association cortex, multimodal cortex)
      1. Hallucinations
         a. Simple
         b. Complex
      2. Visual agnosia
         a. Apperceptive
         b. Associative
         c. Color blindness—color agnosia

TABLE 19-2 (continued)

    d. Prosopagnosia
    e. Visual simultanagnosia (Balint syndrome)
  3. Alexia
    a. Pseudo-alexia
    b. Literal alexia
    c. Alexia without agraphia
    d. Alexia with agraphia
D. Auditory information (primary auditory area and association cortex of the temporal lobe and inferior parietal lobule)
  1. Hallucinations
  2. Auditory agnosia
  3. Pure word deafness
  4. Sensory amusia
  5. Sensory (posterior) aphasias
    a. Wernicke's aphasia
    b. Conduction aphasia
    c. Transcortical sensory aphasia
    d. Semantic anomia
    e. Word selection anomia
E. Somatosensory perception
  1. Simple somatosensory disturbances
    a. Decreased perception
    b. "Increased" perception, objectless perception (paresthesias)
  2. Complex somatosensory disturbances
    a. Disturbances of "body schema" and spatial relationships
      (1) Nondominant hemisphere
        (a) Anosognosia
        (b) Autotopagnosia
        (c) Spatial disorientation
        (d) Hemispatial neglect
        (e) Constructional apraxia
        (f) Dressing apraxia
      (2) Dominant hemisphere
        (a) Finger agnosia
        (b) Right-left disorientation
    b. Somatosensory varieties of agraphia
    c. Somatosensory varieties of acalculia

V. *Disturbances of Sensorimotor Integration and of Movement Execution (Parietal, Frontal)*
A. Apraxias
  1. Parietal apraxia
  2. Callosal apraxia
  3. Frontal apraxia
  4. Apraxia of gait (often with urinary incontinence)
  5. Limb-kinetic apraxia
B. Other disturbances of limb or face movements
  1. "Pyramidal" weakness
  2. Paratonia ("Gegenhalten")

TABLE 19-2 (continued)

---

    3. Primitive reflexes
      a. Grasp
      b. Palmomental
      c. Sucking, snout, rooting
      d. Corneomandibular
    4. Opercular syndrome, pseudo-bulbar palsy
  C. Oculomotor disturbances
    1. Supranuclear gaze palsy
    2. Lateral eye deviation on forcible eye closure
    3. Gaze apraxia (Balint syndrome)
  D. Motor disturbances of symbolic behavior
    1. Motor (anterior) aphasias
      a. Pure word anarthria (phonetic disintegration syndrome)
      b. Broca's aphasia
      c. Transcortical motor aphasia
    2. Pure agraphia
  E. Disturbances of goal-oriented behavior

VI. *Disturbances Related to Interhemispheric Disconnection (Callosal Syndrome)*
  A. Lack of kinesthetic transfer
    1. Inability to mimic position of the contralateral hand
    2. Left hand apraxia?
    3. Left hand agraphia
    4. Right hand constructional apraxia
    5. Intermanual conflict (alien left hand)
  B. Perplexity (and confabulation) elicited by right hand activity
  C. Double hemianopia

VII. *Dementia*

---

cal damage, or with metabolic encephalopathies, which in addition impair the subcortical alerting mechanisms. When a focal cortical lesion is responsible, it usually affects the mesial aspect of both frontal lobes [21]. Large lesions in this location cause akinetic mutism, a state of motionlessness and speechlessness with regular sleep-wake cycles. Medial diencephalo-mesencephalic lesions can also cause this syndrome.

Emotional Disturbances. The word *emotion* is usually taken to mean an inner feeling of well-being or, more often, of unrest. This inner feeling colors all the actions that the person performs and is thereby outwardly expressed. It depends on the satisfaction of the instinctive appetites and personal wishes. External or internal events are felt as agreeable or disagreeable to the integrity of the person and of the species. Emotions induce action: The uncomfortable feeling caused by soiled bed linen induces the patient to demand angrily immediate help from the nursing service. This is a normal emotional response. Neurologic disorders may cause blunting, exaggeration, or perversion of emotional responses.

The experience of emotion can be modulated by pharmacologic intervention. Normal subjects placed in a stressful situation experience a subjective feeling of anxiety. This subjective feeling can be enhanced by the injection of adrenalin. The injection of adrenalin without a concomitantly stressful situation causes many of the vegetative correlates of anxiety (pupillary dilation, tachycardia, cutaneous vasoconstriction) but not the inner feeling of anxiety [93]. Whether a situation is stressful or not depends to a great extent on the conscious or unconscious remembrance of a similar previous experience that was harmful to the subject or to the species.

The hypothalamus mediates some of the most primitive emotional responses, matching the ongoing metabolic variables with the parameters set for the individual species. When a deviation occurs, or when the circumstances are ripe for an action that would favor the survival of the individual or the species, a preset behavioral response occurs. Such relatively simple behavioral responses can be modified by phylogenetically newer structures, such as the cortex. Some cortical regions are involved in the recording and retrieval of stimuli that proved to be noxious to the individual (limbic cortex). Others allow him to communicate with other human beings semantically (language areas of the dominant hemisphere) or through facial expressions and other forms of "body language" (nondominant hemisphere). Still others mediate the complex balance of emotional responses needed for the survival and development of a social community (frontal lobes; temporal lobes ?). Finally, the outward expression of emotion uses the motor system.

Therefore, emotions and their expression depend on the following factors:

1. The state of arousal of the individual (alertness) mediated by the reticular activating system, including some thalamic structures, and the medial frontal cortex.
2. Vegetative functions, mediated in part by the hypothalamus.
3. A previous-experience retrieval system (memory) mediated by the hippocampus and other portions of the so-called limbic system.
4. The ability to perceive stimuli that carry an affective component, such as a friendly face. Aphasic patients with lesions in the left inferior parietal lobule and superior temporal gyrus, for example, are unimpressed when told "I will kill you" in a matter-of-fact tone but react to a threatening pitch of voice or an angry face. In contrast, right parietotemporal damaged individuals understand the semantic meaning of a verbal threat, but their perception of the emotional overtones that ac-

company the utterance is impaired [89]. Right parietooccipital lesions lessen the ability to perceive facial expression [33].

5. The ability to evaluate properly the importance of internal and external stimuli for the survival and well-being of the subject. For patients with bilateral orbitofrontal destructive lesions, most social nuances are trivial; however, they may go into a rage when some basic instinctive drives are not satisfied. By contrast, for patients with temporal lobe epilepsy even trivia become transcendental issues. Patients with small bilateral anterior cingulate (area 24) lesions may be unconcerned in the presence of painful stimuli. Those with bilateral anterior temporal lesions have a bland affect. Lesions of the septal region cause enhanced irritability and rage reactions. Patients with epileptogenic foci in the left temporal lobe tend to be paranoid and have antisocial behavior, whereas those with right temporal foci show emotional extremes (elation, sadness) and denial [94]. Some patients with acute medial temporooccipital lesions become not only disoriented but also agitated and abusive (syndrome of agitated delirium) [72].

6. The ability to express emotion, which requires more than a grossly intact motor system. Right frontal hemispheric lesions may cause impairment of the voluntary emotional intonation of speech [89]. Lack of voluntary control of the emotional expression may adopt another form, namely, accentuated emotional expression, to the point of irrepressible laughing or crying unaccompanied by the corresponding inner feeling. Pathologic laughing or crying results from bilateral internal capsular lesions that also involve the basal ganglia, from lesions in the substantia nigra, cerebral peduncles, and hypothalamus, and from pronounced involvement of the corticobulbar fibers, such as occurs in severe suprabulbar amyotrophic lateral sclerosis [84]. It has been postulated that lesions that affect mainly the left hemisphere tend to induce pathologic crying, whereas laughter appears more often after right hemispheric damage [92]. Likewise, patients with left hemispheric damage tend to show depression more often than those with right hemispheric damage. A large subset of the latter are somewhat unaware of their deficit, and such a denial may prevent the negative effect that the handicap might otherwise have on their mood.

7. An intact "baseline" affective situation (mood), which is disturbed in endogenous depression and mania. The anatomic substrate of these syndromes has not been elucidated, but rostral brainstem and basal midline diencephalic structures are probably involved.

Memory Disturbances.. Bilateral mesial temporal lesions cause amnesia. The memory loss includes those events that took place sometime before the injury (retrograde amnesia) and new information (data-based learning) afforded the patient after the injury (anterograde amnesia). Skill-based learning (e.g., how to use a tool) may be unaffected by these lesions [105]. General intelligence and complex perceptual abilities remain intact. Patients with cortical amnesia tend to confabulate less and to be more aware of their deficit than patients with Korsakoff's psychosis, for which mesial thalamic damage seems to be crucial. Lesions of the left temporal lobe impair mainly the storage of language-related information, whereas those on the right side affect the storage of nonverbal patterned materials, such as a geometric or tonal pattern [22]. Because verbal tasks are most often used to test memory, such hemispheric "specialization" may explain why memory deficits have been reported after unilateral lesions of the left temporal lobe but not of the right temporal lobe [44, 96].

In regard to the exact medial temporal structure responsible for amnesia, the traditional teaching pointing to the hippocampus has been recently challenged. Horel [57] has postulated that damage to temporothalamic connections running in the temporal stem (white matter linking the temporal lobe with the rest of the hemisphere) rather than hippocampal damage would account for the amnesia. His interpretation of some clinico-pathologic studies [82], and some new data [103, 105], seem to weaken his postulate. On the other hand, recent anatomic studies in the rat have shown that the subiculum, rather than the hippocampus, provides most of the fornical fibers and all of the ones destined for the hypothalamus, whereas fibers from the hippocampus proper end in the septal nuclei [95]. Better anatomico-clinical correlation is needed to define further the role of the temporal lobe in mnestic processes. Bilateral cingulate gyrus lesions may also impair memory. Memory loss caused by thalamic or hypothalamic lesions was discussed in the corresponding chapters. Bilateral lesions of any of the structures of the Papez circuit (hippocampus, fornix, mammillary body, mammillothalamic tract, anterior and dorso-medial thalamic nuclei, cingulate gyrus, and cingulum, Fig. 19-7) have been reported to cause amnesia [57].

Sensory Disturbances

SMELL AND TASTE. Olfactory nerve disturbances are discussed in Chapter 5. Epileptogenic lesions in the region of the temporal uncus may give rise to hallucinations of smell or taste. They are often accompanied by mouthing or chewing movements. Ageusia (lack of taste) may occur after bilateral insular lesions [20].

VISION. Calcarine cortex (primary visual area) lesions causing impaired visual acuity are discussed in Chapter 6. This chapter will deal with

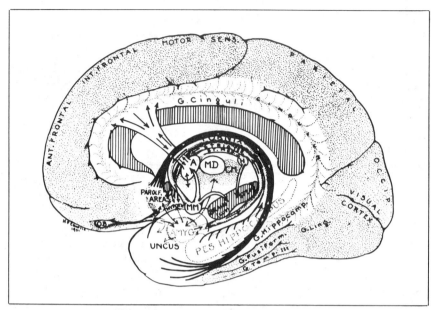

FIG. 19-7. *The limbic structures and some of their connections (according to Penfield and Jasper [81])*
are highlighted in this medial view of the right hemisphere.

more complex disturbances that reflect damage to the visual association
cortex or to other regions of the cerebral hemispheres involved in the acquisition and processing of visual information.

VISUAL HALLUCINATIONS AND DELUSIONS. These may be related to
poor visual acuity in elderly people (Charles Bonnet syndrome), in
which case the small, brightly colored people or objects that constitute
the hallucination have a cartoonlike appearance, and the patient is usually aware of their unreality [48].

Simple visual hallucinations, consisting in flashes of light (photopsias) or
lines of different colors that adopt simple patterns (zigzag, circle, fortifi-
cation pattern) often accompany a defective field of vision and indicate
inferomedial occipital disease, usually migraine or an epileptogenic lesion.

Complex visual hallucinations such as landscapes or animals are related
to temporal lobe dysfunction. Hippocampal stimulation may evoke visual hallucinations [1]. Among structural lesions, tumors have the greatest
tendency to induce hallucinations. Lesions in the upper midbrain that
also involve the thalamus, often bilaterally, may cause complex visual
hallucinations that have an oneroid (dreamlike) quality (peduncular hallucinosis) [23].

Other visual illusory phenomena include polyopsia (seeing a single target as multiple), palinopsia (persistence or recurrence of the visual image once the object has been removed), and visual allesthesia (transposition of an object seen in a visual field to the contralateral visual field). These illusory phenomena occur on the same side as an impaired but not blind visual field and are associated with occipitotemporal disease, often epileptogenic [58].

Focal seizures arising in the neocortex of the temporal lobe give rise to visual illusions ("déjà vu" [already seen]; "jamais vu" [never seen before]) or to experiential illusions ("déjà vécu" [already lived]; "jamais vécu" [never experienced before]). The patient feels a strong sense of familiarity with scenes or experiential situations that in reality he has never seen or experienced before or, on the contrary, a sense of strangeness about visual stimuli such as the face of a close relative or experiential situations that should be familiar to him.

VISUAL AGNOSIA. Visual agnosia is an impairment of the ability to recognize objects visually in the absence of a loss in visual acuity or general intellectual functions that would account for it [91]. Impaired visual recognition may adopt one or several of the following clinical expressions.

1. *Apperceptive visual agnosia.* Although these patients avoid obstacles when walking, they otherwise behave as if they were blind. They cannot name items presented to them, draw them, or match them to samples. They cannot point to objects named by the examiner. Yet they can distinguish small changes in the intensity or hue of a minute source of light. Their defect lies in an impairment of visual pattern recognition. Some of them complain that still objects are invisible but that they stand out from the background as soon as they move. Bilateral lesions, often ischemic, of the calcarine cortex cause this disturbance, which tends to appear in the process of recovery from cortical blindness. The extrastriatal visual pathway, which includes the pulvinar, superior colliculus, and parietal lobe, may play a role in recognition of light and movement in these patients [15].

2. *Associative visual agnosia.* This term refers to the deficit of patients who cannot recognize objects visually but can draw them or point to them when they are presented in an array of different objects. Picture identification is usually more difficult than the identification of real objects. In the process of recovery, this deficit tends to progress into a milder deficit, *optic aphasia,* which is characterized by inability to name objects that are recognized because their use can be explained.

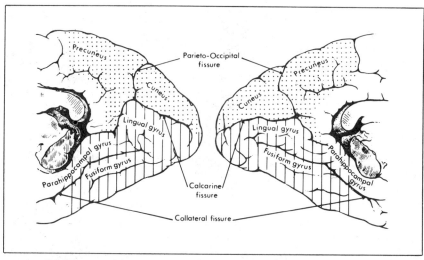

FIG. 19-8. *Medial aspect of the posterior portion of both hemispheres. Prosopagnosia and other visual agnosias result from bilateral temporooccipital lesions (vertical hatching), whereas visual simultanagnosia tends to follow bilateral parietooccipital lesions (stippling). Unilateral lesions of either hemisphere may cause a contralateral field defect and hemiachromatopsia. Unilateral left occipitotemporal lesions that also involve the splenium of the corpus callosum result in the syndrome of alexia without agraphia. (Modified from A. R. Damasio, H. Damasio, and G. W. van Hoesen [29].)*

These two disturbances are often associated with right homonymous hemianopia, pure alexia, and color-naming deficits. They usually occur following lesions affecting the mesial aspect of the left occipital lobe and the splenium of the corpus callosum.

COLOR AGNOSIA. Patients with cortical *color blindness* (achromatopia) cannot read Ishihara plates or sort colors according to hue. These tasks are well performed by patients with *color agnosia*, who, however, cannot name colors or point to a color named by the examiner but perform well in verbal-verbal tasks (e.g., "tell me the color of the sky"). Dominant hemispheric lesions that involve the inferomesial aspect of the occipital and temporal lobes are most probably responsible for color agnosia. Acquired achromatopia appears with bilateral inferior occipitotemporal lesions [27]. Bilateral inferooccipitotemporal lesions also cause inability to identify faces visually *(prosopagnosia)* or objects that are visually similar, such as a specific car in a parking lot (Fig. 19-8) [29].

VISUAL SIMULTANAGNOSIA. This phenomenon may underlie some of the agnostic deficits described above. The term refers to an inability to appreciate the meaning of the whole, though the elemental parts are well recognized. Patients with this deficit often have other components

of the so-called Balint [6] syndrome, which follows bilateral parietooccipital lesions in the convexity of the hemispheres and is characterized
by (1) failure to shift gaze on command (apraxia of gaze); (2) optic ataxia,
manifest by clumsiness of object-bound movements of the hand performed under visual guidance [26, 27]; and (3) decreased visual attention, affecting mainly the peripheral visual fields and resulting in constriction of the fields to "tunnel vision." Such a patient failed to see a
match offered him a few inches away from the tip of the cigarette he was
concentrating on [47].

Formal visual field testing in these patients is difficult because they fail
to keep their eyes focused on a target. When successful, it reveals full
visual fields. Failure of analysis of the different visual items and integration in a whole is partially mediated by a disruption of the normal exploratory eye movements that allow the identification of an assembly of
objects in space. When all of the elements of the syndrome are present,
bilateral posterior watershed lesions in the convexity of the hemispheres
(usually related to carotid artery disease) [27] or diffuse cortical processes with a posterior parietal preponderance (some cases of Alzheimer's disease) are most often to blame.

ALEXIA. The ability to read can be impaired by lesions in very different areas of the cerebral hemispheres [10]. Those that cause *aphasia*, discussed below, often affect to some extent the ability to understand written language. Anterior perisylvian lesions that cause Broca's aphasia
may particularly affect the patient's ability to read letters (*literal anomia* or
literal alexia) despite the preserved ability to read and comprehend whole
familiar words [7]. These patients also have difficulty understanding
sentences when the meaning depends on syntax (e.g., "He showed her
the girls' hats"). Left supramarginal gyrus damage may be critical for
such impairment of syntactic comprehension [90]. Most patients with
Wernicke's aphasia fail to understand both spoken and written language, although they may read aloud quite fluently. Patients with lesions restricted to the superior temporal gyrus can comprehend written
language much better than spoken language [52].

Patients with impaired saccadic eye movements and an attentional
disorder, which is most often due to large right frontoparietal infarcts or
hemorrhages, may complete the beginning or end of a word or sentence
they have scanned imperfectly by adding a high-frequency beginning or
ending. Thus, "Thursday" becomes "today" for a right hemispheric
damaged patient, and "latent" becomes "later" for a left hemispheric
damaged patient. More often, these patients will read only the words to
the right or to the left of a printed paragraph. Such *paralexias* may occur
with cortical or diencephalic disease.

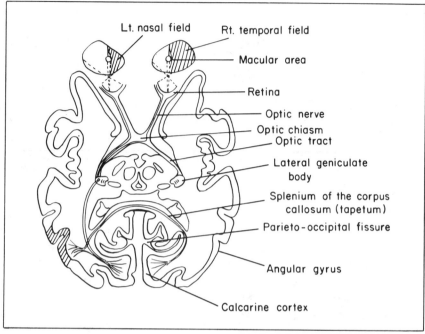

FIG. 19-9. *Representation of the visual pathways in a low horizontal section of the brain. Alexia with agraphia results from lesions that involve the left angular gyrus (oblique hatching). Alexia without agraphia occurs with lesions affecting the left medial occipitotemporal cortex and the fibers that reach the angular gyrus from the right occipitotemporal cortex. These fibers are often damaged in the splenium of the corpus callosum but may also be destroyed as they sweep lateral to the parietooccipital fissure. (Modified from J. Dejerine [32].)*

Alexia due to parietooccipital lesions may or may not be associated with impaired writing ability (agraphia).

Alexia without agraphia. These patients cannot read but are able to write on dictation. Visual identification of individual letters may be possible in some cases. In contrast to their marked difficulty in identifying visual patterns, these patients may identify the word by tracing the letters (kinesthetic "reading"). They can also read digits and multidigit numbers but often have color agnosia. Alexia without agraphia follows lesions of the dominant medial occipital region (particularly lesions involving the cortex around and below the calcarine fissure) and the inferior fibers of the splenium of the corpus callosum (Fig. 19-9) [2].

Alexia with agraphia. In addition to the reading and writing disturbance, these patients usually have acalculia, finger agnosia, right-left disorientation, and difficulty with spelling words and understanding spelled-out words. A lesion in the angular gyrus is most likely if the patient does not have a Wernicke's aphasia. Patients with sensory aphasia often have alexia with agraphia, and their lesion extends to the superior temporal gyrus.

ANTON'S SYNDROME (DENIAL OF BLINDNESS). Patients with acute, bilateral, and extensive medial occipital lesions that render them blind may deny having any difficulty with seeing and confabulate about what they "see." Such a phenomenon often appears in the setting of a generalized metabolic encephalopathy. When it is related to discrete lesions, these are likely to extend to the lateral aspect of the occipital lobes and reach the parietal lobes [38]. It is unclear whether thalamic involvement in the case of posterior circulation infarcts may be instrumental in the genesis of Anton's syndrome in some patients.

DISTURBANCES IN THE PROCESSING OF AUDITORY INFORMATION

AUDITORY HALLUCINATIONS. This "positive" symptom has little localizing value because it can occur with lesions anywhere between the ear and the temporal cortex. Auditory hallucinations occasionally follow impaired hearing, particularly when there is an attentional defect due to a metabolic brain disease [50]. About 20 percent of temporal lobe tumors may be accompanied by auditory hallucinations, which are most common as a symptom of schizophrenia and accompany infrequently the alcohol withdrawal syndrome.

HEARING LOSS. Lesions in the auditory pathways as far as the cortex are discussed in Chapter 10. Unilateral lesions restricted to the primary auditory cortex (transverse gyrus of Heschl, in the floor of the Sylvian fissure) remain asymptomatic, but they can be detected with dichotic stimulation and other methods. Bilateral lesions cause impairment in sound discrimination (auditory agnosia), but pure tone audiometry remains normal or reflects slight impairment. Different sounds, such as ringing of the phone or clapping of hands, cannot be distinguished or localized. Some sounds of a normal intensity may be perceived as having an annoying quality. The spoken word cannot be identified either (pure word deafness), though these patients may read and speak quite normally, if loudly on occasion [79]. When the defect is severe, they may complain that people sound as if they were speaking a foreign language. By using lip reading, these patients can improve their performance, but not by increasing the sound volume. One such patient, unable to understand his wife's normal speech, disliked the sound of the television set and compelled her to turn the volume so low that she herself could not understand what was being said [79]. Rarely, when temporal lobe lesions are asymmetrical, greater impairment of sound and word recognition may be detected in the ear contralateral to the larger lesion [4]. Patients with larger lesions on the left hemisphere may have greater difficulty in distinguishing words, whereas predominantly right hemispheric lesions may cause greater impairment in the discrimination of nonverbal sounds, including music. Poor recognition of words accompanied by almost normal reading and speech may occasionally appear in the process of recovery from a sizable unilateral lesion in the dominant first temporal gyrus involving the auditory association cortex (Wernicke's area). In such cases the receding Wernicke's aphasia gives way to almost normal language ability, tainted by an occasional paraphasic error, but understanding of the spoken word remains markedly impaired, particularly when short sentences of a somewhat complex syntactic structure are given to the patient in a test situation.

SENSORY AMUSIA. This term refers to the inability to appreciate the different characteristics of heard music. Right hemispheric lesions result in impairment of appreciation of pitch, timber, and rhythm, whereas left hemispheric lesions affect mainly appreciation of the lyrics. The degree of musical sophistication of the patient may be reflected in the lateralization of the cortex used to process music [39]. The left hemisphere seems to play a greater role in the appreciation of music by musically trained individuals, who may use a more analytic strategy to identify a musical composition.

POSTERIOR APHASIAS. Most cortical left hemispheric lesions leading to impaired processing of auditory information cause a language disturbance, that is, an aphasia. The type of aphasic disturbance depends on

1. Cortical representation of the analysis of language-related auditory stimuli in a particular patient. In most right-handed persons and in about 50 percent of left handers, the left superior temporal gyrus and the neighboring inferior parietal lobule play the greatest role in this analysis [31].
2. The location of the lesion. Lesions centered in the posterior two-thirds of the superior temporal gyrus (areas 41, 42, and 22, Wernicke's area) tend to cause the greatest impairment of auditory comprehension of language, even when reading may be only mildly affected. The neighboring area of the second temporal gyrus also participates in language processing [77]. The more posterior the location of the lesion, in the angular gyrus region, the more pronounced is alexia and anomia for visually recognized objects. Predominantly inferior parietal lesions give rise to impaired arithmetical skills (acalculia), disturbances of body schema (right-left disorientation, finger agnosia), and agraphia. Lesions circumscribed to the inferior temporal gyrus give rise to *word-selection anomia* [8]. The patient cannot remember the name of an object presented to him, and cueing does not help, but he can consistently choose the appropriate object from an array when he hears its

name. Both name retrieval and name recognition are impaired with lesions of Wernicke's area (*semantic anomia*).

3. The size of the lesion. A large lesion involving the superior and middle temporal gyri and the inferior parietal lobule is most likely to cause a severe deficit in the comprehension of spoken and written language. In such cases, the words the patient hears are devoid of semantic meaning (semantic aphasia); he gathers no information from them. Similarly, the patient's utterances consist of semantically meaningless nonwords (neologisms) or have a thin connection to the object they are meant to signify (paraphasias). This connection may have a phonologic (e.g., "letter" for "ladder") or a categorical character ("table" for "chair"). These patients write nonsensical words or sentences and cannot name objects appropriately (Fig 19-11). Smaller "through" lesions, or lesions such as tumors that, even when large, leave some neuronal elements functionally active, cause the so-called *conduction aphasia*. These lesions tend to be circumscribed to the posterior portion of the superior temporal gyrus and to the supramarginal gyrus [30]. The patient can handle a conversation well, but when confronted with the task of repeating a word or sentence, the utterance is incomplete or marred by phonemic or semantic substitutions. Although fluent, the spontaneous speech of these patients usually contains paraphasic errors.

4. The time allowed for recovery after an acute lesion. The severe impairment of language comprehension (semantic or Wernicke's aphasia) that follows upon a large vascular lesion tends to improve in subsequent weeks and months (Fig. 19-10). More and more words and sentences regain their informative value, and the deficit may end by resembling a conduction aphasia [61].

TRANSCORTICAL SENSORY APHASIA. Some patients can repeat words well but are unable to understand the meaning of the spoken or written word. They may repeat a command from the examiner (echolalia) and yet fail to follow it. Other auditory information is also missed, despite the ability to repeat the very sentence of which the meaning is not quite grasped. This syndrome, termed transcortical sensory aphasia, is most often seen accompanying the attentional disturbance of metabolic encephalopathy. Lesions in the thalamus, left mesial frontoparietal region, or inferolateral aspect of both temporal lobes may cause a similar syndrome [24, 71, 88].

In recent years, an anatomico-clinical classification of aphasias based on the patient's spontaneous speech, comprehension, naming, and repetition has won widespread acceptance (Table 19-3) [11].

POSTERIOR APROSODIA. Recently it has been proposed that just as

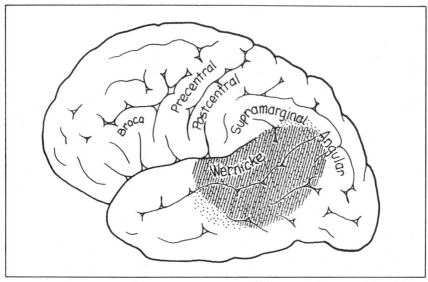

FIG. 19-10. *Clinical manifestations of recent versus old lesions in the posterolateral aspect of the left hemisphere. Vertical hatching indicates the extent of an infarct developed 2 weeks previously in a 57-year-old man. He had a severe word comprehension difficulty, alexia with agraphia, and a semantic anomia. He repeated words inaccurately. His spontaneous speech was uninformative and marred by neologisms. By contrast, the 62-year-old man whose 1-year-old infarct involved the area stippled in the figure understood conversational speech well, could write, and spoke with mild circumstantiality and occasional paraphrasic errors. He still missed the meaning of some dictated words and understood television poorly.*

the left (dominant) hemisphere plays the greater role in the analysis of the syntactic components of language, corresponding areas of the right hemisphere are concerned with the emotional aspects of language (prosody, or affective intonation of spoken language, and emotional gesturing) [89]. Lesions in the right posterior temporoparietal region may result in poor perception of the emotional overtones of spoken language.

DISTURBANCES OF SOMATOSENSORY PERCEPTION

ELEMENTAL SOMATOSENSORY DISTURBANCES. Lesions of the postcentral gyrus cause contralateral impairment in the perception of size and shape by palpation. As a result, the identity of the palpated object remains unknown *(astereognosis)* [87]. Such impairment, which is greatest in the limb represented in the lesioned area (Fig. 19-6), affects also two-point discrimination and graphesthesia (the ability to recognize a letter or digit traced on the patient's skin). Pinprick is also perceived as

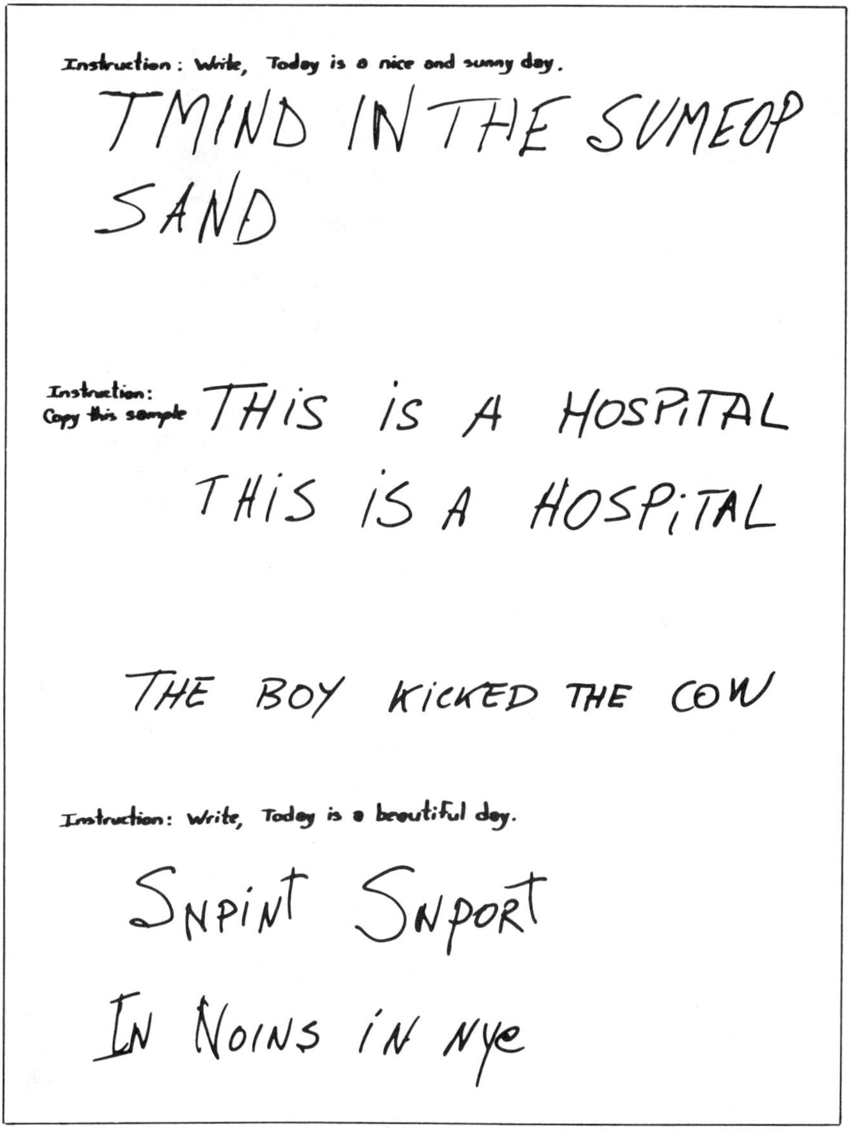

FIG. 19-11. *Jargon writing by a 59-year-old, left-handed man with a large left-hemispheric perisylvian infarct. The dictated text is printed beside the patient's writing. He could copy ("this is a hospital") but not read printed words. His oral language was practically normal.*

TABLE 19-3. *Classification of the Aphasias*

Type of Aphasia	Fluency	Comprehension	Repetition	Naming	Lesion Location
Broca's	↓	Good	↓	↓	Frontoparietal operculum
Wernicke's	Good	↓	↓	↓	Inferoposterior perisylvian (temporal)
Conduction	Good	Good	↓	↓	Posterior perisylvian
Transcortical motor	↓	Good	Good	May be normal	Frontal, striatum
Transcortical sensory	Good	↓	Good	Usually normal	Parietal, temporal, thalamus
Anomic	Good	Good	Good	↓	Depends on type of anomia
Global	↓	↓	↓	↓	Perisylvian (large)

less sharp on the side contralateral to an acute parietal lobe lesion. Sensory loss with parietal lesions tends to be localized to the distal portion of the limbs, which have the largest cortical representation and are almost exclusively innervated by the contralateral hemisphere. Paresthesias, usually of a tingling quality, may occur in the limb represented in an area of the postcentral gyrus affected by ischemia or epileptic activity (sensory seizure). It has been postulated that lesions of the parietal operculum (superior lip of the Sylvian fissure corresponding to the secondary somatosensory area) may cause a pseudothalamic syndrome, with pronounced impairment in the perception of pain and temperature in the acute stage and a delayed "thalamic" type of pain [13, 17]. However, delayed pain and paresthesia frequently occur after deep or large parietal lesions. Lesions in the association cortex of the parietal lobe (areas 7, 39, and 40) cause disturbances in the evaluation of spatial relationships and in the sensorimotor integration of language (aphasia) or other motor acts (apraxia). The former will be considered first.

DISTURBANCES OF "BODY SCHEMA" AND SPATIAL RELATIONSHIPS. Both parietal lobes mediate the orienting response to a sensory stimulus in space. However, the right hemisphere seems to play a greater role in this attentional task, mediating attention to stimuli from both hemispaces, whereas the left parietal lobe is mainly concerned with stimuli delivered to the right hemispace [54, 63]. As a consequence, right hemispheric lesions tend to cause hemineglect much more readily than left-sided lesions. Perhaps on the same basis, large right parietal lesions are often accompanied by anosognosia in which the patient denies an obvious left hemiparesis or even being sick at all. Still other patients fail to recognize the hemiplegic limbs as belonging to them (autotopagnosia) and confabulate when asked whom they belong to (they often ascribe them to the examiner). Sudden onset of confusion without agitation and a pronounced disorientation for place disproportionate to the rest of the patient's behavior have been described as signs of right parietal (or right prefrontal) infarction [36, 73]. Right parietal lesions cause impairment of tasks requiring apprehension of spatial relations, independently of sensory modality. Visual or tactile localization of points in space and judgment of direction and distance are defective. Patients with right parietal lobe lesions tend to misplace the cities on a map and to get lost in unfamiliar surroundings; this last type of topographic disorientation is more common with bilateral parietal lesions.

Some of these perceptual difficulties probably underlie the impaired motor performance (apraxia), which is out of proportion to the primary motor or sensory deficit, of right parietal patients. *Constructional apraxia*, the inability to put together the different parts of a spatial array, is a characteristic disorder. Depending on the degree of their impairment, these patients cannot build a block design that matches a given sample, copy two- or three-dimensional figures, or draw two- or three-dimensional objects. Hemispatial neglect is often conspicuous, for instance, when the patient leaves out all of the left-sided numbers on the face of a clock or the petals on the left side of the daisy he has been asked to draw.

DRESSING APRAXIA. Impaired tactile and visuospatial coordination plus a degree of hemineglect may explain why some patients with right parietal lesions have a striking difficulty donning their clothes. Hemineglect is obvious when they leave the left side of the body uncovered and dishevelled.

FINGER AGNOSIA, RIGHT-LEFT DISORIENTATION, AGRAPHIA, AND ACALCULIA. Gerstmann described the association of these four signs (Gerstmann syndrome) as characteristic of lesions in the angular gyrus of the dominant hemisphere [41]. However, cases have been reported in which patients with all four components of the syndrome proved on necropsy examination to have an intact angular gyrus [55]. Other studies have shown a strong correlation of finger agnosia and right-left disorientation with impairment of language comprehension in unilateral lesions. This holds not only for performances in which understanding of the labels *right* and *left* is required, but also for nonverbal performances such as imitation [12]. Nondominant parietal lesions may give rise to some forms of right-left disorientation, specifically misidentification of body parts of a confronting person and failure to imitate crossed movements of the examiner (e.g., *left* hand on *right* ear). Impairment in these tasks may be based on visual-spatial disability [12].

AGRAPHIA. Inability to write properly (agraphia) accompanies all other language disturbances. The characteristics of these forms of agraphia are described in the paragraphs dealing with aphasia. The association of agraphia with alexia in angular gyrus lesions affecting the dominant hemisphere was discussed in the section on alexia. This writing disturbance has been called parietal agraphia because it results from lesions of the inferior parietal lobule. Marked difficulty with spelling out and putting together spelled-out words accompanies this type of agraphia. Apraxia is almost always present; anomia is common. Parietal agraphia is characterized by impairment in the drawing of letters, relative preservation of the syntactic structure of sentences, and parallel impairment of all writing modalities (spontaneous writing, writing to dictation, copying). By contrast, in aphasic agraphia copying ability is usually preserved. Parietal agraphia is not merely a direct expression of hand apraxia because spelling using block letters is also impaired. The relative severity of agraphia and alexia varies with the location of the lesion; alexia predominates with temporooccipital lesions, and agraphia is more prominent with parietooccipital lesions [68].

ACALCULIA. Left parietooccipital lesions that cause aphasia often cause difficulty in performing simple arithmetic calculations. Anterior frontal lesions impair the ability to solve problems in which more than one step is involved (e.g., distribute six books between two shelves in such a way that one shelf contains twice as many books as the other) or calculations in an open-ended series, in which the patient utters perseverations after an accurate answer (e.g., $100 - 7 = 93$, $- 7 = 83$, $- 7 = 73$).

Simple calculations may be impaired because of

1. Alexia or agraphia for numbers. One such patient stated that $4 + 5$ added up to 8; his written answer was 5, but he chose the correct amount when given a multiple choice. As with most of these patients, his lesion affected the left inferior parietal lobule. Patients with left temporal lesions may be able to calculate as long as they can use a paper to write down the calculations, but they cannot handle calculations given orally or those that require verbal carryover, even silent, of numbers.
2. Impaired spatial organization of numbers, reflected by misalignment of digits, visual neglect (e.g., 252 read as 52), inversion of digits (e.g., 9 interpreted as 6), reversal errors (e.g., 12 interpreted as 21), and inability to maintain the decimal place. In a patient without generalized mental deterioration or aphasia, this type of spatial acalculia suggests a postrolandic lesion in the right hemisphere [65]. Patients with parietooccipital lesions of either hemisphere may understand the value of single digits, yet be unable to read and write compound numbers. They read 19 as 1 and 9. They may estimate the size of a figure from the value of the individual numbers, thus they consider 2989 larger than 5010.
3. Pure anarithmetria, the inability to calculate despite intact number reading and in the absence of spatial deficits, appears most often with bilateral hemispheric or dominant retrorolandic lesions. Impairment of analytic memory and attention plays a role in many of these cases. Multiplication and division are usually most impaired.

Disturbances of Sensorimotor Integration and of Movement Execution (Parietal, Frontal)

APRAXIAS

PARIETAL APRAXIA. Apraxia has been defined as a disorder of skilled movement that is not caused by weakness, sensory loss, abnormality of tone or posture, abnormal movements, intellectual deterioration, or poor comprehension [42, 66]. The deficit becomes most obvious when the patient is asked to perform a pantomime, such as to make believe he is lighting a cigarette or combing his hair. Patients with dominant hemispheric lesions in the neighborhood of the intraparietal sulcus become befuddled or perform the wrong sequence of movements on command. For movements such as the ones mentioned above, which require the use of the hand, they often use the hand as an object (e.g., as a comb). However, they perform normally when given the actual object. This type of apraxia, which has been termed *ideomotor apraxia*, appears also with lesions of the premotor area of the frontal lobe (areas 6 and 8 of Brodmann). Clinically, these two locations of apraxia can be distinguished because parietal apraxia is accompanied by a greater degree of difficulty in recognizing that a motor performance (by the patient or others) was poor [53]. Traditionally, it has been thought that, just as one hemisphere is dominant for language, one is dominant for the performance of "object-free" motor acts. In right-handed persons, the left hemisphere would be dominant for praxis and speech. In left handers these functions may be represented in opposite hemispheres. Thus, after a high parietal lesion on the right hemisphere, a left-handed man developed apraxia without aphasia, but this was accompanied by an inability to discriminate well-performed from poorly performed acts [53].

In patients with therapeutic callosotomies (section of the corpus callosum) the right hemisphere can organize relatively simple sequences of left-handed movements without the participation of the left hemisphere [99]. It can probably also organize object-free movements, because callosal section does not induce apraxia [40]. Apraxia of the left hand has been reported in clinical cases in which the corpus callosum had been involved by ischemia or tumors (callosal apraxia) [43, 67]. These cases, however, are compounded by damage to the mesial aspect of the frontal lobe that by itself may interfere with the performance of bimanual coordination tasks [16, 46].

Patients with bilateral lesions in the neighbohood of the intraparietal sulcus have the greatest difficulty in performing object-free movements and often exhibit impairment of more elementary movements as well. They may miscalculate reaching for a fork under visual guidance or using it to bring food to the mouth. Proximal, less elaborate movements, like ambulation, are unimpaired. Dressing and constructional apraxia were discussed among the disorders of spatial relationships.

ANTERIOR (FRONTAL) APRAXIAS. We have just considered the impairment of motor performance derived from parietal or premotor lesions (ideomotor apraxia). Unilateral lesions of the supplementary motor area impair the performance of tasks in which bimanual coordination is required [16]. Also, tasks of reciprocal coordination such as repetitively making a fist with one hand while opening the other are impaired. This is also reflected by an inability to draw alternating patterns and by constructional perseveration (Fig. 19-12). Writing is often impaired, more so with lesions of the left hemisphere [3, 70]. The hand contralateral to the lesion has a tendency to grasp when the palm is stimulated (grasp reflex) and may perform seemingly purposeful movements (such as reaching for an object or imitating what the other hand is doing) that are unwilled by the patient (alien hand sign) [46].

Lesions in the pathways originating in the mesial frontal cortex are often accompanied by a characteristic gait (apraxia of gait)—the patient appears to be stuck to the floor (magnetic gait) and has difficulty lifting up each foot to take the next step [74]. As a result, the feet drag along, and steps are short. Turns are particularly difficult. The resultant gait thus resembles that of patients with Parkinson's disease, due to bilateral nigral degeneration. Patients with frontal apraxia of gait perform clumsily when asked to kick an imaginary ball or to outline a circle with the foot. The most common causes of apraxia of gait include bilateral subcortical infarcts in the centrum semiovale and stretching by hydrocephalus of the fibers projecting from the mesial aspect of the frontal lobe as they sweep around the ventricles.

Seizures originating in the supplementary motor area induce head turning to the opposite side and raising of the contralateral hand to the level of the head, in such a way that the patient seems to be performing a military salute.

Lesions of the mesial aspect of the frontal lobe cause akinesia (paucity of movement). The contralateral limbs are used sparingly, although when used they appear strong. Bilateral lesions cause paucity of movement and of speech (akinetic mutism) [21, 60, 70]. Some patients with bilateral mesial frontal lesions (and perhaps also those with bilateral pallidal pathology) have a remarkable disorder of movement. They can be fully oriented and move well the limbs on command, yet they will not use them to take care of their needs. Such a patient requested water, but did not even attempt to reach for the cup offered him, while he could raise either arm on command. This disorder contrasts with most of the apraxias described above, in which object-bound actions are generally performed better and more easily than object-free actions (e.g., a pantomime on command). These patients also fail to perform movements that require a preferential use of the axial muscles, such as pushing themselves up in bed, shifting their position, or getting up. This abnormality of movement may be a minor degree of the syndrome described above as akinetic mutism, usually present with large bilateral lesions in the medial frontal or medial thalamo-diencephalic regions.

Lesions in the perirolandic cortex cause impairment of fine distal

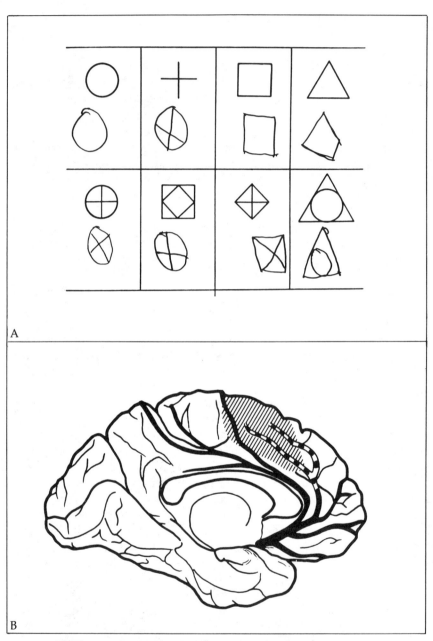

FIG. 19-12. (A) Perseveration is evident in this copying task by a 76-year-old woman with a recent infarct in the distribution of the left anterior cerebral artery (B). (B reproduced from J. C. Masdeu, W. C. Schoene, and H. Funkenstein [70]. Copyright © 1978 by Harcourt, Brace, Jovanovich, Inc.)

movements of the contralateral hand. Picking up small objects by apposing the index and thumb, or handling a small coin may become impossible. This type of apraxia has been termed limb-kinetic apraxia. Because separate fine movements of each finger are unavailable these patients pick up a pen or a coin by pressing it against the palm with the proximal portion of the thumb, much as infants do before they develop pincer grip.

OTHER MOTOR DISTURBANCES OF THE EXTREMITIES OR FACE

"PYRAMIDAL" WEAKNESS. Lesions of the motor strip or fibers therefrom induce impairment in the voluntary control of the limb represented in the affected portion of the cortex (Fig. 19-6). Sometime after the lesion occurs, spasticity develops in the affected limb. Brisk muscle stretch reflexes usually precede the onset of spasticity.

Clumsiness in the use of the arm was discussed above. Lesions of the medial aspect of the frontal lobe in the area of representation of the legs (paracentral lobule) give rise primarily to weakness of foot dorsiflexion and of alternating movements of the toes. A Babinski sign and, if the lesion involves the mesial aspect of the first frontal gyrus, a grasp response may be present. Such lesions often affect both hemispheres, causing urinary incontinence with uninhibited emptying of the bladder.

PARATONIA (GEGENHALTEN). This type of increased muscle tone results from rather extensive bilateral dysfunction of the mesial cortex and superior convexity of the frontal lobes (premotor cortex, area 6). When a patient with paratonia is asked to relax a joint (elbow, knee) so that the examiner may move it freely, the involved muscles tense up instead, and the patient appears to the examiner to be trying to actively oppose any movement of the joint by the examiner. The tone of the involved muscles increases in proportion to the speed and strength with which the examiner tries to move the joint.

"PRIMITIVE" REFLEXES. These motor responses, present during infancy, disappear during childhood and tend to reappear with aging. They can be elicited in hydranencephalic infants lacking suprastriatal brain structures. Thus, it is considered that as the infant cortex matures and myelination proceeds, these primitive signs are inhibited. Cortical or subcortical damage, particularly damage affecting the frontal lobes, would release them. However, up to 25 percent of normal adults have a palmomental reflex, which becomes a very common finding in normal elderly individuals [59]. The grasp and suck reflexes are more specific indicators of extensive frontal lobe disease. The grasp and snout reflexes often accompany impaired performance of cognitive tests [97].

Grasp Reflex. The grasp reflex is elicited by stroking lightly the palm of the patient's hand with the radial aspect of the index finger and then rubbing the palm and the volar aspect of the fingers with a gentle forward motion. The patient's fingers hook around the hand of the examiner, who can then pull from the flexed fingers of the patient, who is unable to release the grip (forced grasping reflex). For the reflex to be most reliable, the patient should be told not to grab the examiner's fingers. Patients with mild loss of cortical inhibition may be able to release the grip voluntarily, particularly at the beginning of the eliciting maneuver, before strong tension on the finger flexors is applied. Distracting the patient with a task such as giving his address will allow the reflex to reappear. Damage to the contralateral area 6, particularly in the mesial aspect of the hemisphere, accounts for the release of the grasp reflex.

Palmomental Reflex. The palmomental reflex consists of a brief contraction of the ipsilateral mentalis muscle when the palm of the hand is briskly stroked with a blunt object. When pronounced, this reflex may be elicited by stroking the arm or even the chest. This finding indicates damage of the contralateral paracentral cortex or the fibers from it.

Sucking, Snout, Rooting Reflexes. When tapping on the upper lips elicits a pursing-pouting movement of the lips, the patient is said to have a snout reflex. Curving of the lips around a round object applied to them represents a suck reflex, which when accentuated may be expressed by a sucking position of the lips and turning of the mouth toward a round object that approaches the patient's mouth or gently strokes his cheek (rooting reflex). The snout reflex may reflect impairment of the corticobulbar projection, whereas the suck reflex correlates better with diffuse frontal premotor disease.

Corneomandibular Reflex; Eye-Jaw Synkinesis. A corneomandibular reflex occurs when the patient's jaw deviates to the side opposite a stimulated cornea. A synkinesis, which is probably accentuated by loss of corticobulbar inhibition, consists of ipsilateral movement of the jaw when the patient voluntarily looks sideways.

OPERCULAR SYNDROME. PSEUDO-BULBAR PALSY. In addition to dysarthria (and aphasia when on the dominant hemisphere), acute lesions of the frontoparietal operculum cause difficulty in swallowing liquids (dysphagia), which tend to come back through the nose [20]. When the lesions involving the operculum or corticobulbar pathways are bilateral, dysphagia tends to last longer and may be permanent. In those cases, saliva accumulates in the mouth, aspiration of food may cause repeated bouts of pneumonia, and the patient may be aphonic. This array of symptoms resembles the clinical picture produced by involvement of the bulbar muscles themselves (e.g., by dermatomyositis) or by involvement of the neuromuscular junction (myasthenia gravis), peripheral nerve (Guillain-Barré syndrome, diphtheria), or medullary neurons (motor neuron disease, medullary lesions). Thus it has been termed pseudo-bulbar palsy because, unlike actual bulbar palsy, the bulbar muscles themselves are not affected and lack atrophy. The jaw jerk is brisk in these patients, who often have emotional incontinence with uninhibited crying and laughter.

Oculomotor disturbances related to frontal or parietal lesions are discussed in Chapter 7.

MOTOR DISTURBANCES OF SYMBOLIC BEHAVIOR

MOTOR (FRONTOPARIETAL) APHASIAS. Lesions involving the anterior portion of the frontoparietal operculum cause language disturbances in which production of language is altered and reduced (nonfluent aphasia), but comprehension of spoken language is preserved. As in the posterior (sensory) aphasias, the degree and quality of language impairment in anterior aphasias depends on several factors. First, it depends on the cortical representation of motor sequences (frontal association cortex) and of the integration of kinesthetic and motor information (parietal association cortex) that mediate speed production. *Unilateral* lesions of the "face area" of the precentral gyrus (area 4, see Fig. 19-6) cause transient dysarthria. The verbal utterances contain a correct set of words, disposed in a grammatically correct order (phonemic and morphosyntactic levels), yet the articulation of each sound by the oral muscles is clumsy. The patient speaks slowly and effortfully. Because of oral muscle incoordination, voiced consonants such as *b*, become their devoiced counterparts ($b \rightarrow p$), occlusive consonants are abnormally strong, and fricative consonants adopt the related occlusive sound (e.g., $z \rightarrow d$). Vowels are abnormally long and hesitant, sounding like pseudo-diphthongs. As a result, the patient's speech resembles that of someone with a foreign accent [64]. Lesions of the precentral gyrus or fibers therefrom cause contralateral facial weakness involving the lower facial muscles, which is most noticeable when the patient speaks; the affected orbicularis oris then shows reduced speed and range of movements. *Bilateral* lesions of the corticobulbar fibers originating in the face region of area 4 cause lasting dysarthia, which may be severe (pure anarthria or phonetic disintegration syndrome, aphemia). Such a syndrome is most often caused by bilateral infarcts in the corticobulbar fibers as they course in the anterior portion of the posterior limb of the internal capsule. This explains why this disturbance of speech was termed *subcortical motor aphasia*. However, these patients, even when mute, can write correctly and do not have any difficulty in the production of verbal sequences as long as they do not have to articulate them [64].

By contrast, unilateral left-sided lesions in the strip of cortex immediately anterior to the primary motor cortex for the face—that is, the cortex in the posterior portion of the third (and second?) frontal gyri (*Broca's area*) [32], cause a true language disturbance. Although the patient knows what he wants to say and can recognize an appropriate sentence, he cannot produce the appropriate sounds or write a meaningful sequence of letters [49, 69, 75]. Speech and writing are impaired to the point of mutism and complete agraphia, in which the patient can copy but cannot write spontaneously or on dictation (Fig. 19-13). Repetition is also impaired, but with smaller lesions or when the patient begins to improve, repetition is usually better than spontaneous speech. The speech of these patients has an agrammatical character; function words, such as articles, are omitted, and verbal endings are dropped. Nouns and verbs ("content" words) fare better than adjectives, adverbs, and other "filler" words. Thus, these patients convey much information using few words (telegraphic speech). Sound substitution, usually by including a stressed syllable of a word that comes later in the sentence, gives rise to literal and phonemic paraphasias. These are recognized by the patient as paraphasic errors, unlike the situation that occurs when paraphasias are uttered as a result of posterior lesions. Naming of objects is also impaired, but, unlike patients with temporal lobe lesions, these patients benefit from cueing (e.g., by the examiner's mouthing the beginning of the object's name) [8]. Lesions restricted to the frontal lobe cause a transient aphasia, which, except for decreased spontaneity of the patient's speech (transcortical motor aphasia), clears completely in the course of a few days or weeks [19, 75, 76].

Lasting aphasia of the type described above, with pronounced agrammatism and markedly reduced fluency (*Broca's aphasia*), corresponds to lesions extending across the frontoparietal operculum, including the postcentral and supramarginal gyri [76]. Patients with this type of Broca's aphasia have difficulty understanding sentences whose meaning depends on syntax (e.g., "the boy was kicked by the cow" versus "the boy kicked the cow"). This impairment may be related to damage to the supramarginal gyrus, which is part of the auditory association cortex [90]. However, cortical stimulation studies suggest a more critical participation of the motor sequencing areas of the frontoparietal perisylvian operculum in the decoding of the phonemes that constitute the syntactic changes [77]. Patients with large perisylvian lesions are mute or have a nonfluent, agrammatical speech accompanied by impaired comprehension and repetition (*global aphasia*).

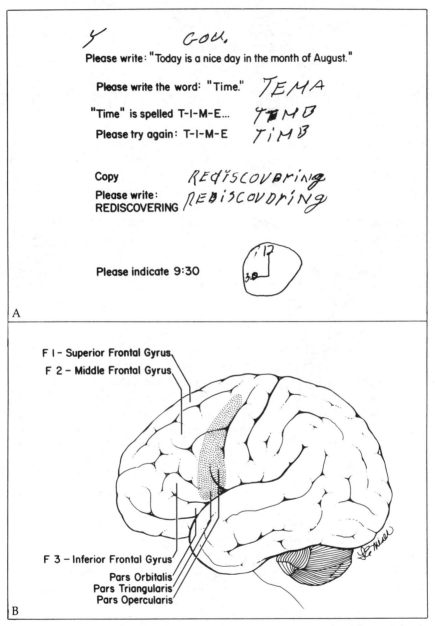

FIG. 19-13. *(A) Writing sample of a 43-year-old man with an embolic infarct of a cortical strip (Broca's area) anterior to the primary motor cortex for the mouth and hand. (B) Outline of the infarct area. (Reproduced from J. C. Masdeu and R. J. O'Hara [69]. Copyright © 1983 by Harcourt, Brace, Jovanovich, Inc.)*

In most right-handed people the left hemisphere is dominant for speech [31]. Only left hemispheric lesions cause the disturbances of symbolic behavior outlined above. Among left-handers, language dominance is less clear-cut than among right-handers. Left hemispheric lesions may leave oral language unaltered, whereas writing and reading may be severely impaired (Fig. 19-11). About 50 percent of left-handers will develop a language deficit, often transient, after lesions of the left hemisphere. Hemispheric dominance appears early in life. Complete transfer of language capabilities to the right hemisphere when the left hemisphere suffers a lesion is unlikely to occur in children older than 6 years [85, 104].

In addition to the location of the lesion and the pattern of cortical representation, the amount of time spent since an acute cerebral insult (usually infarction or trauma) determines the type of language disturbance. The initial difficulty producing and understanding language (global aphasia) often evolves into Broca's aphasia because comprehension of spoken language improves. Anomia may remain as the only language deficit in patients who months previously had a language deficit ranging from Broca's aphasia to transcortical sensory aphasia [61].

PURE AGRAPHIA. Writing disturbances often accompany language deficits and have similar characteristics. However, the degree and type of impairment can differ widely from the patient's performance with oral material. The extreme case, in which the patient writes poorly, even though oral language, reading, and praxis are normal, is termed *pure agraphia*. It has been related to affection of the posterior part of the second frontal gyrus (Exner's area) or of the superior parietal lobule. Lesions of the nondominant hemisphere may cause letter reduplication, slanted lines, and crowding of the words to the right side of the paper [68].

DISTURBANCES OF GOAL-ORIENTED BEHAVIOR. Patients with bilateral lesions affecting the anterior (so-called prefrontal) portion of the frontal lobes and orbitofrontal cortex (areas 9, 10, and 11) have impaired ability to plan their future. Even when they voice their desire to pursue personal endeavors, such as finding a job, they fail to carry out the steps necessary to achieve them. When the damage is restricted to the frontal lobes, these patients may be perfectly well oriented and obtain normal scores in the ordinary battery of cognitive tests. However, they tend to perform poorly on open-ended tasks such as naming items that begin with a particular letter. They tend to manifest perseveration and, when the lesion is greater on the dominant frontal lobe, have sparse language with verbal intrusions, which are segments of speech with little or no relevance to the context that have been picked from external stimuli (such as a sign) or from previous segments of speech.

Disturbances Related to Interhemispheric Disconnection (Callosal Syndrome). Nonsurgical lesions (trauma, infarction, tumor) that destroy the corpus callosum usually involve the medial aspect of the frontal, parietal, or occipital lobes. Thus it becomes difficult to assign any particular clinical deficit to the callosal lesion itself. Knowledge of the deficit that follows upon callosal lesions themselves derives mainly from the study of epileptic patients who underwent section of the corpus callosum and anterior commissure in order to reduce interhemispheric propagation and kindling [40]. The interhemispheric disconnection does not interfere with most activities of daily living but becomes apparent in the failure, by a left-hemispheric-dominant individual, to perform tasks such as the following [14]: (1) Name an object briefly presented to the left hemifield, although the same can be chosen by the left hand from an array of different objects. Lack of visual transfer may also be evident at the bedside by testing the visual fields with the usual confrontation method, which will reveal a "double hemianopia." The patient is asked to point to the moving target first with his left hand (when a right homonymous hemianopia is recorded) and then with his right hand (which fails to point to stimuli in the left hemifield). (2) Imitate with one hand the position of the contralateral hand, which is kept hidden from view. (3) Name objects, kept from view, palpated by the left hand (unilateral anomia). (4) Write with the left hand (unilateral agraphia) or perform with the left hand commands that involve objectless activity, such as "Pretend that you are turning a knob." (5) Copy a somewhat complex design with the right hand, which is clearly outdone in the same task by the performance of the left hand.

Lack of intermanual coordination and even a situation in which the left hand acts independently from the patient's volition (alien hand sign) may result from both callosal and mesial frontal damage [16, 46].

Dementia. Dementia has recently been defined as a loss of intellectual habilities of sufficient severity to interfere with social or occupational functioning [5]. More relevant to the scope of this chapter, dementia refers to deterioration of mental function due to diffuse or disseminated disease of the cerebral hemispheres [101]. Brainstem lesions give rise to weakness, sensory loss, poor coordination, or lethargy, but they are usually unattended by cognitive loss. Bilateral lesions of the medial hypothalamus or thalamus, which are discussed in Chapters 16 and 17, may cause severe memory loss and attentional disorders. The resultant behavior of the patient may be such that the label of *dementia* is applied to his condition. A patient with bilateral frontal disease may have a rather good memory and yet his ability to plan in the future and to stick with a task is so impaired that it interferes seriously with his social or occupational functioning. These two instances exemplify the heterogeneity of the conditions known as dementias as far as cerebral localization is concerned [25a, 71a]. The onset of dementia can be sudden, as when it follows severe head trauma, or insidious, as with Alzheimer's disease. In either case, the demented patient has a clinical presentation that corresponds to *bilateral*, rather extensive, damage of the cerebral cortex, subcortical structures, or, very often, of both.

When the lesions are predominantly *cortical*, the clinical findings depend on the part of the cortex that bears the brunt of the pathology. The entity known as senile dementia of the Alzheimer type (which accounts for about half of the cases of slowly progressive dementias) has an important subcortical component but also tends to affect roughly symmetrical areas of the cortex, resulting in a different topographic predominance in different patients. Because the medial aspect of the temporal lobes is often involved, memory loss becomes obvious in many patients with dementia. Involvement of the lateral aspect of the temporal lobes and of the parietal lobes gives rise to aphasias, visual spatial deficits, and apraxias. When the frontal lobes are primarily affected (as in Pick's disease, in normal aging, and in some cases of Alzheimer's), the patient lacks drive, neglects social nuances, and may have the primitive signs, motor aphasia, and other frontal lobe findings described above. The clinical picture in cortical dementias reflects extensive damage of the association areas [9]. Elementary motor and sensory disturbances, such as limb weakness or loss of position sense, never occur until late in the clinical course.

By contrast, dementias like progressive supranuclear palsy or others with preferential involvement of the subcortical nuclei are often accompanied by abnormalities of movement and overall slowing of psychomotor function, with prominent attentional deficits and forgetfulness. Speech may be dysarthric, but language is normal—that is, aphasia is absent. It has been argued that this type of dementia does not differ neuropsychologically from the cortical dementias [71b]. Memory loss may be the major determinant of social or occupational disability. These patients, with medial thalamic or hypothalamic pathology, are often considered to be "amnesic" rather than "demented."

Depression and other psychiatric disorders may mimic dementia ("pseudo-dementia"). Because their treatment differs from that of dementia, this distinction is important. Some helpful differential findings are listed in Table 19-4.

TABLE 19-4. *Clinical Features Differentiating Pseudo-dementia from Dementia*

Pseudo-dementia	Dementia
CLINICAL COURSE AND HISTORY	
Family aware of dysfunction	Family often unaware of degree of dysfunction
Onset can be dated with some precision	Insidious, onset can dated only within broad limits
Rapid progression of symptoms after onset	Often slow progression
History of previous psychiatric dysfunction common	History of previous psychiatric dysfunction unusual
COMPLAINTS AND CLINICAL BEHAVIOR	
Patients usually complain much of cognitive loss	Patients usually complain little of cognitive loss
Patients emphasize disability	Patients conceal disability
Patients make little effort to perform even simple tasks	Some patients struggle to perform
Patients usually communicate strong sense of distress	Patients often appear unconcerned
Affective change often pervasive	Affect labile and shallow
Behavior often incongruent with severity of cognitive dysfunction	Behavior usually compatible with severity of cognitive dysfunction
Nocturnal accentuation of dysfunction uncommon	Nocturnal accentuation of dysfunction common
"Don't know" answers typical	"Near miss" answers frequent
Memory loss for recent and remote events equally severe	Memory loss for recent events more severe than for remote events

TABLE 19-5. *Consequences of Localized Cerebral Hemispheric Lesions*

I. *Occipital Lobe*
  A. Mesial
    1. Visual field defects
    2. Visual agnosia
    3. Visual hallucinations
    4. Alexia without agraphia
    5. Anton syndrome (denial of blindness)
  B. Lateral
    1. Alexia with agraphia
    2. Impaired opticokinetic nystagmus
    3. Impaired ipsilateral scanning

II. *Temporal Lobe*
  A. Inferomedial aspect
    1. Amnesia (impaired storage)
  B. Anterior tip (bilateral lesions)
    1. Kluver-Bucy syndrome
      a. Visual agnosia
      b. Oral-exploratory behavior
      c. Tameness (amygdala)
      d. Hypersexuality
      e. Hypomotility
  C. Lateroinferior aspect
    1. Dominant hemisphere
      a. Transcortical sensory aphasia
      b. Word selection anomia
    2. Nondominant hemisphere
      a. Impaired recognition of facial emotional expression
  D. Laterosuperior aspect
    1. Dominant hemisphere
      a. Pure word deafness
      b. Sensory aphasia
    2. Nondominant hemisphere
      a. Sensory amusia
      b. Sensory aprosodia
    3. Bilateral lesions
      a. Auditory agnosia
    4. Contralateral superior quadrantic anopsia
  E. Nonlocalizing
    1. Auditory hallucinations
    2. Complex visual hallucinations
  F. With epileptogenic lesions (mainly inferomedial)
    1. Interictal manifestations (1–5 below plus a. or b.)
      (1) Deepening of emotions
      (2) Tendency to trancendentalize minutia (cosmic vision)
      (3) Concern with minor details
        (a) Hypergraphia
        (b) Circumstantiality

TABLE 19-5 (continued)

        (4) Paranoid ideation
        (5) Hyposexuality
     a. Left hemispheric foci
        (1) Ideational aberrations
        (2) Paranoia
        (3) Sense of personal destiny
     b. Right hemispheric foci
        (1) Emotional disturbances (sadness, elation)
        (2) Denial
  2. Ictal manifestations
     a. Hallucinations of smell and taste (amygdala)
     b. Visual delusions (déjà vu, jamais vu)
     c. Experiential delusions (déjà vécu, jamais vécu)
     d. Psychomotor seizures (temporal lobe variety of partial complex
        seizures)

III. *Parietal Lobe*
  A. Postcentral gyrus
    1. Simple somatosensory disturbances
     a. Contralateral sensory loss (object recognition > position
       sense > touch > pain and temperature, vibration)
     b. Contralateral pain, paresthesias
  B. Mesial aspect (cuneus)
    1. Transcortical sensory aphasia? (dominant hemisphere)
  C. Lateral aspect (superior and inferior parietal lobules)
    1. Dominant hemisphere
     a. Parietal apraxia (higher lesions)
     b. Finger agnosia
     c. Right-left disorientation
     d. Literal alexia (supramarginal gyrus)
     e. Alexia with agraphia (angular gyrus)
     f. Conduction aphasia?
    2. Nondominant hemisphere
     a. Anosognosia
     b. Autotopagnosia
     c. Spatial disorientation
     d. Hemispatial neglect
     e. Constructional apraxia
     f. Dressing apraxia

IV. *Frontal Lobe*
  A. Precentral gyrus
    1. Face area (unilateral: transient; bilateral: lasting)
     a. Dysarthria
     b. Dysphagia
    2. Hand area
     a. Contralateral weakness, clumsiness, spasticity
    3. Leg area (paracentral lobule)
     a. Contralateral weakness
     b. Gait apraxia
     c. Urinary incontinence (lasting with bilateral lesions)

TABLE 19-5 (continued)

B. Mesial aspect (F_1, cingulate gyrus)
  1. Akinesia
  2. Perseveration
  3. Hand and foot grasp
  4. "Salutatory" seizures
C. Lateral aspect, premotor region
  1. Middle frontal gyrus (F_2)
     a. Impaired contralateral saccades
     b. Pure agraphia?
  2. F_3, dominant hemisphere
     a. Motor aphasia
D. Frontal pole, orbitofrontal area
  1. Blunted affect
  2. Impaired appreciation of social nuances
  3. Impaired goal-directed behavior
  4. Impotence
  5. Facetiousness

V. *Callosal Lesions*
  1. Lack of kinesthetic transfer
     a. Inability to mimic position of the contralateral hand
     b. Left-hand apraxia?
     c. Left-hand agraphia
     d. Right-hand constructional apraxia
     e. Intermanual conflict (alien left hand)
  2. Perplexity (and confabulation) trying to explain left-hand activity
  3. Double hemianopia

In the preceding pages the emphasis has been placed on the *symptoms* and *signs* that result from hemispheric lesions. Table 19-5 lists the different *regions* of the cerebral hemispheres and the clinical manifestations of lesions in each region.

REFERENCES

1. Adams, J. E., and Rutkin, B. B. Visual responses to subcortical stimulation in the visual and limbic system. *Confin. Neurol.* 32:158, 1970.
2. Ajax, E. T., Schenkenberg, T., and Kosteljanetz, M. Alexia without agraphia and the inferior splenium. *Neurology* 27:685, 1977.
3. Alexander, M. P., and Schmitt, M. A. The aphasia syndrome of stroke in the left anterior cerebral artery territory. *Arch. Neurol.* 37:97, 1980.
4. Allard, T., Woods, B. T., and Hebben, N. Asymmetrical word deafness. *Neurology* 32:A190, 1982.
5. American Psychiatric Association. *Diagnostic and Statistical Manual of Mental Disorders* (3rd ed.). Washington, D.C.: American Psychiatric Association, 1980.

6. Balint, R. Seelenlähmung der "Schauens," optische Ataxie, raümliche Störung der Aufmerksamkeit. *Monatsschr. Psychiat. Neurol.* 25:51, 1909.
7. Benson, D. F. The third alexia. *Arch. Neurol.* 34:327, 1977.
8. Benson, D. F. *Aphasia, Alexia and Agraphia.* New York: Churchill Livingstone, 1979.
9. Benson, D. F. Subcortical Dementia: A Clinical Approach. *In* Mayeux, R., Rosen, W. G. (Eds.). *The Dementias.* New York: Raven Press, 1983. Pp. 185–194.
10. Benson, D. F., and Geschwind, N. The Alexias. *In* Vinken, P. J., and Bruyn, G. W. (Eds.). *Handbook of Clinical Neurology,* Vol. 4. New York: American Elsevier, 1969. Pp. 112–140.
11. Benson, D. F., and Geschwind, N. The Aphasias and Related Disturbances. *In* Baker, A. B., and Baker, L. H. (Eds.). *Clinical Neurology.* Hagerstown, Md.: Harper & Row, 1980.
12. Benton, A. Visuoperceptive, Visuospatial, and Visuoconstructive Disorders. *In* Heilman, K. M., and Valenstein, E. *Clinical Neuropsychology.* New York: Oxford University Press, 1979.
13. Biemond, A. The conduction of pain above the level of the thalamus opticus. *Arch. Neurol. Psychiat.* 75:231, 1956.
14. Bogen, J. E. The Callosal Syndrome. *In* Heilman, K. M., and Valenstein, E. *Clinical Neuropsychology.* New York: Oxford University Press, 1979.
15. Botez, M. I. Two visual systems in clinical neurology: Readaptive role of the primitive system in visual agnostic patients. *Eur. Neurol.* 13:101, 1975.
16. Brinkman, C. Lesions in supplementary motor area interfere with a monkey's performance of a bimanual coordination task. *Neurosci. Lett.* 27:267, 1981.
17. Brodal, A. *Neurological Anatomy in Relation to Clinical Medicine* (3rd ed.). New York: Oxford University Press, 1981.
18. Brodmann, K. *Vergleichende Lokalisationlehre der Grosshirnrinde in ihren prinzipien Dargestellt auf Grund des Zellenbaues.* Leipzig: J.A. Barth, 1909. 1909.
19. Brown, J. W. Language Representation in the Brain. *In* Steklis, H. D., and Raleigh, M. G. (Eds.). *Neurobiology of Social Communication in Primates.* New York: Academic Press, 1979. Pp. 133–195.
20. Bruyn, G. W., and Gathier, J. C. The Operculum Syndrome. *In* Vinken, P. J., and Bruyn, G. W. (Eds.). *Handbook of Clinical Neurology.* Vol. 2, *Localization in Clinical Neurology.* New York: American Elsevier, 1969.
21. Buge, A., et al. Mutisme akinétique, et ramollissement bicingulaire. Trois observations anatomocliniques. *Rev. Neurol.* 131:121, 1975.
22. Butters, N. Amnesic Disorders. *In* Heilman, K. M., and Valenstein, E. *Clinical Neuropsychology.* New York: Oxford University Press, 1979.
23. Caplan, L. R. "Top of the basilar" syndrome. *Neurology* 30:72, 1980.
24. Cappa, S. F., and Vignolo, L. A. "Transcortical" features of aphasia following left thalamic hemorrhage. *Cortex* 15:121, 1979.
25. Carpenter, M. B. *Human Neuroanatomy* (7th ed.). Baltimore: The Williams & Wilkins Co., 1976. Pp. 21–36, 547–599.
25a. Cummings, J. L., and Benson, D. F. *Dementia: A Clinical Approach.* Boston: Butterworth, 1983.
26. Damasio, A. R., and Benton, A. L. Impairment of hand movements under visual guidance. *Neurology* 29:170, 1979.

27. Damasio, A. R., and Damasio, H. The anatomic basis of pure alexia. *Neurology* (Cleveland) 33:1573, 1983.
28. Damasio, A. R., Damasio, H., and Chui, H. C. Neglect following damage to frontal lobe or basal ganglia. *Neuropsychologia* 18:123, 1980.
29. Damasio, A. R., Damasio, H., and Van Hoesen, G. W. Prosopagnosia: Anatomic basis and behavioral mechanisms. *Neurology* 32:331, 1982.
30. Damasio, H., and Damasio, A. R. The anatomical basis of conduction aphasia. *Brain* 103:337, 1980.
31. Davis, A. E., and Wada, J. A. Speech dominance and handedness in the normal human. *Brain Lang.* 5:42, 1978.
31a. Dawson, R. G. Recovery of function: Implications for theory of brain function. *Behav. Biol.* 8:439, 1973.
32. Dejerine, J. *Sémiologie des Affections du Système Nerveux.* Paris: Masson et Cie, 1926.
33. DeKosky, S., et al. Recognition and discrimination of emotional faces and pictures. *Brain Lang.* 9:206, 1980.
34. Von Economo, C. F. *The Cytoarchitectonics of the Human Cerebral Cortex.* London: Oxford Medical Publications, 1929.
35. Falzi, G., Perrone, P., and Vignolo, L. A. Right-left asymmetry in anterior speech region. *Arch. Neurol.* 39:239, 1982.
35a. Finger, S., and Stein, D. G. *Brain Damage and Recovery.* New York: Academic Press, 1982.
36. Fisher, C. M. Disorientation for place. *Arch. Neurol.* 39:33, 1982.
37. Galaburda, A. M. La règion de Broca: Observations anatomiques faites un siècle après la mort de son découvreur. *Rev. Neurol.* 136:609, 1980.
38. Gassel, M. M., and Williams, D. Visual function in patients with homonymous hemianopia. Part III. The completion phenomenon; insight and attitude to the defect; and visual functional efficiency. *Brain* 86:229, 1963.
39. Gates, A., and Bradshaw, J. L. The role of the cerebral hemispheres in music. *Brain Lang.* 4:403, 1977.
40. Gazzaniga, M. S., LeDoux, J. E., and Wilson, D. H. Language, praxis, and the right hemisphere: clues to mechanisms of consciousness. *Neurology* (Minn.) 27:1144, 1977.
41. Gerstmann, J. Some notes on the Gerstmann syndrome. *Neurology* (Minn.) 7:866, 1957.
42. Geschwind, N. Disconnexion syndromes in animals and man. *Brain* 88:237, 585, 1965.
43. Geschwind, N., and Kaplan, E. A human cerebral disconnection syndrome. *Neurology* (Minn.) 12:675, 1962.
44. Geschwind, N., and Fusillo, M. Color-naming defects in association with alexia. *Arch. Neurol.* 15:137, 1966.
45. Geschwind, N., and Levitsky, W. Human brain: Left-right asymmetries in temporal speech region. *Science* 161:186, 1968.
46. Goldberg, G., Mayer, N. H., and Toglia, J. U. Medial frontal cortex infarction and the alien hand sign. *Arch. Neurol.* 38:683, 1981.
47. Hécaen, T., and de Ajuriaguerra, J. Balint's syndrome (psychic paralysis of visual fixation) and its minor forms. *Brain* 77:373, 1954.
48. Hécaen, H., and Albert, M. L. *Human Neuropsychology.* New York: John Wiley & Sons, 1978. Pp. 144–166.
49. Hécaen, H., and Consoli, S. Analyse des troubles du language au cours des lésions de l'aire de Broca. *Neuropsychologia* 11:377, 1973.

50. Hécaen, H., and Ropert, R. Hallucinations auditives au cours de syndromes neurologiques. *Ann. Med. Psychol.* 117:257, 1959.
51. Heilman, K. M. Neglect and Related Disorders. *In* Heilman, K. M., and Valenstein, E. *Clinical Neuropsychology.* New York: Oxford University Press, 1979.
52. Heilman, K. M., et al. Wernicke's and global aphasia without alexia. *Arch. Neurol.* 36:129, 1979.
53. Heilman, K. M., Rothi, L. J., and Valenstein, E. Two forms of ideomotor apraxia. *Neurology* 32:342, 1982.
54. Heilman, K. M., and Valenstein, E. Mechanisms underlying hemispatial neglect. *Ann. Neurol.* 5:166, 1979.
55. Heimburger, R. F., Demyer, W., and Reitan, R. M. Implications of Gerstmann's syndrome. *J. Neurol. Neurosurg. Psychiat.* 27:52, 1964.
56. Hernández-Peón, R. Neurophysiologic Aspects of Attention. *In* Vinken, P. J., and Bruyn, G. W. (Eds.). *Handbook of Clinical Neurology.* Vol. 3, *Disorders of Higher Nervous Activity.* New York: American Elsevier, 1969.
57. Horel, J. A. The neuroanatomy of amnesia. A critique of the hippocampal memory hypothesis. *Brain* 101:403, 1978.
58. Jacobs, L. Visual allesthesia. *Neurology* 30:1059, 1980.
59. Jacobs, L., and Gossman, M. D. Three primitive reflexes in normal adults. *Neurology* 30:184, 1980.
60. Jonas, S. The supplementary motor region and speech emission. *J. Commun. Disord.* 14:349, 1981.
60a. Kertesz, A. (Ed.). *Localization in Neuropsychology.* New York: Academic Press, 1983.
61. Kertesz, A., and McCabe, P. Recovery patterns and prognosis in aphasia. *Brain* 100:1, 1977.
62. Kirshner, H. S., and Webb, W. G. Word and letter reading and the mechanism of the third alexia. *Arch. Neurol.* 39:84, 1982.
63. Knight, R. T. Decreased response to novel stimuli after prefrontal lesions in man. *Electroencephal. Clin. Neurophysiol.* 59:9, 1984.
64. LeCours, A. R., and Lhermitte, F. The "pure form" of the phonetic disintegration syndrome (pure anarthria); anatomo-clinical report of a historical case. *Brain Lang.* 3:88, 1976.
65. Levin, H. S. Historical Background and Classification of the Acalculias. *In* Heilman, K. M., and Valenstein, E. *Clinical Neuropsychology.* New York: Oxford University Press, 1979.
66. Liepmann, H. Motor aphasia and apraxia. (Transl. by G. H. Eggert.) *Aphasia Apraxia Agnosia* 1:53, 1979.
67. Liepmann, H., and Maas, O. Fall von linksseitiger Agraphie und Apraxie bei rechtsseitiger Lähmung. *J. Psychol. Neurol.* 10:214, 1907.
68. Marcie, P., and Hecaen, H. Agraphia: Writing Disorders Associated with Unilateral Cortical Lesions. *In* Heilman, K. M., and Valenstein, E. *Clinical Neuropsychology.* New York: Oxford University Press, 1979.
69. Masdeu, J. C., and O'Hara, R. J. Motor aphasia unaccompanied by faciobrachial weakness. *Neurology* (N.Y.) 33:519, 1983.
70. Masdeu, J. C., Schoene, W. C., and Funkenstein, H. Aphasia following infarction of the left supplementary motor area. A clinico-pathologic study. *Neurology* 28:1220, 1978.
71. Masdeu, J., and Shewmon, A. Left parietal lobe and receptive language functions. *Neurology* (N.Y.) 30:1137, 1980.

71a. Mayeux, R., and Rosen, W. G. *The Dementias*. New York: Raven Press, 1983.
71b. Mayeux, R., et al. Is "subcortical dementia" a recognizable clinical entity? *Ann. Neurol.* 14:278, 1983.
72. Medina, J., Rubino, F., and Ross, E. Agitated delirium caused by infarction of the hippocampal formation and fusiform and lingual gyri. *Neurology* (Minn.) 24:1181, 1974.
73. Mesulam, M. M. Acute behavioral derangements without hemiplegia in cerebrovascular accidents. *Primary Care* 6:813, 1979.
74. Meyer, J. S., and Barron, D. W. Apraxia of gait: A clinico-physiological study. *Brain* 82:261, 1960.
75. Mohr, J. P. Broca's Area and Broca's Aphasia. *In* Whitaker, H., and Whitaker, H. A. (Eds.). *Studies in Neurolinguistics*. New York: Academic Press, 1976. Pp. 201–235.
76. Mohr, J. P., et al. Broca aphasia: Pathologic and clinical. *Neurology* 28:311, 1978.
77. Ojemann, G., and Mateer, C. Human language cortex: Localization of memory, syntax, and sequential motor-phoneme identification systems. *Science* 205:1401, 1979.
78. Ojemann, G. A., and Whitaker, H. A. Language localization and variability. *Brain Lang.* 6:239, 1978.
79. Oppenheimer, D. R., and Newcombe, D. M. F. Clinical and anatomic findings in a case of auditory agnosia. *Arch. Neurol.* 35:712, 1978.
80. Pandya, D. N., and Seltzer, B. Intrinsic connections and architectonics of posterior parietal cortex in the rhesus monkey. *J. Comp. Neurol.* 204:196, 1982.
81. Penfield, W., and Jasper, H. Epilepsy and the Functional Anatomy of the Human Brain. Boston: Little, Brown, 1954.
82. Penfield, W., and Mathieson, G. Memory. Autopsy findings and comments on the role of hippocamus in experiential recall. *Arch. Neurol.* 31:145, 1974.
83. Penfield, W., and Perot, P. The brain's record of auditory and visual experience. *Brain* 86:595, 1963.
84. Poeck, K. Pathophysiology of Emotional Disorders Associated with Brain Damage. *In* Vinken, P. J., and Bruyn, G. W. (Eds.). *Handbook of Clinical Neurology*. Vol. 3, *Disorders of Higher Nervous Activity*. New York: American Elsevier, 1969.
85. Rasmussen, T., and Milner, B. The role of early left-brain injury in determining lateralization of cerebral speech functions. *Ann. N.Y. Acad. Sci.* 299:355, 1977.
86. Rockel, A. J., Hiorns, R. W., and Powell, T. P. S. The basic uniformity in structure of the neocortex. *Brain* 103:221, 1980.
87. Roland, P. E. Astereognosis. *Arch. Neurol.* 33:543, 1976.
88. Ross, E. D. Left medial parietal lobe and receptive language functions: Mixed transcortical aphasia after left anterior cerebral artery infarction. *Neurology* 30:144, 1980.
89. Ross, E. D. The aprosodias. Functional-anatomic organization of the affective components of language in the right hemisphere. *Arch. Neurol.* 38:561, 1981.
90. Rothi, L. J., McFarling, D., and Heilman, K. M. Conduction aphasia, syntactic alexia, and the anatomy of syntactic comprehension. *Arch. Neurol.* 39:272, 1982.

91. Rubens, A. B. Agnosia. *In* Heilman, K. M., and Valenstein, E. *Clinical Neuropsychology.* New York: Oxford University Press, 1979.
92. Sackeim, H. A., et al. Hemispheric asymmetry in the expression of positive and negative emotions. Neurologic evidence. *Arch. Neurol.* 39:210, 1982.
93. Schacter, S. The Interaction of Cognitive and Physiological Determinants of Emotional State. *In* Berkowitz, L. (Ed.). *Advances in Experimental Social Psychology.* Vol. 1. New York: Academic Press, 1970.
94. Sherwin, I., et al. Prevalence of psychosis in epilepsy as a function of the laterality of the epileptogenic lesion. *Arch. Neurol.* 39:621, 1982.
95. Swanson, L. W., and Cowan, W. M. An autoradiographic study of the organization of the efferent connections of the hippocampal formation in the rat. *J. Comp. Neurol.* 172:49, 1977.
96. Torch, W. C., Hirano, A., and Solomon, S. Anterograde transneuronal degeneration in the limbic system: Clinical-anatomic correlation. *Neurology* 27:1157, 1977.
97. Tweedy, J., et al. Significance of cortical disinhibition signs. *Neurology* (N.Y.) 32:169, 1982.
98. Valenstein, E., and Heilman, K. M. Emotional Disorders Resulting from Lesions of the Central Nervous System. *In* Heilman, K. M., and Valenstein, E. *Clinical Neuropsychology.* New York: Oxford University Press, 1979.
99. Volpe, B. T., et al. Cortical mechanisms involved in praxis: Observations following partial and complete section of the corpus callosum in man. *Neurology* (N.Y.) 32:645, 1982.
100. Weinberger, D. R., et al. Asymmetrical volumes of the right and left frontal and occipital regions of the human brain. *Ann. Neurol.* 11:97, 1982.
101. Wells, C. E. *Dementia.* (2nd ed.) Philadelphia: F.A. Davis, 1977.
102. Wells, C. E. Pseudodementia. *Am. J. Psychiat.* 136:895, 1979.
103. Woods, B. T., Schoene, W., and Kneisely, L. Are hippocampal lesions sufficient to produce lasting amnesia? *Neurology* 29:587, 1979.
104. Woods, B. T., and Teuber, H. L. Changing patterns of childhood aphasia. *Ann. Neurol.* 3:273, 1980.
105. Zola-Morgan, S., Squire, L. R., and Mishkin, M. The neuroanatomy of amnesia: Amygdala-hippocampus versus temporal stem. *Science* 218:1337, 1982.

Chapter 20

VASCULAR SYNDROMES
OF THE CEREBRUM

José Biller

VASCULAR SUPPLY
OF THE CEREBRAL HEMISPHERES

Anatomically, the aortic arch gives rise to three major vessels: the *brachiocephalic,* the *left common carotid,* and *the left subclavian arteries* [58]. The brachiocephalic in turn gives rise to the *right subclavian* and the *right common carotid arteries.* The two common carotid arteries run upward lateral to the trachea to approximately the level of the fourth cervical vertebra, where each bifurcates into the *external* and *internal carotid arteries.* The *two vertebral arteries* arise from their respective subclavian arteries medial to the anterior scalene muscle and join to form the *basilar artery.* The basilar artery runs rostrally on the ventral surface of the pons and bifurcates into its two terminal branches, the right and left *posterior cerebral arteries,* at the level of the interpeduncular cistern. The blood supply of the upper spinal cord, brainstem, cerebellum, and posterior cerebrum originates from the vertebral-basilar system. The carotid and vertebral artery systems join at the base of the brain to form the circle of Willis.

The Internal Carotid Artery. The internal carotid artery (ICA) may be divided into three main segments: *cervical, petrosal, and intracranial.* The *cervical segment* of the ICA has no branches. It ascends vertically in the neck, extending from the common carotid bifurcation to the base of the skull. It then enters the base of the skull through the carotid canal in the petrous portion of the temporal bone. The artery crosses the foramen lacerum and enters the cavernous sinus. The *petrosal segment* gives off a caroticotympanic branch and sometimes a pterygoid branch. The *intracranial segment* begins distal to the petrous segment and proximal to the anterior clinoid process. A presellar and juxtasellar portion of this vessel are distinguished. The juxtasellar portion lies within the cavernous sinus in close proximity to the oculomotor, trochlear, and abducens nerves (cranial nerves III, IV, and VI) and the ophthalmic and maxillary divisions of the trigeminal nerve (cranial nerve V). Meningohypophyseal branches arise from the presellar and juxtasellar portions to supply the adjacent meninges and posterior lobe of the hypophysis. The ICA then pierces the dura mater medial to the anterior clinoid process, where it becomes supraclinoid. The *ophthalmic artery,* the first major branch of the ICA, arises at the level of the anterior clinoid process. This vessel runs initially intracranially, then traverses the optic canal en route to the orbit. The ophthalmic artery gives off orbital, extraorbital, and ocular branches; the most important of the ocular branches is the *central retinal artery.* Other ocular branches include the long and short posterior ciliary arteries and the anterior ciliary arteries. Rich anastomoses exist between the ophthalmic and the external carotid artery branches.

After giving off the ophthalmic branch, the internal carotid artery gives rise to the *posterior communicating artery* and then to the *anterior choroidal artery*. The posterior communicating artery joins the posterior cerebral artery to form the posterolateral portion of the circle of Willis. The posterior communicating arteries may be large or threadlike and provide a link between the anterior and posterior circulations and between the two cerebral hemispheres. Penetrating branches from the posterior communicating artery supply the anterior and posterior hypothalamus, the optic tract and posterior portion of the optic chiasm, and the anterior and ventral thalamic nuclei. The *anterior choroidal artery* passes posterolaterally to reach the optic tract and supplies the choroid plexus of the temporal horn, the hippocampus and dentate gyri, the amygdaloid nucleus, the piriform cortex and uncus of the temporal lobe, the lateral geniculate body, the optic tract and origin of the optic radiations, the genu and inferior and medial parts of the posterior limb of the internal capsule, the basal ganglia, and the upper brainstem.

After giving off the anterior choroidal artery, the ICA then bifurcates to form the *anterior cerebral* and *middle cerebral arteries*.

The Anterior Cerebral Artery. The anterior cerebral artery (ACA) arises below the anterior perforated substance and runs anteromedially to the interhemispheric fissure, where it joins the opposite ACA by way of the *anterior communicating artery*, closing the rostral portion of the circle of Willis. The ACA supplies the medial surface of the cerebrum and the upper border of the frontal and parietal lobes [5]. It gives origin to (1) *medial lenticular branches*, (2) *pericallosal branches* to the corpus callosum, and (3) *hemispheric branches*. The *medial lenticular branches* include basal branches, which supply the dorsal apect of the optic chiasm and hypothalamus, and the medial striate artery (recurrent artery of Heubner), which supplies blood to the anteroinferior limb of the internal capsule and the anterior aspects of the putamen and caudate nuclei. The callosal branches arise from the *pericallosal artery*, which is that portion of the ACA distal to the anterior communicating artery. Others reserve the term *pericallosal artery* for the segment beyond the origin of the callosomarginal artery. The ACA and the pericallosal arteries also supply the septum pellucidum and the fornix. The *hemispheric branches* supply the medial surface of the hemisphere and include the orbitofrontal, frontopolar, internal frontal (anterior, middle, and posterior), paracentral, and internal parietal (superior and inferior) branches.

The Middle Cerebral Artery. The middle cerebral artery (MCA), the largest branch of the ICA, arises below the medial part of the anterior perforated substance. It supplies most of the lateral surface of the cerebral hemisphere and the deep structures of the frontal and parietal lobes

[49]. Three segments of the MCA are recognized: *proximal, Sylvian,* and *distal.* From the posterosuperior aspect of the *proximal segment* arise the lenticulostriate arteries, which nourish the adjacent corona radiata, external capsule, claustrum, putamen, part of the globus pallidus, body of the caudate nucleus, and superior portion of the anterior and posterior limbs of the internal capsule. Other branches that may arise from the horizontal segment are the orbitofrontal and the anterior temporal arteries, but many variations occur. The *Sylvian segment* consists of all the branches on the insula of Reil and in the Sylvian fissure. Shortly after the take-off of the anterior temporal artery, the main trunk of the MCA bifurcates, one branch giving rise to the *anterior or proximal group* of arteries and the other branch giving rise to the *posterior or distal group.* The *anterior group* includes the orbitofrontal, precentral, central, and anterior parietal arteries. The *posterior group* includes the posterior parietal, posterior temporal, and the angular or terminal arteries.

The Posterior Cerebral Artery. The posterior cerebral arteries (PCA) are the terminal branches of the basilar artery. They arise from the rostral end of the basilar artery within the interpeduncular cistern and supply the occipital lobes and the inferomedial portions of the temporal lobes. Numerous other branches supply the mesencephalon, thalamus, and other structures. The branches of the PCA have been divided into three groups [29]: (1) the *penetrating arteries* to the brainstem, thalamus, and other deep structures, (2) the *dorsal callosal artery,* and (3) the *cortical branches.* From the origin of the PCA (as it surrounds the midbrain) numerous *perforating branches* are given off. Mesencephalic branches include the interpeduncular perforators and the short and long circumferencial arteries. The arterial supply to the anterior thalamus arises from the posterior communicating arteries, whereas the medial ventral thalamus receives blood from the thalamoperforators. The lateral ventral thalamus is supplied by the thalamogeniculate branches, and the posterior and superior thalamus is supplied by the posterior choroidal branches. Other branches from this group include the hippocampal branches that supply the hippocampal formation, fornices, and the psalterium. The dorsal callosal artery or splenial branch anatomoses with distal branches of the anterior cerebral artery. The PCA has four main cortical branches: the anterior temporal, posterior temporal, parietoccipital, and calcarine arteries.

Collateral Circulation. There are three main sources of collateral circulation to the brain: (1) the circle of Willis, which connects the internal carotid and vertebrobasilar arterial systems with each other; (2) anastomoses between branches of the extracranial and intracranial arteries;

and (3) leptomeningeal anastomoses between the terminal branches of the major arteries of the cerebrum and cerebellum [2]. Unusual carotid-basilar anastomoses may occur, such as a persistent trigeminal artery, a persistent otic artery, or a persistent hypoglossal artery [6]. A persistent trigeminal artery [18] is the most frequent of the three and may maintain significant collateral flow.

SYNDROMES OF THE CEREBRAL ARTERIES

A *stroke* indicates the relatively abrupt onset of a focal neurologic deficit resulting from disease of the arteries or veins that serve the central nervous system. However, the etiologic factors that may give rise to a stroke are multiple. The key word is *focal*, whether the deficit is transient or permanent, static or progressive, and whether the lesion is located in the cerebral cortex, subcortical areas, brainstem, or cerebellum. The neurologic deficit reflects the location and size of the lesion. Cerebrovascular disease may take the form of an infarct or a hemorrhage. An infarct may be pale, hemorrhagic, or mixed and is usually due to either thrombosis from atherosclerotic lesions or embolism from the heart or extracranial vasculature. Hemorrhage may be subarachnoid, intraparenchymal, or intraventricular, and may have various etiologies including arterial hypertension, saccular aneurysms, arteriovenous malformations, blood dyscrasias, vasculitis, drugs, trauma, or neoplasms.

More than 50 percent of strokes can be attributed to a thrombotic mechanism involving the extracranial or intracranial vessels. Lacunar infarction related to arterial hypertension affecting the small penetrating vessels of the basal ganglia or brainstem accounts for approximately 20 percent of all strokes. Embolism is responsible for about 30 percent of strokes. Intracerebral hemorrhage comprises about 10 percent of all strokes, and subarachnoid hemorrhage accounts for about another 6 percent [47, 54]. Cerebral embolism involves predominantly the MCA, followed by the PCA territory; the ACA and basilar artery are involved less frequently. In addition to extracranial occlusive cerebrovascular disease, sources of cerebral embolism include recent myocardial infarction with a mural thrombus, atrial fibrillation and other arrhythmias, valvular heart disease, prosthetic heart valves, mitral valve prolapse, congenital heart disease, prosthetic heart valves, cardiac tumors, and infective and marantic endocarditis.

The following temporal patterns of the stroke syndrome are recognized: *transient ischemic attacks, "completed" stroke,* and *stroke in evolution.*

Transient Ischemic Attacks (TIAs). TIAs are defined as sudden episodes of focal, nonconvulsive neurologic dysfunction that completely resolve within 24 hours. They are thought to be vascular in etiology and commonly last 2 to 15 minutes [59]. To qualify as a TIA, the episode should be followed by a *complete* recovery, and no neurologic residua should be detected after 24 hours. TIAs involving the anterior or carotid circulation should be separated from those involving the posterior or vertebrobasilar circulation, although such a distinction is not always feasible [43]. The following symptoms are considered typical of TIAs in the carotid system: ipsilateral amaurosis fugax, contralateral motor or sensory dysfunction limited to one side of the body, aphasia, contralateral homonymous hemianopia, or any combination of these. The following symptoms represent typical TIAs in the vertebrobasilar system: bilateral or shifting motor or sensory dysfunction, complete or partial loss of vision in both homonymous fields (bilateral homonymous hemianopia), or any combination of these. Isolated diplopia, dysphagia, dysarthria, or vertigo should not be considered a TIA when it occurs alone. However, in combination with one another or with any of the other symptoms just listed, they should be considered as vertebrobasilar TIAs.

"Completed" Stroke. A completed stroke is the term applied to the temporal profile of the stroke syndrome in which the deficit is prolonged and often permanent. Most completed strokes reach the maximum of neurologic dysfunction within an hour of onset [10].

Stroke in Evolution. This term describes the temporal profile in which the neurologic deficit occurs in a stepwise or progressive fashion, culminating in a major deficit in the absence of treatment. Should the site of ischemia be the carotid arterial distribution, 24 hours without progression is enough time to establish that further progression is unlikely. However, if the site of ischemia is the vertebrobasilar arterial system, the deficit may progress for up to 72 hours [44].

The Carotid Artery Syndrome. The only feature distinguishing the carotid syndrome from the middle cerebral artery syndrome is amaurosis fugax or transient monocular blindness [19, 48]. The patient with amaurosis fugax often describes the sudden onset of loss of vision either as a "curtain" or "shade" effect that progresses from the top, the bottom, or the sides of the visual fields, or as an iris diaphragm [20, 33, 52, 53]. The former presentation is most likely embolic, whereas the latter is most probably related to hypotension causing diminished blood flow to the eye. The episode usually lasts 2 to 10 minutes. During attacks there is an amaurotic pupil and collapse of the retinal vessels. Ophthalmoscopy may disclose three main types of retinal microemboli (Table 20-1) [34].

Patients with carotid artery occlusive disease may present with recur-

TABLE 20-1. *Microemboli in Carotid Artery Syndrome*

Microemboli	Appearance	Vessel Occlusion	Origin	Composition
White plug	White, nonrefractile	Often	Carotid thrombus	Fibrin platelets
Bright plaque (Hollenhorst)	Bright, glistening, refractile	Rarely	Eroded atheroma	Cholesterol crystals
Calcific emboli	Refractile, larger than bright plaques	Yes	Heart valve or calcified plaque	Calcium

rent TIAs, an apoplectic or stepwise onset, or a slowly progressive neurologic deficit (pseudotumoral form) [21]. Occlusion of the ICA in the neck may be totally asymptomatic in the presence of adequate collateral circulation, particularly if the occlusion develops slowly. Infarction of the homolateral hemisphere may occur when the collateral circulation is inadequate. According to location, infarcts may involve the entire territory of the MCA (total), the areas of supply nearest the ICA or MCA (proximal), the border zone between the ACA and MCA (watershed), or only the white matter supplied by peripheral branches of the MCA (terminal). Patients may initially complain of localized or generalized headaches, and focal seizures may occur. Contralateral hemiplegia, hemianesthesia, homonymous hemianopia, and aphasia (if the dominant hemisphere is compromised) or apractagnosia (if the nondominant hemisphere is involved) may ensue. The association of amaurosis fugax with contralateral hemiplegia is rarely seen. Careful examination may reveal an ipsilateral partial Horner syndrome, usually transient, which is due to compromise of the sympathetic fibers coursing along the ICA. Ipsilateral optic atrophy seldom occurs. The neurovascular examination may disclose a well-localized bruit in the midcervical area. If it extends throughout systole, it indicates stenosis of at least 50 percent; if the bruit goes through systole and enters diastole, it indicates a 90 percent or greater stenosis of the carotid vessel. The bruit may disappear when the stenosis is greater than 90 percent, and therefore the absence of a bruit has little diagnostic value. A thrill may be felt over a partially occluded vessel. Lowering of retinal artery pressures in the ipsilateral eye may be noted by ophthalmodynamometry.

The Anterior Cerebral Artery Syndrome. This syndrome will vary according to the point at which occlusion occurs. The extent of signs also depends upon the patency of the collateral circulation [13].

The syndrome of infarction in the ACA territory *(hemispheric branches)* consists of the following signs:

1. Contralateral weakness affecting primarily the lower extremity and to a lesser extent the arm
2. Contralateral sensory loss affecting primarily the lower extremity
3. Disorders of sphincter control
4. Gait and postural disorders
5. Paratonia and abnormal reflexes (grasp, rooting, snout, sucking)
6. Loss of initiative and spontaneity with "adynamia"
7. Transcortical motor aphasia with unilateral left-sided lesions
8. Memory and emotional disturbances
9. Akinetic mutism with bilateral mesiofrontal involvement

Infarction in the territory supplied by the *artery of Heubner (medial striate artery)* results in contralateral face and arm weakness without sensory loss. Infarction of the *basal branches* is characterized by transient memory disorders, anxiety, and agitation. Finally, occlusion of the *pericallosal branches* is characterized by apraxia, agraphia, and tactile anomia of the left hand.

The Middle Cerebral Artery Syndrome. The clinical picture will vary according to the site of occlusion and the availability of collateral circulation. Partial or complete syndromes may occur. Infarction in the distribution of the MCA is characterized by the following [3, 7, 41, 61]:

1. Contralateral hemiplegia affecting the face, the arm, and to a lesser extent the leg
2. Contralateral hemianesthesia involving the face, the arm, and to a lesser extent the leg (touch, pain, temperature, proprioception, vibration, two-point discrimination, stereognosis, and tactile inattention)
3. Nonrepetitive aphasias if the dominant hemisphere for language is involved
4. Contralateral homonymous inferior quadrantanopia or homonymous hemianopia
5. Gerstmann's syndrome (finger agnosia, acalculia, right-left disorientation, pure dysgraphia)
6. Alexia with agraphia (left angular gyrus lesion)
7. Inattention, neglect, denial, and apractic syndromes (mainly with nondominant hemispheric lesions)
8. Paresis and apraxia of conjugate gaze to the opposite side, with transient tonic deviation of the eyes and head toward the side of the lesion

The Posterior Cerebral Artery Syndrome. The clinical picture varies according to the site of the occlusion and the availability of collaterals. Partial syndromes are the rule. Infarction in the distribution of the *hemispheric branches* of the PCA may produce [1, 4, 12, 28, 40]

1. Contralateral homonymous hemianopia with occasional macular sparing
2. Bilateral homonymous hemianopia
3. Cerebral blindness characterized by visual loss in both eyes in the presence of normal pupillary reactivity and funduscopic appearances (with bilateral lesions)
4. Anton syndrome, or denial of blindness (with bilateral lesions extending to the parietal lobe)
5. Visual and color agnosias

6. Agnosia for familiar faces or prosopagnosia (usually with bilateral lesions)
7. Apraxia of ocular movements (bilateral lesions)
8. Acute onset of agitated delirium (bilateral mesiotemporooccipital lesions)
9. Acute amnestic syndrome (bilateral mesiotemporal lesions)
10. Elementary visual hallucinations
11. Balint syndrome, sometimes characterized by optic ataxia, psychic paralysis of fixation with inability to look to the peripheral field and disturbance of visual attention (bilateral lesions)

Infarction in the distribution of the *callosal branches* affecting the left occipital region and splenium of the corpus callosum produces the syndrome of alexia without agraphia (agnosic alexia). Infarction of the distribution of the *penetrating branches to the thalamus* can produce

1. *Dejerine and Roussy's syndrome (thalamic syndrome)*, characterized by contralateral sensory loss to all modalities, transient contralateral hemiparesis, severe dysesthesias in the affected side (thalamic pain), vasomotor disturbances, and choreoathetoid or hemiballistic movements. (Ventral posterolateral and ventral postero-medial nuclei are affected.)
2. Aphasia (left pulvinar nuclei affected)
3. Amnesia (mesial thalamoperforators affected)
4. Akinetic mutism

Infarction in the distribution of the *penetrating branches to the midbrain* may be characterized by [12, 45]:

1. Ipsilateral oculomotor palsy with contralateral cerebellar ataxia *(Nothnagel syndrome)*
2. Ipsilateral oculomotor palsy with contralateral hemiplegia *(Weber syndrome)*
3. Ipsilateral oculomotor palsy with contralateral ataxia and hemichoreoathetosis *(Benedikt syndrome)*
4. Nuclear oculomotor palsy (rare), characterized by (a) unilateral oculomotor palsy with contralateral superior rectus and bilateral partial ptosis, or (b) bilateral oculomotor palsies with sparing of the levator
5. Unilateral or bilateral internuclear ophthalmoplegia *(INO)*
6. Wall eyes bilateral internuclear ophthalmoplegia *(WEBINO syndrome)*
7. Dorsal rostral midbrain syndrome *(Parinaud)*, characterized by (a) supranuclear paralysis of elevation, (b) defective convergence, (c) con-

vergence-retraction nystagmus, (d) light-near dissociation, (e) Collier's sign (lid retraction), (f) skew deviation

8. Pseudoabducens palsy
9. Midbrain corectopia
10. Peduncular hallucinations, usually silent, mobile, and colorful and frequently pleasurable
11. Decerebrate rigidity
12. Locked-in syndrome (bilateral)
13. Disturbances of consciousness

LACUNAR INFARCTS

Lacunes are small ischemic infarcts that range in diameter from 0.5 to 15 mm and result from occlusion of the penetrating arteries, chiefly from the anterior choroidal, middle cerebral, posterior cerebral, or basilar arteries. Lacunes usually occur in patients with longstanding arterial hypertension and evidence of cerebral atherosclerosis [24, 42, 46]. The most frequent sites of involvement are the putamen, basis pontis, thalamus, posterior limb of the internal capsule, and caudate nucleus, in that order. However, they may also occur in the anterior limb of the internal capsule, subcortical cerebral white matter, cerebellar white matter, and corpus callosum. Although they generally carry a good prognosis, multiple lacunes may lead to pseudo-bulbar palsy or dementing states. Shortly before onset of a lacunar stroke, transient ischemic attacks may occur. Associated headaches are infrequent.

The four best recognized clinical syndromes related to lacunar strokes can be described as follows:

1. *Pure motor hemiparesis* is due to an internal capsule or basis pontis lacune and is characterized by a unilateral motor deficit involving the face, arm, and to a lesser extent, the leg. There should be no aphasia or apractagnosia, and there are no sensory, visual, or higher cortical disturbances.
2. *Pure sensory stroke,* also known as pure paresthetic stroke, is due to a lacune involving the ventral lateral nucleus of the thalamus. It is characterized by numbness, paresthesias, and a unilateral hemisensory deficit involving the face, arm, trunk, and leg. Subjective symptoms often predominate over objective findings in this syndrome.
3. *Homolateral ataxia and crural paresis (ataxic hemiparesis)* is due to a lacune affecting either the contralateral posterior limb of the internal capsule or the contralateral basis pontis. It is characterized by weakness, predominantly in the lower extremity, and ipsilateral incoordination of the arm and leg. There is usually an extensor plantar response and no dysarthria or facial involvement.

4. *Dysarthria—clumsy hand syndrome* is due to a lacune involving the depth of the basis pontis and is characterized by supranuclear facial weakness, deviation of the protruded tongue, dysarthria, and a loss of fine motor control of the hand.

CEREBRAL HEMORRHAGE SYNDROMES

Arterial hypertension is the most common cause of spontaneous hemorrhage into the brain parenchyma. Because the pathogenesis is not clearly understood, the term *primary* may be used to distinguish this type of bleeding from bleeding secondary to known causes such as aneurysms, arteriovenous malformations, or bleeding diatheses. The hemorrhage arises mainly in the arterial territories of the lenticulostriate, thalamoperforators, and paramedial branches of the basilar artery [11, 23, 39].

Other etiologic factors of nontraumatic intracerebral hemorrhage include primary or metastatic brain tumors, vasculitis, cortical vein or dural sinus thrombosis, and congophilic angiopathy.

The relative frequency of intracerebral hemorrhages by location is as follows: putamen, 55%; thalamus, 20-30%; cerebellum, 10%; subcortical white matter, 10%; and pons, 5-7.5%.

The clinical manifestations of spontaneous intracerebellar hemorrhage depend on the location, size, direction of spread, and rate of development of the bleeding [22].

General Features of the Clinical Syndrome

HISTORY

1. The onset is usually sudden but may be gradual.
2. Headache is present in about half of the patients.
3. Vomiting occurs in slightly more than half.
4. Seizures rarely occur.
5. Prodromal attacks are unusual.
6. There is a previous history of arterial hypertension in about 80 to 90 percent.
7. The level of alertness may be variable.

EXAMINATION. A syndrome of meningeal irritation can be seen if the bleeding extends to the subarachnoid space. Ophthalmoscopy may reveal retinal hemorrhages.

Specific Signs by Location

PUTAMINAL HEMORRHAGE. Putaminal hemorrhage [31] is characterized by

1. Hemiparesis or hemiplegia and, to a lesser degree, hemisensory deficit
2. Transient global aphasia with dominant hemispheric lesions
3. Apractagnosia or unilateral neglect with nondominant hemispheric lesions
4. Homonymous hemianopia
5. Contralateral gaze palsy: the patient looks to the side of the hemorrhage and away from the hemiplegia (superior Foville syndrome)

THALAMIC HEMORRHAGE. Thalamic hemorrhage [62] is characterized by

1. Hemisensory deficit and, to a lesser degree, hemiparesis
2. Nonfluent, anomic aphasia with intact repetition and comprehension with lesions of the dominant thalamus
3. Convergence-retraction nystagmus, impairment of vertical gaze, and pupillary light-near dissociation
4. Downward-inward deviation of the eyes (depression-convergence syndrome)
5. Unilateral or bilateral pseudo-sixth nerve paresis
6. Skew deviation
7. Conjugate gaze palsy to the side of the lesion ("wrong side") or conjugate horizontal gaze deviation as seen in putaminal cases

CEREBELLAR HEMORRHAGE. The clinical presentation of cerebellar hemorrhage [8, 25] may be acute, subacute, or chronic. Only the acute form will be described. Patients present suddenly with occipital headache, dizziness, vertigo, nausea, repeated vomiting, and difficulty in walking. Examination of cerebellar function is not complete unless the patient's gait has been evaluated. The findings on examination may include

1. Variable degrees of alertness
2. Small reactive pupils
3. Skew deviation
4. Ipsilateral gaze palsy
5. Usually gaze-paretic nystagmus; occasionally ocular bobbing
6. Ipsilateral peripheral facial weakness
7. Ipsilateral absence of corneal reflex
8. Slurred speech may be present
9. Gait or truncal ataxia more common than limb ataxia
10. Bilateral hyperreflexia and Babinski signs

CORTICOSUBCORTICAL HEMORRHAGE. This type of hemorrhage [51] can occur in the frontal lobe or, more frequently, in the parietotemporooccipital region. *Frontal lobe hemorrhage* may be associated with abulia and contralateral arm weakness. *Parietotemporooccipital hemorrhage* may be associated with homonymous hemianopia, hemisensory-motor syndromes, and dysphasia or apractagnosia.

PONTINE HEMORRHAGE. Pontine hemorrhage [27] may cause

1. Coma
2. Hyperthermia
3. Respiratory abnormalities
4. Pinpoint reactive pupils
5. Eyes in central position, with absence of oculocephalic and oculovestibular reflexes
6. Ocular bobbing possible
7. Quadriplegia

SYNDROMES RELATED TO CEREBRAL ANEURYSMS

The overall incidence of intracranial saccular aneurysms is about 2 percent of autopsies. Over 85 percent involve the anterior portion of the circle of Willis, and 15 percent involve the vertebrobasilar circulation. Aneurysms are multiple in approximately 20 percent of cases. The three most frequent sites of aneurysms are (1) the junction of the anterior communicating artery with the anterior cerebral artery [60], (2) the junction of the internal carotid artery and the posterior communicating artery, and (3) the main division of the middle cerebral artery. Vertebrobasilar aneurysms that rupture are usually more than 0.5 cm in diameter; however, once an aneurysm reaches "giant" proportions (2.5 cm or larger) it behaves more like a space-occupying lesion [9, 14, 57]. The clinical manifestations of the unruptured aneurysm depend on the location, size, and projection. A discussion of some aneurysmal syndromes follows [50].

Intracavernous Aneurysms of the Internal Carotid Artery. Aneurysms arising from the internal carotid artery in the region of the cavernous sinus may rupture, causing a carotid-cavernous fistula [36], or expand, causing regional syndromes [32]. They occur especially in middle-aged women.

RUPTURED ANEURYSM: CAROTID-CAVERNOUS FISTULA. This lesion is associated with

1. Ocular pain
2. Pulsating exophthalmos (unilateral or bilateral)

3. Cephalic or ocular bruit, which can be diminished by digital carotid compression in the neck
4. Chemosis and redness of the conjunctiva
5. Diplopia, caused either by cranial nerve palsy or mechanical restriction of the globe (abducens palsy is the most common cause)
6. Decreased visual acuity due to pressure on the optic nerve, glaucoma, or retinal and optic nerve hypoxia

UNRUPTURED ANEURYSM. Typically, unruptured intracavernous ICA aneurysms are characterized by

1. Ocular pain
2. Abducens, oculomotor, or trochlear nerve palsies (in decreasing order) with small pupil due to oculosympathetic dysfunction
3. Pain and numbness in the distribution of the ophthalmic division of the trigeminal nerve; all three divisions can be occasionally affected
4. Bilateral ophthalmoplegia (rare)

If there is anterior extension of the aneurysm, the patient may have (1) exophthalmos, (2) chemosis, or (3) optic atrophy. If there is posterior extension of the aneurysm, the patient may have (1) deafness or (2) facial palsy.

Posterior Communicating Artery Aneurysms. The clinical distinction between internal carotid and posterior communicating artery aneurysms can be exceedingly difficult [55]. Classically, unruptured aneurysms of the posterior communicating artery may present with (1) headache, (2) ocular pain, or (3) oculomotor palsy with pupillary involvement. If rupture occurs, compromise of the trochlear, abducens, and ophthalmic division of the trigeminal nerve may be present.

Middle Cerebral Artery Aneurysms. Middle cerebral artery aneurysms lack a well-defined clinical syndrome [26]. The following may be seen:

1. Headache.
2. Seizures, either partial seizures with elementary symptomatology, complex partial seizures, or generalized tonic-clonic seizures. There is an increased incidence of right-sided aneurysms in patients with "uncinate" fits.
3. Aphasia.
4. Transient sensorimotor deficits.

Basilar Artery Aneurysms. Vertebrobasilar artery aneurysms may arise in the basilar, superior cerebellar, anterior inferior cerebellar, vertebral, posterior inferior cerebellar, or posterior cerebral artery, in that order of frequency [16, 64]. Unruptured basilar artery aneurysms may present with

1. Vertebrobasilar TIAs
2. Cerebellopontine angle syndrome
3. Alternating hemiplegia with cranial nerve palsies
4. Ataxia
5. Atypical facial pain
6. Abducens or facial palsies
7. Occasional oculomotor palsy
8. Nonhemorrhagic thalamic infarctions

SUBARACHNOID HEMORRHAGE

Subarachnoid hemorrhage (SAH) can be either primary, due to blood invading the subarachnoid space from a ruptured artery or vein, or secondary, caused by an intracerebral hemorrhage leaking into the ventricular system and subarachnoid space after dissection through the brain substance [15, 63]. Intracranial saccular aneurysms are the main cause of nontraumatic SAH [30, 35, 56]. Aneurysms commonly rupture near the fundus of the sac. The blood extends into the subarachnoid space, sometimes into the brain parenchyma, and rarely into the subdural space. Other etiologic factors of nontraumatic SAH include arteriovenous malformations, blood dyscrasias, vasculitis, cortical thrombophlebitis, bacterial meningitis, and intracranial spinal cord tumors. In some cases of spontaneous SAH, no etiology can be found even at autopsy. SAH is one of the few neurologic conditions that can cause sudden unexpected death.

Premonitory symptoms occur in a significant proportion of cases. The commonest premonitory symptom is headache. An aneurysm should be suspected when the following occur:

1. Late onset of migraine headache with no family history of migraine
2. Change in the headache pattern in a known migraineur
3. Severe localized and persistent headache
4. Migrainous headaches refractory to conventional therapy

Other premonitory symptoms may include episodes of neck stiffness, diplopia, nausea, and photophobia that are associated with headache.

Hemorrhage into the subarachnoid space is often accompanied by the development of excruciating headaches, vomiting, and meningismus. However, many variations to the clinical picture occur depending on the severity of the hemorrhage, the presence of an associated hematoma, the occurrence of vasospasm, or the development of hydrocephalus.

The clinical diagnosis of SAH is determined from the symptomatology and verified by lumbar puncture or cranial computerized tomography, and by cerebral angiography [17, 65].

The *symptoms* of SAH include headache, which is usually severe and suboccipital or generalized; less frequently it is frontal, retroocular, frontotemporal, or frontooccipital. Unilateral headaches rarely occur, and when they do they are not indicative of the aneurysmal site. Nausea, vomiting, and photophobia are common complaints. Disturbances of consciousness of variable severity and duration may follow the onset of bleeding. Seizures, either focal or generalized, may occur. The patient may complain of severe neck stiffness or backache.

Meningismus, with nuchal rigidity and Kernig's sign, is a common *sign.* However, it may be absent in a third of the cases. Ophthalmoscopic findings include papilledema, and vitreous, subhyaloid, or preretinal hemorrhage. Ptosis or diplopia is most frequently caused by oculomotor palsy secondary to hemorrhage from an internal carotid or posterior communicating artery aneurysm. However, the oculomotor palsy may result from ruptured aneurysms at the distal end of the basilar artery or from uncal herniation. Unilateral or bilateral abducens palsies may reflect increased intracranial pressure and therefore lack localizing value. Visual field defects or sudden loss of vision may occur when an aneurysm ruptures near the visual pathways. The presence of other focal findings such as aphasia, hemiparesis, sensory impairment, and abnormal reflexes depends on the location of the lesion.

The effect of subarachnoid hemorrhage on hypothalamic function may result in life-threatening cardiac arrhythmias, myocardial infarction, or hyponatremia with inappropriate secretion of antidiuretic hormone (SIADH). A transient rise in blood pressure and minimal elevation of temperature can be present.

Clinical deterioration following SAH may reflect rebleeding, development of hydrocephalus, or vasospasm. Vasospasm or delayed cerebral ischemia is usually seen 3 days after onset. The clinical syndrome of vasospasm is characterized by decreased alertness and focal neurologic deficits that correspond to the region of the brain supplied by the arteries with spasm, usually near the territory of distribution of the artery affected by the aneurysm.

Repeated hemorrhages into the subarachnoid space can give rise to the *subpial siderosis syndrome.* The clinical picture is characterized by ataxia, dementia, decreased hearing, anosmia, and corticospinal tract signs.

REFERENCES

1. Ajax, E. T., Schenkenberg, T., and Kosteljanetz, M. Alexia without agraphia and the inferior splenium. *Neurology* 27:685, 1977.

2. Azar-Kia, B., and Palacios, E. Collateral Circulation of the Brain. *In* Fein, J. M., and Reichmann, O. H. (Eds.). *Microvascular Anastomosis for Cerebral Ischemia.* New York: Springer-Verlag, 1978. Pp. 132–144.
3. Benson, F. D. *Aphasia, Alexia, and Agraphia.* New York: Churchill-Livingstone, 1979.
4. Benson, F. D., Marsden, D. C., and Meadows, J. C. The amnesic syndrome of posterior cerebral artery occlusion. *Acta Neurol. Scand.* 50:133, 1974.
5. Berman, S. A., Hayman, L. A., and Hinck, V. C. Correlation of C.T. cerebral vascular territories with function: I. Anterior cerebral artery. *A.J.N.R.* 135:253, 1980.
6. Bingham, W. G., and Hayes, G. J. Persistent carotid-basilar anastomosis. Report of two cases. *J. Neurosurg.* 18:398, 1961.
7. Boller, F. Strokes and behavior disorders of higher cortical functions following cerebral disease. *Curr. Concepts Cerebrovascular Dis. – Stroke* 16(1):1, 1981.
8. Brennan, R. W., and Bergland, R. M. Acute cerebellar hemorrhage. Analysis of clinical findings and outcome in 12 cases. *Neurology* 27:527, 1977.
9. Bull, J. Massive aneurysms at the base of the brain. *Brain* 92:535, 1969.
10. Buonanno, F., and Toole, J. F. Management of patients with established ("completed") cerebral infarction. *Progr. Cerebrovascular Dis. – Stroke* 12(1):7, 1981.
11. Caplan, L. R. Intracerebral Hemorrhage. *In* Tyler, H. R., and Dawson, D. M. (Eds.). *Current Neurology* (Vol. 2). Boston: Houghton Mifflin, 1979. Pp. 185–205.
12. Caplan, L. R. "Top of the basilar" syndrome. *Neurology* 30:72, 1980.
13. Critchley, M. Anterior cerebral artery and its syndromes. *Brain* 53:120, 1930.
14. Crompton, M. R. Mechanism of growth and rupture in cerebral berry aneurysms. *Br. Med. J.* 1:1138, 1966.
15. Crompton, M. R. The pathology of subarachnoid hemorrhage. *J. R. Coll. Physicians (Lond.)* 7:235, 1973.
16. Drake, L. G. The Treatment of Aneurysms of the Posterior Circulation. *In* Carevel, P. W. (Ed.). *Clinical Neurosurgery.* Baltimore: The Williams & Wilkins Co., 1979. Pp. 96–144.
17. Drake, L. G. Management of cerebral aneurysm. *Progr. Cerebrovascular Dis. – Stroke* 12(3):273, 1981.
18. Fields, W. S. The significance of persistent trigeminal artery. *Radiology* 91:1096, 1968.
19. Fisher, C. M. Occlusion of the internal carotid artery. *Arch. Neurol. Psychiat.* 69:346, 1951.
20. Fisher, C. M. Observations of the fundus oculi in transient monocular blindness. *Neurology* 9:333, 1959.
21. Fisher, C. M. Clinical Syndromes in Cerebral Arterial Occlusion. *In* Fields, W. S. (Ed.). *Pathogenesis and Treatment of Cerebrovascular Disease.* Springfield, Ill.: Charles C Thomas, 1961. Pp. 151–181.
22. Fisher, C. M. Clinical Syndromes in Cerebral Hemorrhage. *In* Fields, W. S. (Ed.). *Pathogenesis and Treatment of Cerebrovascular Disease.* Springfield, Ill.: Charles C Thomas, 1961. Pp. 318–338.
23. Fisher, C. M. Pathological observations in hypertensive cerebral hemorrhage. *J. Neuropathol. Exp. Neurol.* 30:536, 1971.
24. Fisher, C. M. Lacunar strokes and infarcts: A review. *Neurology* 32:871, 1982.
25. Fisher, C. M., et al. Acute hypertensive cerebellar hemorrhage: Diagnosis and surgical treatment. *J. Nerv. Ment. Dis.* 140:38, 1965.

33333

26. Frankel, K., and Alpers, B. J. The clinical syndrome of aneurysm of the middle cerebral artery. *Arch. Neurol. Psychiat.* 74:46, 1955.
27. Goto, N., et al. Primary pontine hemorrhage: Clinicopathological correlations. *Stroke* 11(1):84, 1980.
28. Greenblat, S. H. Alexia without agraphia or hemianopsia. *Brain* 96:307, 1973.
29. Hayman, L. A., Berman, S. A., and Hinck, V. C. Correlation of C.T. cerebral vascular territories with function: II. Posterior cerebral artery. *A.J.N.R.* 2:219, 1981.
30. Hayward, R. D. Subarachnoid hemorrhage of unknown etiology. A clinical and radiological study of 51 cases. *J. Neurol. Neurosurg. Psychiat.* 40:926, 1977.
31. Hier, D. B., et al. Hypertensive putaminal hemorrhage. *Ann. Neurol.* 1:152, 1977.
32. Hirano, A., Barron, K. D., and Zimmerman, H. M. Ruptured aneurysms of the supraclinoid portion of the internal carotid and of the middle cerebral arteries. *J. Nerv. Ment. Dis.* 129:35, 1959.
33. Hooshmand, H., et al. Amaurosis fugax: Diagnostic and therapeutic aspects. *Stroke* 5(5):643, 1974.
34. Hoyt, W. F., and Beeston, D. *The Ocular Fundus in Neurologic Disease.* St. Louis: C.V. Mosby, 1966.
35. Locksley, H. B. Report on the cooperative study of intracranial aneurysms and subarachnoid hemorrhage: Evaluation of conservative management of ruptured intracranial aneurysms. *J. Neurosurg.* 25:574, 1966.
36. Madsen, P. H. Carotid-cavernous fistulae. A study of 18 cases. *Acta Ophthalmol.* 48:731, 1970.
37. McCormick, W. F. Problems and Pathogenesis of Intracranial Arterial Aneurysms. *In* Toole, J. F., Moosy, J., and Janeway, R. (Eds.). *Cerebral Vascular Disease.* New York: Grune & Stratton, 1971. Pp. 219–231.
38. McCormick, W. F. Intracranial arterial aneurysms: A pathologist's view. *Curr. Concepts Cerebrovascular Dis.—Stroke* 8:15, 1973.
39. McCormick, W. F., and Rosenfield, D. B. Massive brain hemorrhage: A review of 144 cases and an examination of their causes. *Stroke* 4:946, 1973.
40. Medina, J. L., Chokroverty, S., and Rubino, F. A. Syndrome of agitated delirium and visual impairment: A manifestation of medial temporo-occipital infarction. *J. Neurol. Neurosurg. Psychiat.* 40:861, 1977.
41. Mesulam, M. M., et al. Acute confusional states with right middle cerebral artery infarction. *J. Neurol. Neurosurg. Psychiat.* 39:84, 1976.
42. Miller, V. T. Lacunar stroke—A reassessment. *Arch. Neurol.* 40:129, 1983.
43. Millikan, C. H., and McDowell, F. H. Treatment of transient ischemic attacks. *Progr. Cerebrovascular Dis.—Stroke* 9(4):299, 1978.
44. Millikan, C. H., and McDowell, F. H. Treatment of progressive stroke. *Progr. Cerebrovascular Dis.—Stroke* 12(4):397, 1981.
45. Minor, R. H., et al. Ocular manifestations of occlusive disease of the vertebral-basilar arterial system. *Arch. Ophthalmol.* 62:112, 1959.
46. Mohr, J. P. Lacunes. *Stroke* 13(1):3, 1982.
47. Mohr, J. P., et al. The Harvard cooperative stroke registry: A prospective registry. *Neurology* 28:754, 1978.
48. Pessin, M. S., et al. Mechanisms of acute carotid stroke. *Ann. Neurol.* 6:245, 1979.
49. Ring, B. A. Middle cerebral artery: Anatomical and radiographic study. *Acta Radiol.* 57:289, 1982.

50. Robertson, E. G. Cerebral lesions due to intracranial aneurysms. *Brain* 72:150, 1949.
51. Ropper, A. H., and Davis, K. R. Lobar cerebral hemorrhages: Acute clinical syndromes in 26 cases. *Ann. Neurol.* 8:141, 1980.
52. Russell, R. W. R. Observations of the fundus oculi in transient monocular blindness. *Neurology* 9:333, 1959.
53. Russell, R. W. R. The source of retinal emboli. *Lancet* 2:789, 1968.
54. Sacco, R. L., et al. Survival and recurrence following stroke. The Framingham Study. *Stroke* 13(3):290, 1982.
55. Soni, S. R. Aneurysms of the posterior communicating artery and oculomotor paresis. *J. Neurol. Neurosurg. Psychiat.* 37:475, 1974.
56. Sundt, T. M., and Whisnant, J. P. Subarachnoid hemorrhage from intracranial aneurysms. Surgical management and natural history of disease. *N. Engl. J. Med.* 299:116, 1978.
57. Suzuki, J., and Ohara, H. Clinicopathological study of cerebral aneurysms. Origin, rupture, repair, and growth. *J. Neurosurg.* 48:505, 1978.
58. Toole, J. F., and Patel, A. N. *Cerebrovascular Disorders* (2nd ed.). New York: McGraw-Hill, 1974. Pp. 12–34.
59. Toole, J. F., et al. Transient ischemic attacks: A prospective study of 225 patients. *Neurology* 28:746, 1978.
60. Vihlein, A., Thomas, R. L., and Cleary, J. Aneurysms of the anterior communicating artery complex. *Mayo Clin. Proc.* 42:73, 1967.
61. Waddington, M. M., and Ring, A. B. Syndromes of occlusions of middle cerebral artery branches. Angiographic and clinical correlation. *Brain* 91:685, 1968.
62. Walshe, T. M., Davis, K. R., and Fisher, C. M. Thalamic hemorrhage. A computed tomographic-clinical correlation. *Neurology* 27:217, 1977.
63. Walton, J. N. *Subarachnoid Hemorrhage.* Edinburgh: E.S. Livingstone Ltd., 1956.
64. Weibel, J., Fields, W. S., and Campos, R. J. Aneurysms of the posterior cervicocranial circulation: Clinical and angiographic considerations. *J. Neurosurg.* 26:223, 1967.
65. Weir, B. Medical aspects of the preoperative management of aneurysms: A review. *Can. J. Neurol. Sci.* 6:441, 1979.

Chapter 21

THE LOCALIZATION OF LESIONS CAUSING COMA

Joseph C. Masdeu

Most causes of coma speedily threaten life or recovery of neurologic function. Thus, they must be promptly identified and removed. Unfortunately, patients with a depressed level of alertness cannot give an account of the events leading to their situation, and often no one is available to provide such information. Thus the physician has to rely on examination of the patient not only to localize the damaged anatomic structures but also to identify the offending agent. Diagnosis of stupor and coma is well reviewed in the most recent edition of an excellent monograph [14]. These pages will draw heavily from that source.

In the clinical setting, the diagnostic evaluation of the comatose patient must proceed side by side with measures that will restore or ensure the proper functioning of vital organs. Adequate oxygenation must be secured by intubation and mechanical ventilation. Maximal oxygenation and injection of 0.6 mg of atropine before intubation help prevent cardiac arrhythmias induced by intubation. If the patient has sustained a neck injury that contraindicates intubation, ventilation may be restored through emergency tracheotomy or insertion of a no. 14 needle in the trachea. The circulation should be maintained and any blood loss replenished; the mean arterial pressure should be kept at about 110 mm Hg. Besides obtaining blood chemistries, 50 ml of a 50% solution of glucose and 100 mg of thiamine should be given to any comatose patient unless the history clearly precludes the possibility of hypoglycemia or the risk of thiamine deficiency (the latter condition may be aggravated by the infusion of glucose). Naloxone (in a slow intravenous injection of 0.4 mg diluted in 10 ml of physiologic saline solution) can reverse coma induced by narcotic and sedative drugs.

COMA, AKINETIC MUTISM, AND THE LOCKED-IN SYNDROME

Different terms such as *coma, stupor, lethargy,* and the like indicate a depressed level of alertness. These terms, however, fail to convey vital information needed for neurologic localization and management. Rather than using one of these terms, a description of the patient's level of consciousness (incorporating some detail of the patient's responses to diverse reproducible stimuli) facilitates communication among members of the health care team, enhances consistency in successive evaluations of the patient, and sets the basis for a rational diagnostic assessment. For instance, stating that "the patient was stuporous" provides little information. Instead, the real situation can be much better conveyed by explaining in everyday English that "Mr. Z lay motionless in bed unless called loudly by name, when he opened his eyes briefly and looked to the left. He failed to answer any questions or to follow instructions."

Two terms have gained acceptance among neurologists and are widely used. *Akinetic mutism* refers to a state in which the patient, although seemingly awake, remains silent and motionless. Only the eyes dart in the direction of moving objects, such as the examiner approaching the patient's bed. The examiner, attempting to converse with a patient in this state, does not apparently arouse (and gets the distinct impression of lacking) the patient's attention and interest. Despite the lack of movement, there are few signs indicative of damage to the descending motor pathways. Instead, "frontal release signs," such as grasp or sucking, may be present. Patients who remain completely motionless are not seen as often as those who move one side or one arm in a stereotyped fashion, but in every other respect they fit into the syndrome of akinetic mutism. In such cases, the paralyzed side may display signs of corticospinal tract involvement, such as hyperreflexia and Babinski sign.

If a history is available, akinetic mutism can usually be distinguished from psychogenic (often catatonic) unresponsiveness. Otherwise, the diagnosis may be difficult. Particularly when exposed to painful stimuli (such as those caused by soiled linen or a decubitus ulcer) or to infection, patients with akinetic mutism appear excited and tachycardic and perspire heavily, thus superficially resembling a catatonic patient. Signs of frontal release or corticospinal tract damage favor the diagnosis of akinetic mutism. In the catatonic patient, the electroencephalogram (EEG) is normal (usually desynchronized, with low-voltage fast activity), but in the patient with akinetic mutism the EEG shows slow wave abnormalities.

Lesions that cause akinetic mutism affect bilaterally the frontal region or the reticular formation of the posterior diencephalon and adjacent midbrain. The most common causes are severe acute hydrocephalus, cerebral infarction, and direct compression by tumors. When the cerebral hemispheres have sustained severe and widespread damage (such as that due to severe trauma, anoxia, or encephalitis), the patient may, after some weeks of complete unresponsiveness, evolve into a situation similar to akinetic mutism, with the return of sleep-wake cycles. These patients, however, demonstrate obvious signs of pronounced bilateral corticospinal tract damage. This situation, in which the patient's functions are restricted to the autonomic sphere, may persist for years and has been termed the *chronic vegetative state*.

The *locked-in syndrome* refers to a condition in which the patient is mute and motionless but remains awake and alert and capable of perceiving sensory stimuli. Although horizontal eye movements are often impaired due to involvement of the paramedian pontine reticular formation (PPRF), the patient's level of alertness can be gleaned from his response

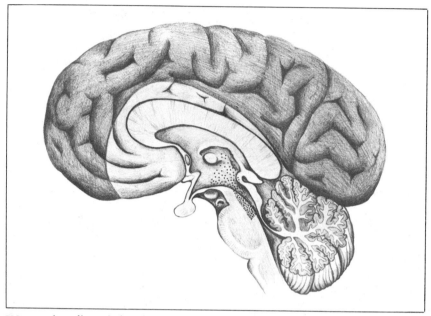

FIG. 21-1. *Ascending reticular activating system (ARAS). The dotted area in this midsagittal section of the brain corresponds to the approximate location of the ARAS in the upper brainstem and diencephalon.*

to commands involving vertical eye movements. The EEG reflects the patient's state of wakefulness. The locked-in syndrome is usually due to ventral pontine infarction, pontine hemorrhage or tumor, or central pontine myelinolysis (lesions that damage the descending motor pathways bilaterally in the basis pontis but spare the more dorsal reticular formation). Ventral midbrain lesions [5, 10], severe polyneuropathies, or myasthenia gravis may rarely cause this syndrome.

ANATOMIC SUBSTRATE OF ALERTNESS

Damage to the ascending reticular activating system (ARAS), described in animals by Moruzzi and Magoun in 1949 [11], induces a state of coma in which the animal becomes unresponsive and its EEG shows sleep patterns despite vigorous sensory stimulation. In humans, this critical area lies in the paramedian tegmental region of the posterior portion of pons and midbrain. It extends from the superior half of the pons through the midbrain to the posterior portion of the hypothalamus and to the thalamic reticular formation (Fig. 21-1). Sedative drugs act, at least in part, by interfering with the synaptic network of the ARAS, which is played upon by sensory stimuli.

The medial longitudinal fasciculus, which connects the abducens and oculomotor nuclei, and the oculomotor and trochlear nuclei themselves are situated amid the neurons of the pontine and midbrain portions of the ARAS. Thus, when unresponsiveness is caused by brainstem lesions, their location can often be determined by the abnormal patterns of ocular motility.

Bilateral cerebral hemispheric lesions may cause transient coma, particularly when they involve the mesial frontal region. Large unilateral lesions of the dominant hemisphere may occasionally cause transient unresponsiveness, even in the absence of a mass effect.

In the diencephalon, posterior hypothalamic lesions induce prolonged hypersomnia. Acute bilateral damage of the paraventricular thalamic nuclei is attended by transient unresponsiveness, followed by severe amnestic dementia (see Chap. 17).

SIGNS WITH LOCALIZING VALUE IN COMA

In a comatose patient, the respiratory pattern, pupillary response, eye movements, and position or movements of the limbs provide important clues to the anatomic site and nature of the injury.

Respiratory Patterns. Although the respiratory pattern of a patient in coma may be helpful in localizing the level of structural dysfunction in the neuraxis, metabolic abnormalities may affect the respiratory centers of the pons and medulla and result in patterns resembling those due to neurologic disease (Fig. 21-2). Caution and a thorough evaluation of the metabolic status of the patient must thus guide the interpretation of respiratory changes.

POSTHYPERVENTILATION APNEA. This condition reflects mild bilateral hemispheric dysfunction. Because demonstration of this respiratory abnormality requires the patient's active cooperation, this sign is mentioned here mainly to clarify the genesis of other respiratory patterns. To elicit this phenomenon, the patient is simply asked to take five deep breaths. This maneuver normally decreases arterial pCO_2 by about 10 mm Hg and, in the healthy patient, is followed by a very brief period of apnea (less than 10 seconds). The stimulus for rhythmic breathing when the pCO_2 is lowered probably originates in forebrain structures because sleep, obtundation, or bilateral hemispheric dysfunction abolish it. Thus, when bilateral hemispheric lesions are present, the posthyperventilation apnea lasts for as long as 20 or 30 seconds.

CHEYNE-STOKES RESPIRATION. This type of respiration consists of brief periods of hyperpnea alternating regularly with even shorter periods of ap-

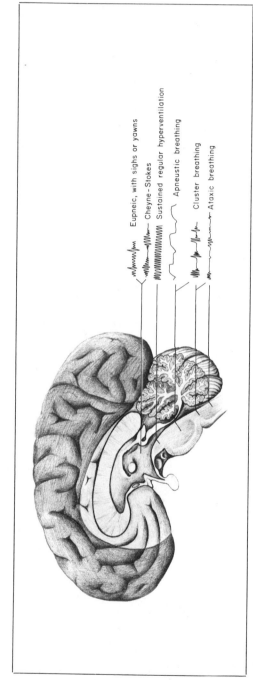

FIG. 21-2. *Respiratory patterns characteristic of lesions at different levels of the brain.*

Eupneic, with sighs or yawns
Cheyne-Stokes
Sustained regular hyperventilation
Apneustic breathing
Cluster breathing
Ataxic breathing

nea. After the apneic phase, the amplitude of respiratory movements increases gradually to a peak and then slowly wanes to apnea. Not only does ventilation fluctuate periodically, but during the hyperpneic stage the patient becomes more alert, the pupils may dilate, and the motor behavior reflects control by higher centers (e.g., decorticate posturing yields to semipurposeful movements).

Cheyne-Stokes respiration represents a more severe degree of posthyperventilation apnea in which the respiratory drive becomes more closely dependent on the pCO_2. Because the "smoothing effect" provided by forebrain structures has been removed, pCO_2 accumulation causes hyperpnea, which in turn induces a drop in pCO_2. With this drop the respiratory stimulus ceases, and a period of apnea ensues.

This respiratory pattern may follow bilateral widespread cortical lesions but is more likely to be associated with bilateral thalamic dysfunction and has also been described with lesions of the descending pathways anywhere from the cerebral hemispheres to the level of the upper pons. Metabolic disturbances, such as uremia and diffuse anoxia, often underlie this breathing disorder.

HYPERVENTILATION WITH BRAINSTEM INJURY. Patients with lesions of the midbrain and pons often have prolonged and rapid hyperpnea. Because most of these patients are relatively hypoxic despite the excessive ventilatory effort, this type of breathing cannot be truly called "neurogenic hyperventilation." In a few cases where pulmonary or metabolic causes of hyperventilation were absent, brainstem tumors were found at autopsy. In these cases, tumoral metabolism may have lowered the pH of the local cerebrospinal fluid, thereby providing a stimulus to the respiratory center of the medulla [13].

APNEUSTIC BREATHING. Apneustic breathing is characterized by a long inspiration, after which the air is retained for several seconds and then released. This abnormality appears with lesions of the lateral tegmentum of the lower half of the pons.

CLUSTER BREATHING. Breathing with a cluster of breaths following each other in an irregular sequence may result from low pontine or high medullary lesions.

ATAXIC BREATHING. This type of breathing has a completely irregular pattern in which inspiratory gasps of diverse amplitude and length intermingle with periods of apnea. This respiratory abnormality, often present in agonal patients, heralds complete respiratory failure and follows damage of the dorsomedial medulla. The most common etiologies for this pattern include cerebellar or pontine hemorrhages, trauma, and posterior fossa tumors. Less often, a paramedian medullary infarct (usually due to severe atherosclerosis of a vertebral artery) may cause this syndrome. The classic breathing pattern described by Biot was ataxic breathing in patients with severe meningitis [14].

"ONDINE'S CURSE." *Ondine's curse* refers to the loss of automatic breathing during sleep. This respiratory pattern, obviously absent in comatose patients, is mentioned here because it occurs with lower brainstem dysfunction. Responsible lesions have a similar or somewhat lower location than those that cause ataxic breathing but are smaller or develop more slowly. This disorder has also been recorded after surgical section of the ventrolateral spinal cord for pain relief, probably because of reticulospinal tract interruption.

The Pupils. Pupillary shape, size, symmetry, and response to light provide valuable clues to brainstem and third cranial nerve function. Because the pupillary light reflex travels over few synapses, it is very resistant to metabolic dysfunction to the point that abnormalities of this reflex, particularly when unilateral, indicate structural lesions of the midbrain or oculomotor nerve. A few exceptions are noteworthy. Atropinic agents, instilled on the eyes, applied on the skin (transdermal scopolamine) [2], ingested, or given during resuscitation, may cause fixed and dilated pupils. In these cases, a solution of 1% pilocarpine applied to the eye will fail to constrict the pupils, whereas in the case of anoxic pupillary dilation, this cholinergic agent, acting directly on the constrictor of the iris, produces miosis. Because many patients in coma have small pupils, anticholinergic agents are sometimes used to facilitate visualization of the optic fundi, thus eliminating a potentially useful diagnostic indicator. In many cases, a better way to obtain pupillary dilation is by pinching the skin of the neck *(ciliospinal reflex)*. Glutethimide (Doriden) induces unequal pupils that are midsized or slightly dilated and poorly responsive to light. Other agents that cause unreactive pupils include barbiturates, succinylcholine, and, rarely, xylocaine, phenothiazines, methanol, and aminoglycoside antibiotics. Agents other than glutethimide or anticholinergic drugs cause pupillary dilation only when taken in massive amounts, enough to cause absence of respiratory reflexes or, in the case of succinylcholine and aminoglycoside antibiotics, generalized neuromuscular junction blockade. Usually, the amount of sedative drug is insufficient to abolish the pupillary light reflex. Hypothermia and acute anoxia may also cause unreactive pupils, which, if persistent beyond several minutes after an anoxic insult, carry a poor prognosis.

The areas of the brain and anatomic pathways that mediate the pupillary light reflex are reviewed in Chapter 7, in which the origin and course of sympathetic and parasympathetic influences on the iris muscle are described.

Various structural lesions causing coma may be associated with pupillary abnormalities (Fig. 21-3):

1. *Sleep or bilateral diencephalic dysfunction* (metabolic coma), is accompanied by small pupils that react well to light ("diencephalic" pupils).
2. Unilateral *hypothalamic* damage induces miosis and anhidrosis on the side of the body ipsilateral to the lesion.
3. *Midbrain* lesions causing coma usually produce distinct pupillary abnormalities. *Tectal* or *pretectal* lesions affecting the posterior commissure abolish the light reflex, but the pupils, which are midsized or slightly large, may show spontaneous oscillations in size (hippus) and become larger when the neck is pinched (ciliospinal reflex). *Tegmental* lesions, which involve the third nerve nucleus, may cause irregular constriction of the sphincter of the iris with a resultant pear-shaped pupil or displacement of the pupil to one side (midbrain corectopia). The pupils, often unequal, tend to be midsized and lack light or ciliospinal responses.
4. *Pontine tegmental* lesions cause pinpoint pupils, which, when observed with a magnifying glass, may be seen to constrict to light.
5. *Lateral pontine, lateral medullary,* and *ventrolateral cervical cord* lesions produce an ipsilateral Horner syndrome.
6. *Oculomotor nerve* compression and elongation by temporal uncal herniation (through the tentorial opening) affect pupillary function earlier and more noticeably than the extrinsic eye movements subserved by cranial nerve III. The light reflex is sluggish or absent, and, unlike the situation with midbrain involvement, the pupil becomes widely dilated owing to sparing of the sympathetic pathways (Hutchinson's pupil).

Eye Movements. The anatomic pathways subserving eye movements were reviewed in Chapter 7. In the comatose patient the assessment of eye movements helps to determine the level of structural brainstem damage (Fig. 21-4) or the depth of coma induced by metabolic agents. The *corneal reflex* has a higher threshold in comatose patients. Nonetheless, it must be elicited by a gentle and aseptic stimulus to avoid the risk of an infected corneal ulceration in patients with decreased corneal sensitivity (as with cranial nerve V lesions, ipsilateral lateral pontine-medullary lesions, or contralateral parietal lesions) [12], or impaired eye

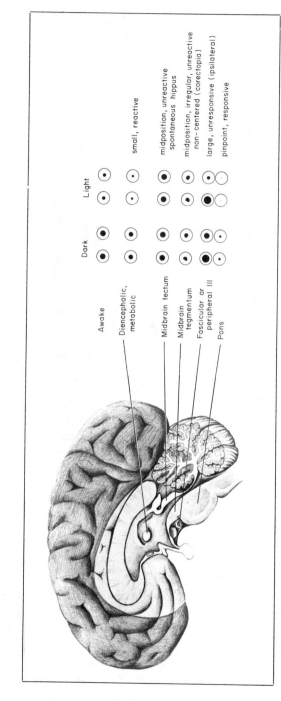

FIG. 21-3. *Pupillary responses characteristic of lesions at different levels of the brain.*

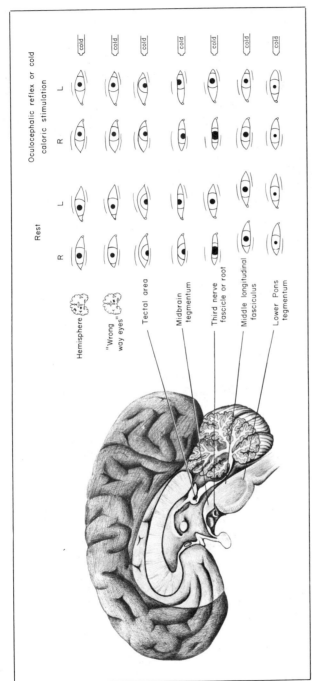

FIG. 21-4. *Eye movement abnormalities characteristic of lesions at different levels of the brain. The responses to cold caloric stimulation are indicated in the right-hand column.*

closure (as with cranial nerve VII lesions and low pontine lesions). In the latter cases, the stimulus may induce deviation of the jaw to the opposite side *(corneopterygoid reflex)*, and, given an intact upper pons and midbrain, the eyes may roll upward *(Bell's phenomenon)*.

In the absence of voluntary eye movements, the assessment of ocular motility in comatose patients relies heavily on reflex eye movements, including the *oculocephalic reflex,* elicited by the doll's eye maneuver, and the *oculovestibular reflex,* elicited by instillation of cold or warm water into the external auditory canal. Caloric testing provides a stronger stimulus than the oculocephalic reflex. If only the latter reflex is present, caloric stimulation has either not been performed adequately (e.g., hindered by the presence of wax in the external auditory canal) or there is damage to the labyrinth (e.g., by streptomycin) or of the vestibular nuclei in the laterosuperior medulla.

Because of the absence of cortical control of eye movements, the comatose patient lacks voluntary saccades, including the quick phase of nystagmus and tracking eye movements. Instead, if the brainstem is intact, the eyelids are closed, and the eyes, slightly divergent, drift slowly from side to side *(roving eye movements).* Spontaneous blinking requires an intact pontine reticular formation. Blinking induced by a bright light is probably mediated by the superior colliculus and remains despite occipital damage. Absence of blinking on one side only is indicative of unilateral nuclear, fascicular, or peripheral facial nerve dysfunction. The eyelids may remain tonically retracted in some cases of pontine infarction.

The roving eye movements of light coma cannot be voluntarily executed and are therefore incompatible with the diagnosis of psychogenic unresponsiveness. As coma deepens, roving eye movements disappear first, followed by the oculocephalic reflex; finally, even cold water instilled in the ear fails to induce eye movements. In metabolic coma, the pupils may still react when eye movements cannot be elicited.

Other spontaneous eye movements seen in comatose patients include periodic alternating gaze, ocular bobbing, and nystagmoid jerks. *Periodic alternating gaze* (Ping-Pong gaze) consists of roving of the eyes from one extreme of horizontal gaze to the other and back. Each oscillatory cycle usually takes 2 to 5 seconds [15]. The few cases reported suggest that this finding indicates bilateral cerebral damage with an intact brainstem. *Ocular bobbing* refers to a conjugate, brisk, downward movement of the eyes, which then return more slowly to the primary position. This phenomenon persists during caloric testing, which may actually enhance it. Ocular bobbing is most often associated with a lower pontine lesion, usually a hemorrhage, but has been described with different pathologic processes resulting in compression of the brainstem and with hepatic encephalopathy [4]. Rarely, a slow downward component may be followed by a quick upbeat *(inverse ocular bobbing)* [9]. *Nystagmoid jerking* of a single eye, in a vertical, horizontal, or rotatory fashion, indicates mid- to lower pontine damage. Pontine lesions occasionally give rise to dis- conjugate rotatory and vertical movements of the eyes, in which one eye may rise and intort as the other falls and extorts. This type of movement should not be confused with see-saw nystagmus, which is very seldom seen in comatose patients.

ABNORMALITIES OF LATERAL GAZE

CONJUGATE GAZE. When both eyes remain deviated toward the same side in a comatose patient, the lesion may be in the cerebral hemi- sphere (most often involving the frontal eye fields) or in the pontine teg- mentum. In the case of a *hemispheric* lesion, unless the patient is having a seizure, the eyes will "look toward the lesion" (away from the hemipa- retic side) but can be brought to the other side with the oculocephalic maneuver, caloric testing, or both. A seizure originating in the frontal or occipital lobes may cause deviation of the eyes and head away from the lesion, but such deviation is brief and usually accompanied by nystag- moid jerks; as soon as the seizure ceases, the eyes return to "look" to- ward the lesion. Thalamic and, very seldom, basal ganglionic lesions, of- ten hemorrhagic, may produce forced deviation of the eyes to the side contralateral to the lesion *(wrong-way eyes)*.

Predominantly unilateral lesions affecting the tegmentum of the *lower pons* cause a horizontal gaze palsy toward the side of the lesion, so that the eyes look toward the hemiparetic side. Another feature differentiat- ing this from a hemispheric cause of gaze palsy is that neither the oculo- cephalic maneuver nor caloric testing overcome a pontine gaze palsy.

DISCONJUGATE GAZE. Isolated failure of ocular adduction, in the ab- sence of pupillary changes and with normal vertical eye movements (elicited by oculocephalic or oculovestibular reflexes), indicates a lesion of the medial longitudinal fasciculus (MLF) in the upper pons ipsilateral to the eye that fails to adduct. MLF involvement is commonly bilateral in comatose patients. Rarely, metabolic coma (such as that due to barbitu- rates, amitriptyline [7], or hepatic failure [1]), may induce a transient MLF syndrome that can usually be overcome by vigorous caloric testing.

Latent strabismus may become apparent when the level of alertness is mildly impaired but disappears in deep coma. Because strabismus in- volves a single muscle, it seldom mimics neurogenic oculoparesis ex- cept, perhaps, when adbuction is reduced.

ABNORMALITIES OF VERTICAL GAZE. In patients in light coma, upward gaze can be tested by holding the eyelids open and gently touching the cor- nea with a wisp of cotton or a similar object. With this stimulus the eyeballs will tend to roll upward *(Bell's phenomenon)*. Unless the patient is intubated or has a neck injury, the doll's head maneuver can be used to elicit the vertical component of the oculocephalic reflex. Irrigation of both ears with cold water induces downward deviation of the eyes; warm water induces upward deviation.

Disconjugate vertical gaze in the resting position *(skew deviation)* indicates a lesion of the brachium pontis or dorsolateral medulla on the side of the depressed eye, or of the MLF on the side of the elevated eye. Persistent deviation of the eyes below the horizontal meridian signifies brainstem dysfunction, which is often due to a structural lesion that affects the tectum of the midbrain but is occasionally caused by metabolic encephalopathy (e.g., hepatic coma). Forced downward deviation of the eyes during caloric testing often occurs in coma induced by sedative drugs. Sustained up-gaze has been reported with severe anoxic encephalopathy [8]. Paresis of upward gaze is usually present with bilateral midbrain tectal damage. Downward gaze is preferentially affected by bilateral lesions of the superomedial perirubral region, in the ventral portion of the origin of the Sylvian aqueduct from the third ventricle. Large midbrain tegmental lesions abolish vertical gaze. At rest, the eyes remain in midposition or may be disconjugately deviated in the vertical plane.

Motor Activity of the Body and Limbs. When examining a patient in coma, observation of the movements and of the tone and reflexes of the limbs supply information that has a less clear-cut localizing value than similar findings in alert patients. Rarely will a metabolic coma (notably hypoglycemic) be accompanied by hemiparesis; however, other motor patterns, widely known as decorticate and decerebrate rigidity, are often produced by metabolic disorders [6] and do not have the structural implications that their denominations, coined during experimental work, would suggest. Of course, structural damage to the origin or course of the motor pathways may give rise to such patterns, which, in these cases, are often asymmetrical. However, the greater frequency of metabolic causes of coma renders them often responsible for the motor patterns discussed below (Fig. 21-5).

In *light coma*, the general motor responses may oscillate between lying quietly in bed and wildly thrashing about. The latter situation occurs when a painful stimulus (such as that caused by a subarachnoid hemorrhage or a full bladder) rouses the patient whose diminished attention prevents any coherent sequence of movements. Such patients, however, try to avoid painful stimuli by appropriately withdrawing a limb or using it to brush off the offending agent. Gently sliding a cotton-tip stick along the patient's forehead often proves enough of a stimulus to obtain

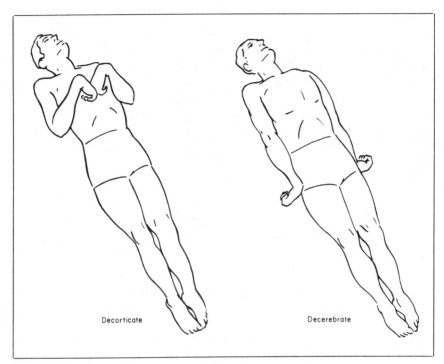

FIG. 21-5. *Decorticate and decerebrate posturing of the limbs in comatose patients.*

such a response. Asymmetrical responses betray a deficit of the motor or sensory pathways, or both.

The tone of the extremities can be checked by lifting the arms from the bed and flexing the patient's knees and releasing them. In light coma, the limbs fall slowly to the resting position. A paretic limb will fall like a "dead weight." Thus, a hemiparesis, or even monoparesis, can be easily detected.

When the level of *coma deepens* or a structural lesion affects a cerebral hemisphere and the diencephalon, *decorticate rigidity* may appear; this rigidity is contralateral to the hemispheric lesion. Decorticate rigidity is characterized by adduction of the arm, *flexion at the elbow,* and pronation and flexion of the wrist; the leg remains extended at the hip and knee (Fig. 21-5).

Severe metabolic (e.g., anoxic) disorders or lesions of the upper brainstem give rise to *decerebrate rigidity,* which is similar to decorticate posturing except for *extension at the elbow* and forcible plantar flexion of the foot (Fig. 21-5). Brought about by painful stimuli, opisthotonos develops periodically with hyperextension of the trunk and hyperpronation of the arms. In experimental animals, decerebrate rigidity results from brainstem transection at the collicular level, below the red nuclei but leaving intact the pontine reticular formation and vestibular nuclei. The action of the vestibular nuclei, unchecked by higher centers, may explain the increased extensor tone characteristic of decerebrate rigidity. Structural lesions that cause this motor pattern usually affect the midbrain and upper pons either directly, as in the case of brainstem infarcts, or indirectly, by pressure effects arising in the supratentorial compartment (downward herniation) or in the posterior fossa.

In a given patient, one side may demonstrate decorticate posturing, whereas the other side, innervated by the motor pathways that have undergone greater damage, displays decerebrate rigidity.

Abnormal extension of the arms with weak flexion of the legs usually indicates damage of the *pontine tegmentum*. With even lower lesions involving the *medulla*, total *flaccidity* ensues.

CLINICAL PRESENTATIONS OF COMA-INDUCING LESIONS DEPENDING ON THEIR LOCATION

Psychogenic Unresponsiveness. The patient may hold the eyes forcibly closed and resist eyelid opening or may keep the eyes open in a fixed stare, interrupted by quick blinks. The pupils, which are of normal size and position, react to light unless a cycloplegic drug has been instilled into them. The doll's head maneuver elicits random or no eye movements. Caloric testing is more helpful because it gives rise to classic vestibular nystagmus with a quick component that requires activity of the frontal eye fields. This quick component is, conversely, absent in comatose patients. Muscle tone and reflexes are normal. The patient may hyperventilate or breathe normally.

Metabolic Encephalopathy (Diffuse Brain Dysfunction). The phylogenetically newer brain structures tend to be more sensitive to metabolic injury. This holds true even though the target of different metabolic abnormalities or toxic agents may vary slightly. For instance, carbon monoxide poisoning causes pallidal necrosis in addition to the widespread cortical damage expected from any hypoxic insult. Functions subserved by complex polysynaptic pathways are affected earlier by metabolic disturbances than those mediated by a few neurons. Thus, higher cortical functions and attention succumb early to metabolic insults, whereas the pupillary light reflex remains to the brink of brainstem death. Survival of other functions ranges between these two extremes. By the time decerebrate posturing appears, the corneal reflexes may be severely depressed, but some eye movements may be elicited by the doll's eye maneuver or caloric stimulation.

Asymmetrical *motor findings* speak against the diagnosis of metabolic encephalopathy. However, downward deviation of the eyes may be occasionally associated with hepatic encephalopathy. Toxic-metabolic disorders often induce *abnormal movements* (tremor, asterixis, myoclonus, and seizures) that seldom accompany focal structural lesions of the brain. But because these two types of etiologic factors often coexist, the diagnostic specificity of these abnormal movements is far from absolute.

The *tremor* of metabolic encephalopathies is coarse and irregular and range between 8 and 10 cycles per second. Its amplitude is greatest when the patient holds his hand outstretched, but in less responsive patients it may be felt by holding the patient's fingers extended.

Asterixis is a sudden, brief loss of postural tone that is translated into a flapping movement when the hand is held in dorsiflexion at the wrist and the fingers are extended and abducted. This hand posture requires some cooperation from the patient, but asterixis can also be elicited by passively extending the patient's fingers and wrist. In any event, asterixis is present with slight stupor and wanes as coma deepens. Unilateral asterixis may appear when a toxic encephalopathy (e.g., phenytoin toxicity) coexists with a structural lesion of the motor pathways that project to the limb with asterixis. Unilateral asterixis may be seen contralateral to lesions of the mesencephalon or parietal lobe [3].

Multifocal myoclonus consists of sudden, nonrhythmic twitching that affects first one muscle, then another, without any specific pattern except a tendency to involve the facial and proximal limb musculature. Causes of multifocal myoclonus include uremic and hyperosmolar-hyperglycemic encephalopathy, carbon dioxide narcosis, and a large dose of intravenous penicillin.

Generalized myoclonus involves mainly the axial musculature, which contracts suddenly, making the patient jump with a certain periodicity. Severe anoxic brainstem damage is the commonest cause of generalized myoclonus, which signifies a poor prognosis.

In addition to symmetrical motor findings, hyperventilation or hypoventilation and the presence of acid-base imbalance are characteristic of metabolic coma.

Supratentorial Structural Lesions. To cause coma, supratentorial lesions must affect both cerebral hemispheres (e.g., massive bihemispheric or bilateral thalamic infarction). The clinical presentation of these lesions and of subarachnoid hemorrhage resembles in many aspects the presen-

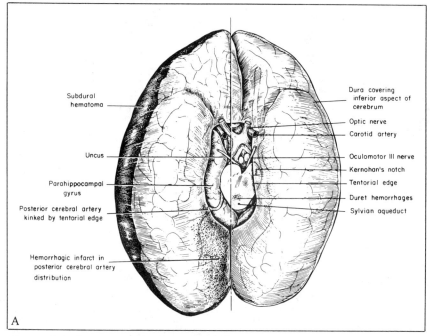

Subdural hematoma

Dura covering inferior aspect of cerebrum

Optic nerve

Carotid artery

Uncus

Oculomotor III nerve

Kernohan's notch

Parahippocampal gyrus

Tentorial edge

Duret hemorrhages

Posterior cerebral artery kinked by tentorial edge

Sylvian aqueduct

Hemorrhagic infarct in posterior cerebral artery distribution

A

FIG. 21-6. *Lateral transtentorial herniation—basal **(A)** and coronal **(B)** views. In this example a subdural hematoma is causing a marked shift of the midline structures and herniation of the hippocampal gyrus through the tentorial notch. Occlusion of the posterior cerebral artery, which is pinched between the herniated hippocampal tissue and the rigid end of the tentorium, has resulted in medial temporooccipital infarction. The midbrain is compressed against the contralateral free tentorial edge, causing a laceration of the crus cerebri (Kernohan's notch). Stretching of the slender perforating branches of the basilar artery has produced petechial hemorrhages in the tegmentum of the midbrain (Duret hemorrhages).*

tation of metabolic disorders. However, cerebral infarcts, even when bilateral, are often staggered, appear more abruptly than metabolic encephalopathies, and cause asymmetrical motor signs, at least early in their course. Sudden onset of severe headache and signs of meningeal irritation separate subarachnoid hemorrhage from metabolic encephalopathies.

This discussion deals mainly with supratentorial lesions that cause mass effects and secondarily impair consciousness by compressing the diencephalic and upper brainstem structures. Prime examples are hemispheric tumors and subdural or intracerebral hemorrhage. Massive infarcts may evolve in a similar manner. When the intracranial pressure of the supratentorial compartment reaches a certain level, the brain substance is squeezed downward through the tentorial opening. Depend-

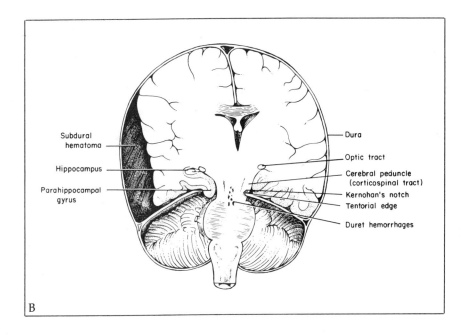

Subdural hematoma

Hippocampus

Parahippocampal gyrus

Dura

Optic tract

Cerebral peduncle (corticospinal tract)

Kernohan's notch

Tentorial edge

Duret hemorrhages

B

ing on the supratentorial location of the mass and the size of the tentorial opening, either one of two different clinical syndromes may result: lateral herniation or central herniation.

LATERAL HERNIATION. In patients with a wide tentorial opening, *lateral extracerebral* or *temporal lobe* masses push the mesial temporal lobe (uncus anteriorly, parahippocampal gyrus posteriorly) between the ipsilateral aspect of the midbrain and the free edge of the tentorium (Fig. 21-6). As the tongue of herniated tissue compresses the posterior cerebral artery and third cranial nerve downward, the ipsilateral pupil becomes progressively dilated and responds sluggishly to light (Fig. 21-7). This stage can be rather brief and, depending on the size and acuteness of the lesion, it may last for a few minutes or several hours. Prompt recognition and removal (often surgically) of the offending agent is mandatory at this stage because the usual progression is deadly. The posterior cerebral artery, pinched against the tentorial edge by the herniated hippocampal gyrus, becomes occluded, giving rise to a hemorrhagic mesial occipital infarct. The herniated hippocampus also pushes the midbrain against the rigid edge of the dura on the opposite side of the tentorial opening. This rigid structure carves out a notch *(Kernohan's notch)* in the lateral aspect of the midbrain, interrupting the cerebral peduncle (particularly those fibers that project to the leg) on the side opposite the orig-

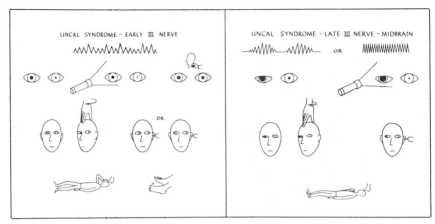

FIG. 21-7. *Clinical findings with lateral transtentorial herniation. (Reproduced from D. E. McNealy and F. Plum. Brainstem dysfunction with supratentorial mass lesions. Arch. Neurol. 7:10, 1962. Copyright © 1962, American Medical Association.)*

inal temporal lobe lesion (Fig. 21-6). This results in a hemiparesis on the same side as the original lesion. If misinterpreted, such hemiparesis may prove to be a false localizing sign. Therefore, when a dilated pupil and hemiparesis appear ipsilaterally, the original lesion is likely to be on the side of the abnormal pupil.

At this point, anteroposterior elongation and downward displacement of the midbrain have already caused tearing of the paramedian perforating vessels that feed the midbrain tegmentum. The consequent infarction and hemorrhages *(Duret hemorrhages)* that involve this structure render recovery almost impossible. The pupil that was larger may become a little smaller as the sympathetic pathway is damaged in the midbrain, while the other pupil becomes midsize and unresponsive. Oculomotor paresis appears, first in the eye originally involved, and shortly afterward in the other eye. Abduction may remain as the only elicitable eye movement.

CENTRAL HERNIATION. Unlike temporal masses, frontal, parietal, or occipital masses first compress the diencephalon, which, as the supratentorial pressure increases, shifts downward and buckles over the midbrain. Subsequent flattening of the midbrain and pons in the rostrocaudal direction causes elongation and rupture of the paramedian perforating arteries feeding these structures, resulting in infarction and hemorrhages in the tegmentum of the midbrain (first) and pons (afterward) (Fig. 21-8).

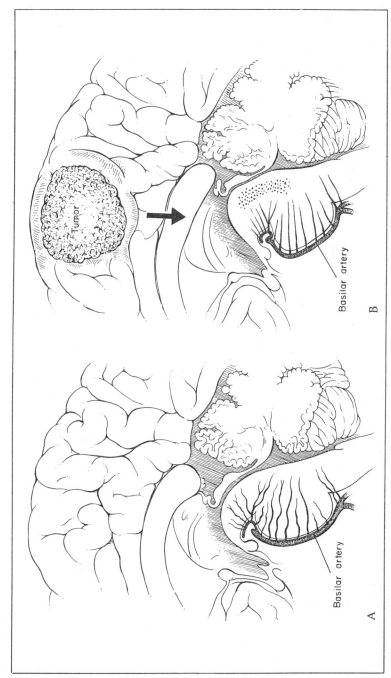

FIG. 21-8. *Central transtentorial herniation. (A) Normal sagittal section of the brainstem. Note the vascular perforators, branches of the basilar artery. (B) Mass effect from a high parietal tumor, resulting in downward displacement and superoinferior flattening of the midbrain and upper pons. The increased cross-sectional diameter of these structures is attended by stretching and rupture of the perforators, with subsequent hemorrhages in the tegmentum of the midbrain and upper pons.*

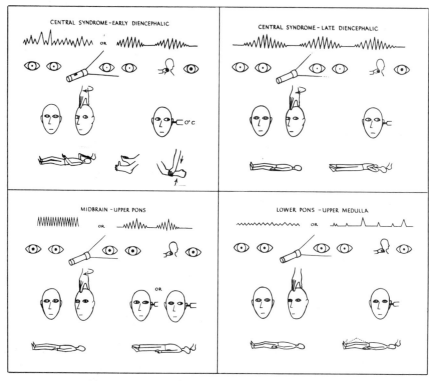

FIG. 21-9. *Clinical findings with central transtentorial herniation. (Reproduced from D. E. McNealy and F. Plum. Brainstem dysfunction with supratentorial mass lesions. Arch. Neurol. 7:10, 1962. Copyright © 1962, American Medical Association.)*

Paralleling the pathologic changes of central herniation, the clinical picture reflects an orderly rostrocaudal progression of brainstem damage. The characteristic evolution of the clinical picture has been termed the *central syndrome of rostrocaudal deterioration.* Description of this syndrome enables one to review the characteristic clinical findings with lesions at the different levels of the brainstem (Fig. 21-9).

EARLY DIENCEPHALIC STAGE. Impaired attention and somnolence appearing in a patient with a supratentorial mass usually herald the beginning of this stage. The respiratory pattern is normal but is punctuated by deep sighs and yawns. In the periods of greater somnolence, the pupils become tiny but react to light, whereas the eyes become slightly divergent, moving slowly from side to side (roving eye movements). Attempts to perform the doll's eye maneuver may provide enough of a stimulus to awaken the patient, and quick eye movements (saccades) are then elicited rather than the slow adversive movements of the oculocephalic reflex. For the same reason, caloric stimulation may induce nystagmus. The patient resists passive motion of the limbs *(paratonia)*, may have grasp reflexes, and brushes off appropriately any noxious stimulus.

LATE DIENCEPHALIC STAGE. At this stage the patient cannot be aroused. Cheyne-Stokes respiration replaces normal breathing. The pupils remain small and reactive. Roving eye movements have disappeared, but the doll's eye maneuver or caloric stimulation easily elicits full and conjugate deviation of the eyes. However, as the process advances, tectal dysfunction may result in restriction of upward gaze. Light painful stimuli fail to elicit any response; heavier ones may induce decorticate posturing, which appears earlier on the side of a previous hemiparesis, opposite the supratentorial lesion. Plantar responses are bilaterally extensor.

Proper diagnosis and treatment at this stage of the syndrome of central herniation may still result in recovery of neurologic function. Once the clinical picture evolves into the next stage (caused by hemorrhages and infarction of the midbrain tegmentum), the prognosis is very poor, except in children.

MIDBRAIN-UPPER PONS STAGE. The patient now breathes rather quickly and evenly. Temperature oscillations are common and an occasional patient may develop diabetes insipidus because of stretching of the median eminence of the hypothalamus. The pupils become midsized, unequal, and irregular, often pear-shaped and eccentric. Terminally, generalized anoxia causes a systemic release of epinephrine, and the pupils may be transiently dilated. The doll's eye maneuver and caloric testing elicit restricted or no vertical eye movements. The eyes often move disconjugately in both the horizontal and the vertical planes. Bilateral impairment of adduction may reflect dysfunction of both third nerve nuclei, of the medial longitudinal fasciculi, or both. Noxius stimuli give rise to decerebrate posturing.

LOWER PONTINE STAGE. Respiration becomes quicker and shallower. Apneustic breathing, common with primary ischemic lesions of this area, is infrequent in patients with transtentorial herniation, perhaps because more medially located structures are preferentially damaged. The pupils remain unchanged from the previous stage, but eye movements are now unobtainable. Decerebrate rigidity decreases. Plantar stimulation may elicit not only bilateral Babinski signs but also withdrawal of the legs with flexion at the knee and hip.

MEDULLARY STAGE. In this agonal stage ataxic breathing soon gives way to apnea. The blood pressure drops, and the pulse becomes irregular.

Large acute supratentorial lesions, particularly massive intraventricular hemorrhage, may cause a quick decompensation of brainstem function leading to respiratory failure. Smaller intraventricular hemorrhages may cause impairment of reflex eye movements in the horizontal and vertical planes while the patient's level of consciousness is only mildly depressed. This phenomenon may be secondary to the action of the blood on the floor of the fourth ventricle.

False localizing signs with supratentorial masses may mislead the observer about the hemisphere involved (e.g., hemiparesis ipsilateral to the lesion due to Kernohan's notch) or falsely localize the primary process to the posterior fossa. The latter occurs mainly with lesions located in the midline (e.g., hydrocephalus) or in areas of the frontal and temporal lobes that are clinically "silent." Extracerebral lesions (e.g., subdural hematoma) in the elderly may behave in a similar manner. These lesions fail to cause focal deficits but raise the pressure of the intracranial contents and produce cranial nerve dysfunction that may be mistaken for evidence of a posterior fossa lesion. Sixth nerve palsy and papilledema are the commonest false localizing signs, but other ophthalmoplegias, trigeminal neuralgia or numbness, unilateral or bilateral deafness, facial palsy, and even weakness in the distribution of the ninth to twelfth cranial nerves may appear as a consequence of raised intracranial pressure with a supratentorial lesion.

Subtentorial Structural Lesions. Destructive lesions (e.g., infarcts, small hemorrhages) of the brainstem can be easily localized clinically. Localization of discrete lesions of the brainstem was discussed in Chapter 14. Compressive lesions that cause coma tend to be associated with brisk involvement of the cerebellum or fourth ventricle. Cerebellar hemorrhage is the prime example. Early in the clinical course, occipital headache, vomiting, and ataxia are usually prominent. In the process of rostrocaudal deterioration characteristic of downward transtentorial herniation, all of the structures at a particular brainstem level tend to be affected at the same time. This does not happen with compressive lesions of the posterior fossa. Unless massive, these latter lesions affect one level more than others, often asymmetrically, giving rise to preferentially unilateral signs.

Lesions that compress the upper brainstem may cause upward transtentorial herniation of the tectum of the *midbrain* and of the anterior cerebellar lobule, giving rise to signs of midbrain dysfunction with coma, hyperventilation, fixed pupils, and vertical ophthalmoplegia. Lower lesions impinge on the *pontine* tegmentum, causing somnolence, pinpoint pupils that react briskly to light, oculoparetic nystagmus on lateral gaze, and truncal ataxia. Appendicular ataxia may be so mild as to pass un-